Fundamentals of

Maternal Anatomy and Physiology

Fundamentals of
Maternal Anatomy and Physiology

EDITED BY

Ian Peate, OBE FRCN EN(G) RGN DipN(Lond) RNT BEd (Hons) MA(Lond) LLM

Editor in Chief, *British Journal of Nursing*; Consultant Editor, *Journal of Paramedic Practice*;
Consultant Editor, *International Journal for Advancing Practice*; Visiting Professor, Northumbria University;
Visiting Professor, St Georges University of London and Kingston University London;
Professorial Fellow, Roehampton University; Visiting Senior Clinical Fellow, University of Hertfordshire.

AND

Claire Leader, MA PGCAP BSc (Hons) RN RM FHEA

Faculty Director of Inter-professional Education and Assistant Professor in Nursing and Midwifery at Northumbria University.
Editorial Board Member for the British Journal of Midwifery.

WILEY Blackwell

Registered Offices
John Wiley & Sons, Inc., 111 River Street, Hoboken, NJ 07030, USA
John Wiley & Sons Ltd, The Atrium, Southern Gate, Chichester, West Sussex, PO19 8SQ, UK

For details of our global editorial offices, customer services, and more information about
Wiley products visit us at www.wiley.com.

Wiley also publishes its books in a variety of electronic formats and by print-on-demand.
Some content that appears in standard print versions of this book may not be available in
other formats.

Library of Congress Cataloging-in-Publication Data
Names: Peate, Ian, editor. | Leader, Claire, editor.
Title: Fundamentals of maternal anatomy and physiology / edited by Ian
    Peate, Claire Leader.
Description: Hoboken, NJ : Wiley-Blackwell, 2024. | Includes index.
Identifiers: LCCN 2023057848 (print) | LCCN 2023057849 (ebook) | ISBN
    9781119864714 (paperback) | ISBN 9781119864721 (adobe pdf) | ISBN
    9781119864738 (epub)
Subjects: MESH: Reproductive Physiological Phenomena |
    Pregnancy–physiology | Maternal-Fetal Exchange–physiology
Classification: LCC RG525 (print) | LCC RG525 (ebook) | NLM WQ 205 | DDC
    618.2–dc23/eng/20240124
LC record available at https://lccn.loc.gov/2023057848
LC ebook record available at https://lccn.loc.gov/2023057849

Cover Design: Wiley
Cover Image: © magicmine/Adobe Stock Photos

Set in 9.5/12.5pt Source sans pro by Straive, Pondicherry, India
Printed and bound by CPI Group (UK) Ltd, Croydon, CR0 4YY
C9781119864714_270324

This text is dedicated my brother, Alan David Peate

Contents

Contributors

Alison Anderson BSc (Hons) PGCE MA Ed RM MSc

Practice Development Midwife and Specialist BAC Midwife, South Tees NHS Foundation Trust, Middlesbrough, UK; Convenor, Virtual International Day of the Midwife Committee

Alison enjoyed 13 years as a secondary science teacher, specialising in biology, before retraining as a midwife through Teesside University and Darlington Memorial Hospital. Alison began her career as a midwife at South Tees NHS Foundation Trust where she became the Specialist Birth After Caesarean Midwife and then Practice Development Midwife. Alison's passions are the humanisation of childbirth and psychological safety in maternity. Alison also has a great interest in global midwifery and is convenor for the Virtual International Day of the Midwife committee and annual 24-hour virtual conference.

Jenny Brewster RM RN BSc Health Studies (OU) PGCe Higher Professional Education (Oxford Brookes University) MEd (OU)

Senior Lecturer in Midwifery, University of West London, UK

Jenny started her training as a nurse at King's College Hospital, London, in 1978 and worked on a male medical ward before moving to St Peter's hospital in Chertsey, where she completed her midwifery training. Having worked in the high-risk environment for several years, she then moved to work in a low-risk midwifery unit before being appointed as a practice development midwife at Wexham Park Hospital in Slough. This led to meeting the teaching team from the University of West London, where Jenny has now been a midwifery lecturer for 13 years. Jenny has written for leading midwifery textbooks. One of her main interests is teaching obstetric emergencies, and especially the support and resuscitation of the newborn baby.

Suzanne Britt RM FHEA ADM BA (Hons) BMedSci Midwifery (Hons) MSc Midwifery Studies PGCHE

Postgraduate Researcher, University of Nottingham, UK

After a teaching career in modern foreign languages, Sue qualified as a midwife in 2002. She has worked in all areas of midwifery practice, beginning her career at Chesterfield Royal Hospital before moving to Sherwood Forest Hospital in 2008 for a community midwifery post. In 2011, she completed her Master's degree and started a secondment as a research midwife at Nottingham University Hospital. In 2013, she moved into midwifery education, working as an Assistant Professor of Midwifery at the University of Nottingham, where she received global and local recognition for teaching. She has delivered on all areas of the curriculum, leading modules on public health, perinatal mental health, and contemporary midwifery care. Her interest and knowledge around the musculoskeletal system spans her personal and professional life, and she has qualifications in both fitness and nutrition. In 2022, she left her teaching role to start a full-time PhD at the University of Nottingham, focusing on healthcare professional response to domestic abuse.

Mel Cameron-Radford MSc BSc (Hons) RM PMA

Maternity Investigator, Healthcare Safety Investigation Branch (HSIB)/Maternity and Newborn Safety Investigations Programme, UK

Mel began her midwifery career at the Royal Victoria Infirmary at Newcastle Upon Tyne Hospitals after graduating from Northumbria University, obtaining a first-class honours degree. She worked as a rotational midwife, intrapartum core team midwife, clinical skills facilitator and later a delivery suite coordinator at the tertiary referral centre. She trained and was appointed as a supervisor of midwives and a professional midwifery advocate. Mel worked as a lead for maternity at NHS England's North East and Cumbria Clinical Network. She studied part time to obtain her MSc in practice development. Mel worked as a lead for the implementation of continuity of carer and Better Births at Newcastle. She joined the Health Care Safety Investigation Branch in 2020 as a maternity investigator. Her key interests are advocacy, intrapartum care, maternal medicine, personalised care and choice.

James Castleman MA MD MRCOG
Consultant in Maternal and Fetal Medicine, Birmingham Women's and Children's NHS Foundation Trust, UK
James is a consultant obstetrician at Birmingham Women's and Children's Hospital, UK. He graduated with distinction from the University of Cambridge and completed foundation training in the East of England before moving home to the midlands for his obstetrics and gynaecology clinical and research training. James has subspecialty accreditation in maternal and fetal medicine from the Royal College of Obstetricians and Gynaecologists. He has a monthly prenatal genomics clinic alongside a clinical geneticist and is part of the regional multidisciplinary team providing this service. His other interests include fetal therapy and obstetric cardiology, as well as maintaining a passion for delivering high quality intra partum care alongside midwifery colleagues.

Claire Ford PGCap PhD FHEA PGDip RN BSc
Assistant Professor, Northumbria University, Newcastle, UK; Co-creator and Leader for Skills for Practice Website
Claire joined the teaching team at Northumbria University in 2013, having spent time working within perioperative care and completing a postgraduate diploma in midwifery. She studied for her BSc (Hons) and PG Dip at Northumbria University and won academic awards for both and the Heath Award in 2009. As an assistant professor, she teaches a range of national/international healthcare programmes and is also a joint programme leader for the MSc Nursing Programme. She has a passion for pain management, clinical skills, women's health, gynaecology, perioperative care, simulation and immersive technologies. She has published many articles and is actively involved in several research projects examining the use of media and technology to facilitate deep learning. She is the co-founder of the 'Skills for Practice' website, which was shortlisted for the Student Nursing Times Awards 2016 – Teaching Innovation of the Year.

Angela Frankland RM MSc FHEA
Senior Lecturer in Midwifery, Kingston University, London, UK
Angela trained as a nurse in 1985 at Kings College Hospital London. After qualifying, she worked as a staff nurse in paediatrics, a neonatal unit and as a nurse educator, where her passion for clinical education started. Since qualifying as midwife in 1990, she has worked various midwifery roles within the NHS, including rotational clinical posts, labour ward coordinator, working in a high-risk midwifery team and then as Practice Development Midwife, before moving in 2018 to Kingston University as a Senior Lecturer in Midwifery.

Clare Gordon RM SCPHN SN BSc (Hons) MSc (S'ton) MSc (UWL) PG Cert Academic Practice FHEA
Senior Lecturer in Midwifery; Programme Leader, Berkshire, Midwifery; University of West London, Reading, UK
Clare began her midwifery career in at the North Hampshire Hospital, becoming a qualified midwife in 2005. She practised as a registered midwife at Frimley Park Hospital, where she gained a wide range of experience before setting up a specialist weight management clinic for pregnant women. She also undertook the Specialist Community Public Health Nurse School Nurse training and was awarded an MSc in Public Health Practice from University of Southampton in 2010. She has always enjoyed learning and educating others and joined the midwifery team at the University of West London in 2013. She has subsequently been awarded an MSc with distinction in professional practice with healthcare education. She is a senior midwifery lecturer and programme lead with a specialist interest in public health, the normality of pregnancy and birth and the foundations for safe midwifery practice.

Rosalind Haddrill PhD MA BSc (Hons) PGCE RM SFHEA
Lecturer in Midwifery, Edinburgh Napier University, UK
Roz trained in Sheffield and qualified as a midwife in 2005, after previous careers as a landscape architect and lecturer. She worked clinically in a variety of midwifery roles until 2019 and has worked as a midwifery lecturer since 2010 in a number of British universities. Her PhD explored delayed access to antenatal care. Her areas of interest include women's perceptions of maternity care, gestational diabetes, postnatal care and infant feeding. Roz is currently programme leader for the Masters in Midwifery programme at Edinburgh Napier University.

Iñaki Mansilla MSc Midwifery (UWL) PGCE RM (Hons) RGN (adult)
Senior Midwifery Lecturer/Practitioner, University of Hertfordshire, Hatfield, UK

Iñaki is a dual registrant for nursing and midwifery. With almost 15 years of experience as a dedicated midwife, he embraces the transformative journey of childbirth, nurturing and empowering women and birthing people. His journey began in Spain in 1999, undertaking adult nursing training, then moved to the UK in 2006 to undertake the BSc (Hons) shortened in midwifery. Along the way, he acquired diverse skills, including complementary therapies, mentorship and advanced management of ankyloglossia. His commitment to improving birthing experiences led him to do his MSc 'Why some women changed their place of birth, from the hospital to home, when they were offered an assessment at home in early labour', a study that is currently being prepared for publication. In 2020, Iñaki became a Senior Midwifery Lecturer at the University of Hertfordshire, sharing his knowledge and inspiring future midwives. He is passionate on his role as a champion for equality, diversity, and inclusion in midwifery. Recognised for his exceptional dedication, Iñaki has been nominated several times for the vice-chancellor's award as Academic and Teaching Staff Member of the Year. In 2022, he won Student's Choice Award.

Claire Leader MA PGCAP BSc (Hons) RN RM FHEA
Faculty Director of Interprofessional Education and Assistant Professor, Adult Nursing, Northumbria University, Newcastle, UK

Claire Leader qualified as a registered nurse from York University in 1998 after which she moved to Leeds, working in the areas of cardiothoracic surgery and emergency nursing. In 2003 she commenced her midwifery education at Huddersfield University where she was awarded a first-class BSc (hons). She worked initially at Sheffield Teaching hospitals, she later moved to the North East, where she commenced her role as a staff midwife, before moving into the area of research as a research nurse and midwife. She was awarded a distinction for the MA in Sociology and Social Research at Newcastle University in 2012. Claire moved to Northumbria University in 2018 and is now Assistant Professor for pre-registration Adult Nursing and Midwifery programmes, while also studying for her PhD in the area of wellbeing for nurses and midwives.

Sarah Malone MBBS MRCOG FRANZCOG CertClinRes DDU (O&G)
Consultant Obstetrician, Royal Women's Hospital, Parkville, Australia

Sarah Malone is an obstetrician with specialist training in maternal and fetal medicine. She began her medical career in North East England and after spending a year working in Auckland, New Zealand, was inspired to complete training in obstetrics and gynaecology in Melbourne, Australia. Sarah undertook additional subspecialty training in maternal and fetal medicine, which included time spent working in Fetal Medicine in Birmingham, UK. Sarah is experienced in the management of complex pregnancy with particular emphasis in diagnostic ultrasound, fetal anomalies, multiple pregnancy and genetics.

Rebecca Murray RM MRes PGCert LTHE FHEA BSc (Hons)
Lecturer (Education) Midwifery, Queen's University Belfast, UK

Rebecca studied biomedical science at Queen's University Belfast, before commencing her midwifery training. She graduated from Queen's University Belfast in 2012 with a BSc (Hons) in midwifery science and moved to London to work as a research midwife, alongside clinical midwifery roles. Rebecca completed an MRes Clinical Research at King's College London in 2017 and began her midwifery education career at London Southbank University and later University of Hertfordshire. Rebecca is an NMC registered teacher and a Fellow of the Higher Education Academy. Rebecca has interests in clinical simulation, medicines management and intrapartum care.

Dr Kate Nash RGN RM BSc (Hons) MSc Practice Educator/Lecturer DClinPrac
Lead Midwife for Education, University of Winchester, UK

Kate began her nursing career at the Royal Free Hospital in 1991 and later trained as a midwife in 2000 at the University of Hertfordshire. Kate is an experienced clinician and professional midwifery advocate having held varied roles and responsibilities within midwifery in London, the Midlands and South East of England. Kate has worked within midwifery education since 2012 and is a passionate advocate for the safe personalised care of women, birthing people, babies and families. Kate is committed to enabling the development of attitudes, skills and knowledge to ensure this.

Elizabeth Routledge MBChB MRCP(UK) BSc(Hons)
Consultant Physician in Acute Medicine, Forth Valley Royal Hospital, Larbert, UK
Beth undertook undergraduate studies at the University of Durham and the University of Glasgow, and went on to complete her postgraduate medical training in the west of Scotland. As a specialist trainee in acute medicine, she developed a subspecialty interest in obstetric medicine, and completed training at Glasgow Royal Infirmary and the Queen Elizabeth University Hospital. She teaches widely in the area of obstetric medicine to medical trainees across Scotland, and has published in this area. She is a standing contributor to the Scottish Government's maternal medicine policy work. She has been a member of the Royal College of Physicians since 2016.

Antonio Sierra RN (Huelva, Spain) RM (London) MSc (London) PGCME (Beds) HEE/ICA Pre-doctoral Programme (UEA)
National Midwifery International Recruitment Adviser, NHS England; Consultant Midwife, West Hertfordshire Hospitals NHS Trust; Visiting Lecturer, University of Hertfordshire, Hatfield, UK
Antonio has been working in healthcare for nearly 20 years. He worked as a stroke nurse in South Wales before relocating to England, where he practised as a midwife in all areas of midwifery services before developing a passion for intrapartum care and clinical education. After working in several hospitals and leading on service development and quality improvement projects across Berkshire, London and Hertfordshire, he was appointed consultant midwife with a focus on midwifery practice and personalisation of care & choice. He is currently leading on international recruitment of midwives for NHS England. His key areas of interest are childbirth research for vulnerable groups, particularly matters affecting the LGBTQ+ community and global majority, as well as leadership and culture in the workplace, alongside clinical and pastoral support for staff.

Joyce Targett RN (Adult) HND Nursing Studies RM BSc (HONS) Midwifery Studies PGC Med Ultrasound
Midwife Sonographer, County Durham and Tees Valley, UK
Joyce started her career as a Medical Assistant in the Royal Air Force before commencing 3 years Nurse training with the University of York in 1994. During her nurse training her exposure to maternity care inspired her to become a midwife, training with the University of Northumbria. On qualifying, Joyce worked as a staff midwife in a consultant led unit and the community setting. In 2005, Joyce completed her training as a sonographer with the University of Teesside and continues to work as a midwife sonographer in a clinical setting. She primarily works within a maternity day unit alongside a midwifery led unit, where Joyce also has an active role as a professional midwifery advocate.

Ashleigh Ward
Consultant Nurse Cancer and Palliative Care and Chair Research and Development Committee, Falkirk Community Hospital, UK; Honorary Clinical Senior Lecturer, School of Medicine, Dentistry and Nursing, University of Glasgow UK
Ashleigh's career focuses on cancer and palliative care. She is a Consultant Nurse and also the Chair of the Research and Development Committee.
As well as her current role Ashleigh holds the position of Honorary Clinical Senior Lecturer at the School of Medicine, Dentistry and Nursing at the University of Glasgow. This role allows her to contribute to the academic community, sharing her expertise and knowledge with the next generation of healthcare professionals.
Ashleigh's contributions, aimed at improving palliative and end-of-life care, have been recognised in numerous publications and reports.

Preface

Understanding maternal anatomy and physiology is essential for any midwifery student who strives to offer women and their families safe and effective care. The *Fundamentals of Maternal Anatomy and Physiology* introduces you to the remarkable processes of human reproduction, pregnancy and childbirth. The *Fundamentals of Maternal Anatomy and Physiology* is a comprehensive exploration of the intricacies and marvels of the female reproductive system and the physiological changes that occur during pregnancy.

Understanding the anatomy and physiology of the maternal body is fundamental to providing quality care to pregnant individuals. Whether you are a student entering the field of midwifery, a healthcare professional specialising in maternal care or simply someone with a keen interest in the wonder of life, this book will serve as your invaluable guide.

There are 16 chapters in the book. In the first chapter, we begin by introducing the reader to the terminology that is used when discussing anatomy and physiology. Chapter 2 offers insight at the cellular level before moving on to the reproductive system and embarking on a fascinating journey through the female reproductive system. We start by delving into the anatomy and physiology of the body systems, unravelling their complex structures and functions. We explore the intricate processes of ovulation, fertilisation and implantation, laying down the groundwork for a deeper understanding of the subsequent stages of anatomy and physiology and how this is related to pregnancy.

We investigate the physiological changes that occur in the maternal body during pregnancy. From the moment of conception, the body undergoes a series of remarkable adaptations to support the growing fetus. We examine the cardiovascular system, respiratory system, endocrine system, immune system and other vital components, discussing and describing the intricate interplay between these systems and the unique demands of pregnancy.

This book pays particular attention to the concept of maternal-fetal exchange – how nutrients, oxygen and waste products are transported between the maternal and fetal circulations via the placenta. We explore the development and functions of the placenta, shedding light on its role in nourishing and protecting the growing fetus.

Throughout the chapters, we emphasise the clinical relevance of maternal anatomy and physiology. Real-life case studies, clinical scenarios and illustrative diagrams enhance the learning experience, allowing readers to apply their knowledge to practical situations. We also highlight common medical conditions and complications that can arise during pregnancy, providing insight into their underlying anatomical and physiological mechanisms.

It is important to note that this book is not meant to replace hands-on clinical experience or professional guidance. Rather, it serves as a companion to enhance your understanding and appreciation of maternal anatomy and physiology. Each chapter is meticulously crafted to present the information in a clear, concise and engaging manner for students, academics and healthcare professionals alike.

The contributors, academics and practitioners, are experts in the field of midwifery and maternal health, who have contributed their extensive knowledge and expertise to make this book a reality. Their dedication and passion shine through these pages and we hope their insights will inspire and empower readers on their journey towards the provision of excellence in maternal care.

We invite you to immerse yourself in the world of maternal anatomy and physiology, as we describe and discuss the complexities of the female reproductive system and the adaptations the body makes to enable new life to flourish. Our wish is that this book becomes a source of inspiration, knowledge and empowerment, guiding you towards providing exceptional care to pregnant individuals and their families and fostering the wellbeing of mother and child.

Finally, a note on language. Inclusive language in health and care is crucial for promoting equality, respecting diversity and ensuring that everyone feels represented and valued. It involves using language that is inclusive of all individuals, regardless of their gender identity, sexual orientation, race, ethnicity, disability or other characteristics. By employing inclusive language, we can foster a more inclusive and accessible environment for readers, patients and professionals alike.

When discussing gender and sex, one of the significant challenges is the complexity and fluidity of the terminology that is and that can be used. The concept of gender is multifaceted and may vary across cultures, communities and individuals. Understanding and navigating this terminology requires sensitivity, open-mindedness and a willingness to learn and adapt to evolving perspectives. It is recognised that not all birthing people will identify with their biological sex and a 'gender additive' approach to language has been advocated in the context of contemporary maternity services. This acknowledges that women may be negatively impacted by reproductive health inequalities. The terms 'woman' and 'women' are used in this book, together with a range of terms to identify and describe those people to whom we have the privilege to offer maternal care.

Ian Peate, London
Claire Leader, Northumbria

Acknowledgements

Ian thanks his partner Jussi for his continued support. Claire would like to thank her husband Gavin for all the support and encouragement over the years. We would like to thank the amazing contributors who gave of their time to help the text come to fruition. We are grateful to the team at Wiley who were receptive and encouraged us to take this project forward.

CHAPTER 1

Learning the Language: Terminology

Joyce Targett

AIM

This chapter aims to provide insight and understanding of the terminology used in the provision of healthcare related to anatomy, physiology and pathophysiology.

LEARNING OUTCOMES

On completion of this chapter you will be able to:

- Discuss the terms and context around anatomy, physiology and pathophysiology.
- Understand prefixes and suffixes used in anatomy, physiology and pathophysiology.
- Understand directional terms.
- Describe the anatomical planes, anatomical regions of the body and the body cavities.

Test Your Prior Knowledge

1. What do you understand by the term 'pathology'?
2. What is the difference between a sign and a symptom?
3. How is the root word altered by a prefix or a suffix?
4. Name and define the nine regions of the abdomen.

Introduction

Science, particularly terms used in the provision of health care, is replete with Latin and Greek terminology. Latin names are used for all parts of the body and Greek terms are also common (the Greeks are said by many to be the founders of modern medicine). Healthcare staff use pathophysiological concepts as they work with people to whom who they offer care and as they offer treatment to those who are experiencing some type of health condition or disease.

Fundamentals of Maternal Anatomy and Physiology, First Edition. Edited by Ian Peate and Claire Leader.
© 2024 John Wiley & Sons Ltd. Published 2024 by John Wiley & Sons Ltd.

Red Flag Alert: Jargon

Like any country with its own language, the medical field also has its own jargon. This is important so communication between healthcare professionals can take place quickly and efficiently without the need for too much explanation. It is a specific language that is not just used by midwives, nurses, doctors and other people who are actively involved in the medical arena. It is important for all others who work in the healthcare arena (e.g. pharmacists, physiologists and dentists). Its correct use can have a significant impact on ensuring the best care. What is important is that we are all speaking the same language; failure to do or making assumptions can lead to error and mistakes.

Anatomy and Physiology

Anatomy discusses the study of the structure and location of body parts, while physiology is the study of the function of body parts. Both these terms are interlinked. Understanding where the body parts are located can help you to understand how they function. As an example, McGuiness (2018) explains that when the various functions of the heart and the four chambers, together with the valves, make up the anatomy. Visualising these many structures can assist in understanding how blood flows through the heart and how the heart beats; this is related to its function and is its physiology.

Anatomy

The Body Map

Learning anatomical terminology is like learning a new language. Developing your learning, understanding more and adding different terms to your vocabulary can help you to talk confidently about the body. The anatomical directional terms and body planes present a universally recognised language of anatomy. When undertaking the study of anatomy and physiology, it is essential that you have key or directional terminology so that you are able to give a precise description as you or others refer to the precise location of a body part or structure.

Reflective Learning Activity

When you are next on placement, identify how many times during a shift you hear the various clinicians describe and discuss anatomy, physiology and pathophysiology. Note the terminology being used and how there is a clearer understanding among the team when using one language – anatomical and physiological terminology.

All parts of the body are described in relation to other body parts and a standardised body position, known as the anatomical position, is used in anatomical terminology. An anatomical position is established from an imaginary central line that runs down the centre or mid-line of the body. When in this position, the body is erect and faces forwards, with the arms to the side; palms face forwards with the thumbs to the side, the feet are slightly apart with the toes pointing forwards.

Orange Flag Alert: Speaking with Patients

While you are encouraged to use the correct anatomical and physiological terms when conversing with other colleagues, caution must be exercised when speaking in front of women and their families. Healthcare professionals can inadvertently use words and jargon that are strange to patients; they may not realise that the meaning is not clear. While there are some concepts that are familiar and obvious to the multidisciplinary team, they may be alien to patients. Try first to establish what the woman knows and understands before launching into a discussion that begins at a level that is either too complex or too simple. Too often, our health-care environments fail to recognise the needs of people with different levels of understanding about their health and this can mean that they may fail to receive the right care at the right time. Using jargon can instil fear, cause confusion and result in poor care.

The standard body 'map' or anatomical position (just like a map) is that of the body standing upright (orientated with the north at the top), with the feet at shoulder width and parallel, toes forward (Figure 1.1). Humans are usually bilaterally symmetrical. This position is used to describe body parts and positions of patients irrespective of whether they are lying down, lying on their side or facing down.

As well as understanding the anatomy and the physiology (the structure and function), understanding directional terms and the position of the various structures is also required. Table 1.1 lists common anatomical descriptive terms that you will need to become acquainted with. This list is not exhaustive; you will come across additional terms as you work through the various chapters. Figure 1.2 depicts anatomical positions.

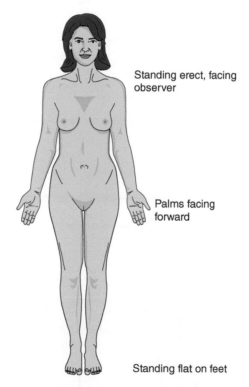

Standing erect, facing observer

Palms facing forward

Standing flat on feet

FIGURE 1.1 Anatomical position: anterior and posterior views of the body. Source: Peate (2017)/John Wiley & Sons.

TABLE 1.1   Anatomical descriptive terms.

Anatomical term	Relationship to the body
Anterior	Front surface of the body or structure
Posterior	Back surface of the body or structure
Deep	Further from the surface
Superficial	Close to the surface
Internal	Nearer the inside
External	Nearer the outside
Lateral	Away from the mid-line
Median	Midline of the body
Medial	In the direction of the mid-line
Superior	Located above or towards the upper part
Inferior	Located below or towards the lower part
Proximal	Nearest to the point of reference
Distal	Furthest away from the point of reference
Prone	Lying face down in a horizontal position
Supine	Lying face up in a horizontal position

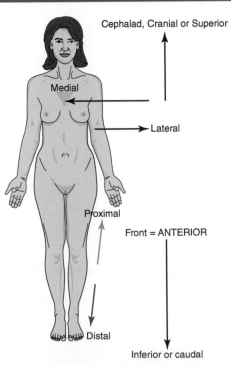

Cephalad, Cranial or Superior

Medial

Lateral

Proximal

Front = ANTERIOR

Distal

Inferior or caudal

FIGURE 1.2   Anatomical positions. Source: Peate (2017)/John Wiley & Sons.

Anatomical Planes of the Body

A plane is an imaginary two-dimensional surface that passes through the body. There are three planes that are generally referred to in anatomy and healthcare (Figure 1.3):

- Sagittal
- Frontal
- Transverse.

The *sagittal plane*, the vertical plane, is the plane that divides the body or an organ vertically into the right and left sides. If this vertical plane runs directly down the middle of the body, it is known as the midsagittal or median plane. If it divides the body into unequal right and left sides, then it is called a parasagittal plane.

The *frontal plane* is the plane dividing the body or an organ into an anterior portion and a posterior portion. The frontal plane is often referred to as a coronal plane (the word *corona* is Latin for crown).

The *transverse plane* divides the body or organ horizontally into the upper (superior) and lower (inferior) portions.

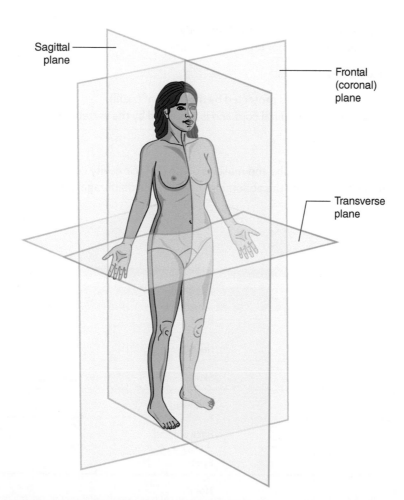

Sagittal plane

Frontal (coronal) plane

Transverse plane

FIGURE 1.3 Anatomical planes. Source: Peate (2017)/John Wiley & Sons.

Anatomical Regions of the Body

The body is divided up into regions, like a map. The anatomical regions of the body refer to a particular area/region of the body, which helps to compartmentalise. The body is divided into:

- The head and neck
- The trunk (thorax and abdomen)
- The upper limbs (arms)
- The lower limbs (legs).

See Tables 1.2–1.5 for a representation of the correct terminology for each region.

Body Cavities

Body cavities are spaces within the body that contain the internal organs. The cavity can be filled with air or with organs. Minor body cavities include the oral cavity (mouth), the nasal cavity, the orbital cavity (eye), middle ear cavity, the uterine cavity and the synovial cavities (these are spaces within synovial joints). There are two main cavities in the body (Figure 1.4):

- The *dorsal cavity* is located in the posterior region of the body.
- The *ventral body cavity* occupies the anterior region of the trunk.

The dorsal cavity is subdivided into two cavities:

- The *cranial cavity* encloses the brain and is protected by the cranium (skull).
- The *vertebral/spinal cavity* contains the spinal cord and is protected by the vertebrae.

The ventral cavity is subdivided into two:

1. The *thoracic cavity* is surrounded by the ribs and muscles of the thoracic cavity containing the lungs, heart, trachea, oesophagus and thymus. Separated from the abdominal cavity by the diaphragm muscle.

TABLE 1.2   Anatomical regions of the head and neck.

Anatomical phrase	Area of body related to
Cephalic	Head
Cervical	Neck
Cranial	Skull
Frontal	Forehead
Occipital	Back of head
Ophthalmic	Eyes
Oral	Mouth
Nasal	Nose

TABLE 1.3 Anatomical regions of the trunk (thorax and abdomen).

Anatomical phrase	Area body related to
Axillary	Armpit
Costal	Ribs
Mammary	Breast
Pectoral	Chest
Vertebral	Backbone
Abdominal	Abdomen
Gluteal	Buttocks
Inguinal	Groin
Lumbar	Lower back
Pelvic	Pelvis/lower part of abdomen
Umbilical	Navel
Perineal	Between anus and external genitalia
Pubic	Pubis

TABLE 1.4 Anatomical regions of the upper limbs.

Anatomical phrase	Area of body related to
Brachial	Upper arm
Carpal	Wrist
Cubital	Elbow
Forearm	Lower arm
Palmar	Palm
Digital	Fingers (also relates to toes)

2. The *abdominopelvic cavity* contains the stomach, spleen, liver, gallbladder, pancreas, small intestine and most of the large intestine. The abdominal cavity is protected by the muscles of the abdominal wall and partly by the diaphragm and ribcage.
   - The female abdominopelvic cavity contains the urinary bladder, uterus, fallopian tubes, ovaries and the rectum. The pelvic cavity is protected by the bones of the pelvis, the sacral promontory posteriorly and the symphysis pubis anteriorly.

TABLE 1.5   Anatomical regions of the lower limbs (legs).

Anatomical phrase	Area body related to
Femoral	Thigh
Patellar	Front of knee
Pedal	Foot
Plantar	Sole of foot
Popliteal	Hollow behind knee
Digital	Toes (also relates to fingers)

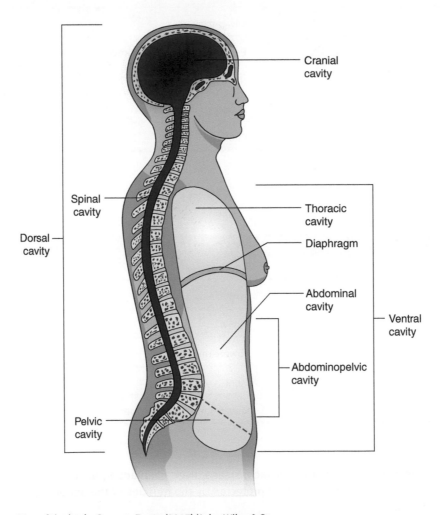

FIGURE 1.4   The cavities of the body. Source: Peate (2017)/John Wiley & Sons.

Snapshot 1.1

Lauren, a 32-year-old multiparous woman presents at the early pregnancy unit complaining of a small amount of vaginal bleeding and a sharp stabbing left iliac fossa pain for two hours. She also reports some shoulder tip and rectal pain. Her pain score is 5/10, she has taken paracetamol (1 g), one hour prior to admission with moderate effect.

History

- Gravida 2 para 1 previous full term normal vaginal delivery.
- Postnatal insertion of an Intrauterine contraceptive device 12 months ago.
- Stopped breastfeeding eight weeks ago.
- Last menstrual period was six weeks ago; positive urine pregnancy test yesterday.
- No significant gynaecological or medical history has been disclosed.

Red Flag Alert: Understanding Anatomy and Physiology

The practitioner caring for Lauren will require an understanding of the anatomy and physiology of the reproductive system.

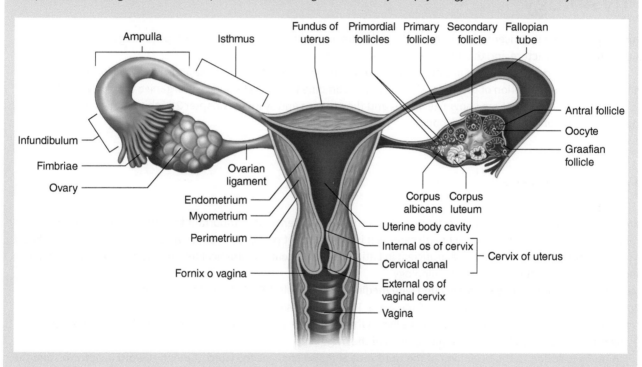

Snapshot 1.2

On Examination

Continuing the story of Lauren from Snapshot 1.1, Lauren is alert and can communicate clearly. She appears pale and clammy; her breathing is regular with no signs of tachypnoea or dyspnoea and her observations reveal she is haemodynamically stable (blood pressure 110/80 mm/Hg, pulse 96 beats/minute and regular, respiratory rate 17 breaths/minute and regular, temperature [tympanic] 36.4°C). There is minimal loss per vagina. On abdominal palpation, obvious guarding but no rebound tenderness is noted in the left iliac fossa.

> **Ultrasound Examination Findings**
> - Anteverted uterus, IUCD sited at the fundus.
> - Right ovary of normal appearance. Left ovary contains a corpus luteum.
> - Adjacent but separate to the left ovary is a mixed echo mass measuring 15 × 12 × 10 mm. The pouch of Douglas contains anechoic free fluid measuring 50 × 30 × 70 mm.
> - Suspected ectopic pregnancy in the left adnexa, with cervical excitation noted on examination.

Reflective Learning Activity

Look through the information provided in Snapshots 1.1 and 1.2 and highlight the information that is associated with anatomy, physiology and pathophysiology. Highlight and find the anatomical and physiological terms and determine their meaning.

Physiology

Human physiology is concerned with the study of the function of the body. Anatomy and physiology therefore relate to the study of the structure and the function of the human body.

The human body is organised in a most precise way whereby atoms combine in appropriate ways forming molecules in the chemical organisation of the body. The molecules combine to form cells and cells organise themselves collectively as functioning masses that are known as tissues and then organs and systems. Chapter 2 of this text describes cells and the organisation of tissues within the body.

10

Terminology

Already in this chapter, you may have come across some complex terms. It is important to learn the language (the terminology) that is used in the provision health care, as it is an important part of safe, effective woman-centred care. While it is not a precourse requirement to be proficient in Latin or Greek to learn anatomical terminology, it is essential that you understand and are able to use the terminology.

There are three basic parts associated with medical terms (Table 1.6). The word root is the core of the word. It provides the basic meaning to the subject of the word. Prefixes and suffixes modify the word. In the word 'hepatitis', for example, the word root is *heap,* which means liver. When the suffix *itis* (which means inflammation) is added, the word changes and it becomes hepatitis – inflammation of the liver.

A prefix is added to the beginning of the word root and also changes the word. If the root word is *nutrition* and the prefix *mal* (meaning bad) is added, then malnutrition means bad or poor nutrition.

TABLE 1.6   Basic components.

Component	Description
Word root	Usually found in the middle of the word – its central meaning
Prefix	Comes at the beginning of the word and usually identifies some subdivision or part of the central meaning
Suffix	Comes at the end of the word and modifies the central meaning as to what or who is interacting with it or what is happening to it

Look at this example:

Hypothermia

The word root is therm (heat)

Hypo means low (this is the prefix), so hypothermia means low heat. Now take a look at this word: myocarditis – let's break it up:

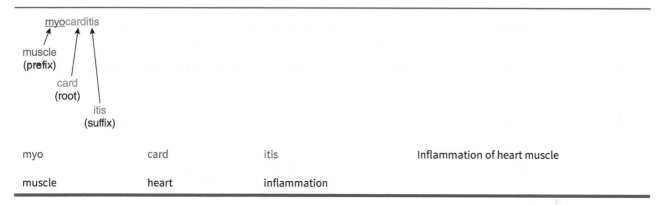

myo	card	itis	Inflammation of heart muscle
muscle	heart	inflammation	

The prefix can change the word:

Myocarditis myo + carditis = inflammation of heart muscle.
Endocarditis endo + carditis = inflammation of the inner layer of the heart.
Pericarditis peri + carditis = inflammation of the outer layer of the heart.

The suffix can also alter the word:

Cardiologist cardi + ologist = a practitioner specialising in the heart.
Cardiomyopathy cardio + myopathy = damage to heart muscle.
Cardiomegaly cardio + megaly = enlargement of the heart.

The prefix can change the word:

Myocarditis myo = inflammation of heart muscle
Endocarditis endo = inflammation of the inner layer of the heart
Pericarditis peri = inflammation of the outer layer of the heart

In these examples, the prefix and suffix can change the word but, the root *card* stayed the same.

Reflective Learning Activity

Explain the difference between polyhydramnios and oligohydramnios.

The suffix can also alter the word:

There are many frequently used prefixes and suffixes; you will already know some of them. See Table 1.7 for a list of some prefixes and suffixes that are used to make up a number of medical terms.

As is the case when learning any language, it can take time to learn all the words and, indeed, the learning will be lifelong. When you are in clinical practice, you will be able to reinforce your learning, using your new vocabulary with confidence. Take your time, seek clarification if needed and be patient with yourself.

Knowing the different anatomical terms can make it easier to understand the various pathophysiological concepts that can help you provide care that is woman centred, safe and effective.

TABLE 1.7   Some prefixes, suffixes, their meaning and examples.

Prefix/suffix	Meaning	Example
a/an	No, not, without, lack of	Anoxia (without oxygen), anuria (without urine), asepsis (without sepsis), asymptomatic (without symptoms), anhydramnios (without amniotic fluid), anencephalic (without parts of brain and skull)
ab	Away from	Abduction (to move away from the midline), abnormal (away from normal)
ad	Towards	Adduction (to move towards the midline), adrenal (towards the kidney), addiction (drawn towards or a strong dependence on a drug or substance)
aemia	Of blood	Leukaemia (cancer of blood cells), anaemia (lack of red blood cells)
algia	Pain	Cephalgia (headache), mastalgia (breast pain), myalgia (muscle pain)
ante	Before/in front of	Antepartum/antenatal (before birth), anterior (to the form of the body), anteprandial (before meals)
arthro	Joint	Arthroscope (an instrument used to look into a joint), arthritis (joint inflammation), arthrotomy (incision of a joint)
baro	Pressure/weight	Isobaric (having equal measure if pressure), bariatrics (the field of medicine that offers treatment to people who are overweight), baroreceptor (a sensor reacting to pressure changes)
brady	Slow/delayed	Bradycardia (slow heart rate), bradykinesia (slowness in movement), bradylalia (abnormally slow speech)
cyto	Cell	Leucocyte (white blood cell), erythrocyte (red cell), cytology (study and function of cells), cytogenetics (study of structure and function of chromosomes)
derm	Skin	Dermatitis (inflammation of the skin), dermatome (a surgical instrument used for cutting slices of the skin), dermatology (the study of skin)
dys	Difficulty/ impaired	Dysphasia (difficulty swallowing), dyspepsia (disordered digestion), dysuria (difficulty in urination), shoulder dystocia
ectomy	To cut out	Appendectomy (removal of the appendix), mastectomy (removal of the breast), prostatectomy (removal of the prostate) hysterectomy (removal of the uterus)
endo	Inner	Endocardium (lining of the heart), endocarditis (inflammation of the heart), endotracheal (within the trachea) endometriosis (a condition where tissue similar to the endometrium grows outside of the uterus)
erythro	Red	Erythrocyte (red blood cell), erythropaenia (reduction in the number of red blood cells), erythema (reddening of the skin)
haem	Blood	Haematogenesis (the formation of blood), haematology (the study of blood), haemarthrosis (bleeding within the joint)
hydro	Water	Hydrophobia (abnormal dread of water), hydrocephalus (accumulation of fluid within the cranium)
hyper	Above/beyond/ excessive	Hypertension (high blood pressure), hyperflexion (movement of a muscle beyond its normal limit), hyperglycaemia (high blood glucose)

TABLE 1.7 (*Continued*)

Prefix/suffix	Meaning	Example
hypo	Below/under/deficient	Hypotension (low blood pressure), hypothermia (low temperature), hypoglycaemia (low blood glucose) hypothyroidism (an underactive thyroid gland), Hypospadias (the opening of the penis is not at the tip)
intra	Within	Intravenous (within the veins), intraocular (within the eye), intracerebral (within the brain), intra-uterine (within the uterus)
ism	Condition/disease	Hirsutism (heavy/abnormal growth of hair), hyperthyroidism (overactivity of the thyroid gland)
itis	Inflammation	Appendicitis (inflammation of the appendix), mastitis (inflammation of the breast) myocarditis (inflammation of heart muscle)
osteo	Bone	Osteoporosis, (a condition that weakens the bones), osteopenia (a generalised reduction in bone mass), osteomalacia (pertaining to soft bones)
otomy	To cut into	Tracheotomy (cutting into the trachea), craniotomy (a hole made into the skull), thoracotomy (cutting into the chest)
ostomy	To make an opening (a mouth)	Colostomy (an opening into the colon), jejunostomy (an opening into the jejunum)
micro	Small	Microscopic (so small can only be seen with a microscope), microcephaly (small brain), microsomia (small body)
macro	Large	Macroscopic (large enough to be seen with the naked eye), macrocytic (an abnormally large cell), macroglossia (an abnormally large tongue). Macrosomia ('fetal macrosomia' large for gestational age)
mega/megaly	Enlarged	Cardiomegaly (enlarged heart), splenomegaly (enlarged spleen), hepatomegaly (enlarged heart)
myo	Muscle	Myocardium (heart muscle), myocyte (muscle cell), myometrium (uterine muscle)
neo	New	Neonate (new born), neoplasm (new growth [tumour])
nephro	Kidney	Nephritis (inflammation of the kidneys), nephrostomy (an incision made into the kidney)
neuro	Nerve	Neuroma (a tumour growing from a nerve), neuralgia (pain felt along the length of a nerve), neuritis (inflammation of a nerve)
ology	Study of	Gynaecology (study of the female reproductive system). Dermatology (study of the skin), neurology (study of the nervous system), cardiology (study of the heart)
oma	Tumour (swelling)	Melanoma (a cancer of melanocytes), carcinoma (a type of cancer), retinoblastoma (tumour of the eye)
ophth	Eye	Ophthalmology (study of the eye), ophthalmoscope (an instrument used to examine the inside of the eye), ophthalmotomy (an incision made into the eye)
osteo	Bone	Osteomyelitis (bone infection), osteosarcoma (bone cancer), osteoarthritis (inflammation of the joints)

(*Continued*)

TABLE 1.7 (*Continued*)

Prefix/suffix	Meaning	Example
oto	Ear	Otology (the study of the ear), otosclerosis (abnormal bone growth inside the ear)
patho	Disease	Neuropathy (disease of the nervous system), nephropathy (disease of the kidney), retinopathy (disease of the retina)
para	Beside/alongside	Para thyroid (adjacent to the thyroid), paraumbilical (alongside the umbilicus)
penia	Deficiency	Leucopoenia (deficiency of white cells), thrombocytopenia (deficiency of thrombocytes)
peri	Around	Pericardium, (the serous membrane around the heart) periosteum, (a covering enveloping the bones), peritoneum (the serous membrane lining the walls of the abdominal and pelvic cavities)
plasm	Substance	Plasma (liquid part of blood and lymphatic fluid), cytoplasm (substance of a cell lying outside of the nucleus)
plasty	Repair	Arthroplasty (surgical repair or replacement of a joint), myoplasty (muscle surgical repair of a muscle)
pneumo	Breathing/air	Pneumonia (a type of chest infection), pneumothorax (a collapsed lung), pneumograph (a device used for recording respiratory movement)
poly	Many/much	Polyhydramnios (increased amniotic fluid in the uterus) Polycystic (many cysts), polyuria (much urine), polyarthritis (arthritis affecting more than four joints)
rhino	Nose	Rhinitis (inflammation of the mucous membrane of the nose), rhinoplasty (surgical repair of the nose)
rrhoea	Discharge	Diarrhoea (frequently discharged faeces), rhinorrhoea (excessive discharge of mucus from the nose), galactorrhoea (excessive production of breast milk)
sclero	Toughen/hard	Sclera (hard/tough layer of the eyeballs), scleroderma (hardening and contraction of the skin and connective tissue), sclerosis (abnormal hardening of body tissue)
sub	Under	Subcutaneous (under the skin) Sublingual (underneath the tongue), subarachnoid (underneath the arachnoid [layer of the brain]), submucosa (tissue below mucus membrane)
tachy	Fast/rapid	Tachycardia (fast heart rate), tachypnoea (fast respiratory rate)
toxo	Poison	Cytotoxic (having a destructive action on cells), toxaemia (blood poisoning resulting from the presence of toxins), ototoxic (being toxic to the ear)
uria	Urine	Proteinuria (protein in urine). Haematuria (presence of blood in the urine), nocturia (passing urine at night), pyuria (pus in the urine)
Vaso	Vessel	Vasovagal syncope (reflex syncope). Vaso constriction (narrowing the vessel), vaso dilation (widening of the vessel), vaso spasm (sudden contraction of a vessel)

Pathophysiology

Pathophysiology brings together a blend of pathology and physiology to consider the connection between disordered physiology and disease or illness. Pathology defines the illness itself and physiology examines how these injuries or diseases change natural biological processes. The study of pathophysiology requires the use of clinical reasoning, which is then used to make a diagnosis and prescribe treatment to address the effects of disease. Learning how pathology, physiology and anatomy interconnect can ensure that the care provided is appropriate, safe and effective.

Pathophysiology, according to Singh et al. (2017), is the study of the changes of normal mechanical, physical and biochemical functions, caused by a disease or resulting from an abnormal syndrome. The chapters in this text address these key pathophysiological concepts. Medical terminology is used to express and describe the various pathophysiological concepts.

Pathophysiology is a key component of practice, enabling the midwife to take on a number of important responsibilities, such as understanding and ordering diagnostic tests, care for and treating women with acute and chronic illnesses, managing medications and managing general health and wellbeing, as well as disease prevention. Midwives who can recognise the pathophysiological signs and symptoms of conditions will be able to provide a higher quality of safe and effective care to women and their families. Asking questions such as 'Why is the woman experiencing this?' helps to understand what is going on in a woman's body at the cellular level, thus helping you to understand how to help them.

Pathophysiology is understanding the progression of disease so as to identify the disease and implement treatment options. Information gathered is used to identify the next course of the disease so that the most suitable mode of action can be provided to deliver the most appropriate care that the woman needs. The medical procedures and medications that are administered will depend very much on the nature of the disease and the needs of the woman. The main objectives when understanding pathophysiology are to assist you to:

- Use critical thinking to understand the pathophysiological principles for care provision.
- Analyse and explain the effects of diseases processes at a systemic and cellular level.
- Discuss the many variables that may be at play affecting the healing of the organ and tissue systems.
- Analyse the environmental risks of the progression and development of particular diseases.
- Explain how compensatory mechanisms can be used to make a response to physiological alterations.
- Compare and contrast the effects of culture, ethics and genetics and how these can have an impact on disease progression, treatment, health promotion and disease prevention.
- Evaluate and review diagnostic tests and determine whether the evaluation and review have any relationship to signs and symptoms that the patient is experiencing.

The Determinants of Health

While it is important to understand the pathophysiological changes that a woman may be experiencing the midwife must also appreciate the socioeconomic and cultural factors that can impact outcomes. These 'non-medical' factors are as important as whether the most appropriate test or diagnostic tool is being used or treatment prescribed. It is important to understand the molecular and genetic determinants of disease; however, non-biological factors also have the potential to influence interactions with women and their families.

There are many factors that come together to impact the health of individuals and communities. Health is determined by a person's circumstances and environment. To a large extent, factors such as where we live, the state of our environment, genetics, our income and education level and our relationships with friends and family all have significant impacts on health. However, the more commonly considered factors, such as access and use of health care services may have less of an impact. The social determinants of health are outlined in Figure 1.5. These factors include political, social, economic, environmental and cultural elements, which shape the conditions in which we are born, grow, live, work and age. Creating a healthy population requires greater action on these factors, not simply on treating ill health.

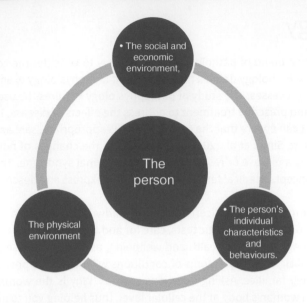

Snapshot 1.3

Ema has attended the maternity day unit complaining of reduced fetal movements. She is a gravida 1 para 0 who booked for routine antenatal care at eight weeks of gestation. The 23-year-old recently moved from Fiji to live with her husband, who is in the army and posted at a local military base. Ema has no significant medical or family history, no known allergies or comorbidities. She is a non-smoker and has a normal body mass index (BMI 27 kg/m²). Ema has accepted all routine antenatal screening as well as combined screening for Down, Edward and Patau syndromes and a glucose tolerance test.

   All routine appointments have been attended by Ema and her husband. Nothing abnormal has been detected at any investigation or examination and no concerns have been expressed. She is 38 weeks' gestation based on her estimated due date from an ultrasound dating scan in the first trimester.

Prior Investigations

- Serology results for HIV, hepatitis, syphilis are negative.
- Blood group A rhesus positive and antibody screen negative.
- No haemoglobinopathy detected.
- All haematology and biochemical markers within normal range.
- Microscopy and culture of the mid-stream urine has no growth.
- Booking blood pressure 110/70 mmHg.
- Routine anomaly scan found no fetal abnormality, with the placenta reported as anterior and not low lying.
- Maternal weight gain of 15 kg since booking.

On Admission

Ema is alert but does not make eye contact. She is mobilising well without any assistance. She states that she is worried as she has not felt baby move for four hours. She reports no abdominal pain or vagial loss. Ema says that her mood is good; she is eating and drinking as normal but has had a headache for 24 hours, which has not been eased by paracetamol. She indicates that the headache is a frontal headache. She has not experienced any visual disturbances or epigastric pain but has swollen ankles.

On Examination

Exposure appropriate for vital signs and palpation. Blood pressure measures 150/95 mmHg, proteinuria in the mid-stream urine. Heart rate 90 beats/minute. Rhythm: regular. Quality: palpable radial pulse. Skin: normal skin temperature, apyrexial with a tympanic thermometer. Capillary refill time: 2 seconds. No evidence of cyanosis. O_2 saturation is 98% in air. Maternal Early Warning Score score 3. Pitting ankle oedema.

On Palpation

Ema is semi-recumbent; the light in the room is ambient and she is comfortable. On palpation, the uterus is soft and non-tender, the symphysis–fundal height measurement is 32 cm, which is static since previously measured at 36 weeks. The fetus presents in a longitudinal lie, cephalic presentation, 4/5th of the presenting part is palpable and the fetal heart is heard, it is regular at 140 beats/minute. The blood pressure is then repeated and recorded at 140/90 mmHg.

Reflective Learning Activity

Looking at the information given in Snapshot 1.1. Determine the symptoms Ema that is experiencing. What are your concerns?

- Reduced fetal movements
- Pregnancy-induced hypertension
- Intrauterine growth restriction
- Social isolation and lack of support

What would be your management plan for Ema?
Consider which investigations you would order and/or perform.

Using a Medical Dictionary, Hints and Tips

Learning to use a medical dictionary and other resources (be these electronic or hard copy) to help find the definition of a term is an important aspect of understanding the correct use of the numerous medical terms. When starting to work with an unfamiliar resource (print or otherwise), spend some time reviewing its user guide. The time spent at this stage can help later when you are looking up unfamiliar terms.

Accuracy in spelling medical terms is extremely important. Changing just one or two letters has the potential to completely change the meaning of a word and the consequences of this can be grave. Some frequently used terms and word parts are confusing because they look and sound alike; however, their meanings can be very different (Table 1.8). Beware, too, that you may encounter alternative spellings used in the United Kingdom, Australia, Canada and the United States.

- If you know how to spell the word:
  - With the first letter of the word, start in the appropriate section of the dictionary. Look at the top of the page for clues (there may be catch words there). The top left word is the first term on the page and the top right word is the last term on that page.
  - Now, search alphabetically for words that begin with the first and second letters of the word you are searching for. Continue looking through each letter until you have found the term that you are looking for.
  - When you think you have found it, be sure to check the spelling, letter by letter, working from left to right. Terms with similar spellings have very different meanings (for example, perineum and peritoneum).
  - When the term has been located, carefully check all of the definitions.
- If you do not know how to spell the word:
  - Listen carefully to the term and then write it down.
  - If you cannot find the word on the basis of your spelling, begin to look for alternative spellings based on the beginning sound, for example, f can sound like f but, the word may begin with ph (such as pharynx, phlegm), k can sound like k but, the word may begin with ch (cholestasis for example) or c (crepitus). Psychologist begins with p but, it sounds like it should begin with an s.

TABLE 1.8   Confusing terminology.

Term/word	Means	Comments
arteri/o	Artery	Endarterial means pertaining to the interior or lining of an artery (end-means within, arteri means artery, and – al means pertaining to)
ather/o	Plaque or fatty substance	An atheroma is a fatty deposit within the wall of an artery (ather means fatty substance, and – oma means tumour)
arthr/o	Joint	Arthralgia means pain in a joint or joints (arthr means joint, and – algia means pain)
-ectomy	Surgical removal	An appendectomy is surgical removal of the appendix (append means appendix, and – ectomy means surgical removal)
-ostomy	Surgical creation of an artificial opening to the body surface	A colostomy is the surgical creation of an artificial excretory opening between the colon and the body surface (col means colon, and – ostomy means the surgical creation of an artificial opening)
-otomy	Cutting or a surgical incision	A colotomy is a surgical incision into the colon (col means colon, and – otomy means a surgical incision)

Source: Adapted from Stansfield et al. (2015).

- Look under categories:
  - Medical dictionaries may use categories such as diseases and syndromes, and may group disorders with these terms in their titles: so venereal disease would be found under 'disease, venereal' and fetal alcohol syndrome would be found under 'syndrome, fetal alcohol'.
- Multiple-word terms:
  - When searching for a term that includes more than one word, begin the search with the last term. If you do not find it there, move forward to the next word. Congestive heart failure, for example, is sometimes listed under 'heart failure, congestive'. In the same way, information pertaining to gestational diabetes may be within a text about diabetes as well as literature pertaining to the complications of pregnancy.

Searching for Definitions on the Internet and Handheld Devices

Internet search engines are helpful resources in locating definitions and details about medical conditions and terms. It is important, however, that you use a site such as the Royal College of Obstetricians and Gynaecologists, National Institutes for Health and Care Excellence (known as NICE) or Scottish Intercollegiate Guidelines Network (known as SIGN), as these bodies are known to be reputable information sources.

Beware of suggested search terms. If you do not spell a term correctly, a website might take a guess at what it is that you are searching for. Be sure to double-check that the term you are defining is the term intended.

Take Home Points

- Use the appropriate anatomical terminology to identify key body structures, body regions and directions in the body.
- A standard reference position for mapping the body's structures is the normal anatomical position.
- The terminology used in anatomy, physiology and pathophysiology can be bewildering; however, the purpose of this language is not to confuse, but rather to increase precision and reduce errors.

- Anatomical terms are very often derived from ancient Greek and Latin words.
- Anatomical terms are made up of roots, prefixes and suffixes.
- Without doubt, it is important to understand the pathophysiological changes. The midwife must also appreciate the socioeconomic and cultural factors that can impact on outcomes – the determinants of health.
- Learning how to use a medical dictionary and other resources to find the definition of a term is an important aspect of understanding the correct use of the numerous medical terms. The time that is spent at this stage can help later when looking up any unfamiliar terms.

Medications Management: Name Confusion

Recent examples of medicine names that have been confused resulting in medication errors include:

- mercaptamine and mercaptopurine
- sulfadiazine and sulfasalazine
- risperidone and ropinirole
- zuclopenthixol decanoate and zuclopenthixol acetate

Some of these errors could result in life-threatening conditions. Be extra vigilant when dispensing medicines with commonly confused drug names to ensure that the intended medicine is supplied.

- If there are any doubts about which medicine is intended, contact the prescriber before dispensing the drug
- Adhere to local and professional guidance in relation to checking the right medicine has been dispensed to the correct person.

Reflective Learning Activity

Drugs are administered in a variety of dosages, preparations and routes. Next time you are in placement, review a drug Kardex® (or drug chart) and pay attention to the prescribed administration of medicines, the route, dose, frequency, its interactions and contraindications.

Take Home Points

- Medical terminology may appear intimidating and complicated.
- A number of terms used in midwifery, healthcare and medicine are derived from Latin and Greek.
- To understand the terminology used it is essential when learning to break it down into its parts. When this is done, you can see how it all fits together – like the carriages of a train.
- In translating medical terms, it is important to understand the word root, the word root (the foundation of the term) can have a prefix and suffix attached to it.
- To communicate safely with other midwives and healthcare professionals, it is imperative that there is a consistency in the language being used so as to reduce any risk of confusion. Learning the language requires practice.
- It is vital to understand the pathophysiological changes so as to provide the most appropriate care intervention. It is equally important to have an understanding of the impact of socioeconomic and cultural factors that can impact on the outcomes, the 'non-medical' factors.

References

McGuiness, H. (2018). *Anatomy and Physiology: Therapy basics*, 5e. London: Hodder Education.

Peate, I. (ed.) (2017). *Fundamentals of Applied Pathophysiology: An essential guide for nursing and healthcare students*. Chichester: Wiley.

Singh, I., Weston, A., Kundur, A., and Dobie, G. (2017). *Haematology Case Studies with Blood Cell Morphology and Pathophysiology*. London: Academic Press.

Stansfield, P., Hui, Y.H., and Cross, N. (2015). *Essential Medical Terminology*, 4e. Chicago, IL: Jones and Bartlett.

World Health Organization (2020). Health impact assessment. https://www.who.int/hia/evidence/doh/en (accessed 20 October 2023).

Further Reading

National Institute for Health and Care Excellence. (2023). Hypertension in Pregnancy: Diagnosis and management. NICE Guideline NG133. London: National Institute for Health and Care Excellence. www.nice.org.uk/guidance/NG133 (accessed 20 October 2023).

Royal College of Obstetricians and Gynaecologists. (2016). *Diagnosis and Management of Ectopic Pregnancy*. Green-top Guideline No. 21. London: Royal College of Obstetricians and Gynaecologists. www.rcog.org.uk/guidance/browse-all-guidance/green-top-guidelines/diagnosis-and-management-of-ectopic-pregnancy-green-top-guideline-no-21 (accessed 20 October 2023).

Online Resources

British National Formulary: https://bnf.nice.org.uk

Health Information and Quality Authority. Safer Better Care: www.hiqa.ie

NHS England. Abbreviations you may find in your health records. https://www.nhs.uk/using-the-nhs/nhs-services/the-nhs-app/abbreviations

NHS England. Saving Babies' Lives Care Bundle: https://www.england.nhs.uk/mat-transformation/saving-babies

Glossary

Aetiology	Study of the cause(s) of disease and/or injury.
Anatomy	The study of the structure of living organisms and their parts.
Auscultation	The act of listening to internal body sounds using a Pinnard stethoscope or other listening device.
Blood pressure	The force of blood against the walls of arteries, expressed in millimetres of mercury (mmHg).
Homeostasis	The body's ability to maintain a stable internal environment despite external changes.
Oedema	Refers to the accumulation of excess fluid in the body's tissues.
Organ	A structure composed of different tissues that work together to perform specific functions.
Palpation	Using the hands and fingers to touch and feel the body, usually to examine its physical characteristics or to assess certain structures or conditions.
Pathology	Study of structural alterations in cells, tissues and organs that help to identify the cause of disease.
Pathophysiology	The study of functional changes in the body occurring in response to disease or injury.
Physiology	The branch of biology that deals with the normal functions and processes of living organisms and their parts.

Multiple Choice Questions

1. What does lymphoedema refer to?
   a. Removal of lymph glands in the neck
   b. Removal of lymph glands during pregnancy
   c. A chronic condition that causes swelling in the body's tissues
   d. Infection of the lymph nodes located in the thorax

2. What is polyhydramnios?
   a. A reduced volume of amniotic fluid in the uterus during pregnancy
   b. Excessive ankle oedema in pregnancy
   c. An excessive amount of fluid in the uterus during pregnancy
   d. A normal amount of fluid in multiple pregnancies

3. What is the meaning of abduct in relation to muscles?
   a. It means the same as adduct
   b. To pull away from the body
   c. Relates to the torso only
   d. To pull towards the body

4. What is the difference between the words 'afferent' and 'efferent'?
   a. Afferent means towards a centre and efferent outward from a centre
   b. Afferent means outward from a centre and efferent towards a centre
   c. Afferent is associated with the kidney only and efferent is associated with the brain only
   d. Afferent refers only to nerves and efferent refers only to blood

5. Which of the following conditions is a multifactorial condition of pregnancy characterised by pruritus in the absence of a rash with abnormal liver function tests, neither of which has an alternative cause, and resolving after birth?
   a. Pre-eclampsia
   b. Eclampsia
   c. Obstetric cholestasis
   d. Hyperemesis gravidarum

6. What is the definition of pathophysiology?
   a. Another term for renal failure
   b. A mental health disorder
   c. The study of functional changes in the body occurring in response to disease or injury
   d. The term used to describe end of life care

7. What does the term 'xerosis' mean?
   a. Liver disease
   b. Abnormal dryness, as seen in the eyes, skin or mouth
   c. Excessive and abnormal production of vaginal discharge
   d. Depleted production of mucous

8. What are determinants of health?
   a. The measures used by physiotherapists to determine prognosis
   b. Determinants of health are only applicable in low income countries
   c. The determinants of health include the social and economic environment, the physical environment and the person's individual characteristics and behaviours
   d. All of the above

9. The sagittal plane divides what from what?
   a. Divides the body top and bottom
   b. Divides the abdomen only left and right
   c. Divides the contents of thoracic cavity top and bottom
   d. Divides the body or an organ vertically into the left and right sides

10. The prefix is added to which part of a word?
    a. The end of the second letter of a sentence
    b. The beginning of a word
    c. The end of a word
    d. Words beginning with a vowel only

CHAPTER 2

Cell Physiology

Rebecca Murray

AIM

The aim of this chapter is to improve your knowledge and understanding of cell physiology and ability to apply this knowledge to midwifery practice.

LEARNING OUTCOMES

After reading this chapter you will be able to:

- Describe the structure and functions of the human cell.
- Describe how the structure of the plasma membrane determines its permeability.
- Describe the ways in which substances move into and out of cells.
- Understand the different types of cells and their function.
- Understand the process of cell division.
- Understand the changes that occur during pregnancy and their impact on the cells and their function.

Test Your Prior Knowledge

1. What is a cell?
2. What are the structures that form a cell?
3. What different types of cells are there?
4. How do substances move across the cell membrane?

Introduction

All living things are composed of cells. These cells are classified as either *eukaryotic* or *prokaryotic* cells. Eukaryotic cells have a distinct nucleus – they are present in all human, animal and plant tissue. Prokaryotic cells, including some bacteria and blue-green algae, do not contain distinct nucleus but the nuclear material is spread within the cytoplasm (the liquid inside a cell).

Fundamentals of Maternal Anatomy and Physiology, First Edition. Edited by Ian Peate and Claire Leader.
© 2024 John Wiley & Sons Ltd. Published 2024 by John Wiley & Sons Ltd.

A cell is the smallest living part of the human body and makes up all living organisms and tissues. Cells are an extremely important part of normal biological function, as they provide structure to the body, convert food to nutrients and energy, and carry out specialised functions to ensure that the body works optimally. Most cells within the human body contain DNA, so they have the ability to replicate themselves and repair via the process of mitosis. Within the cell, there are a number of organelles (little organs), which have specialised functions. While the biological structures of cells are similar, their functions can vary widely. Cells can provide a particular function on their own but more commonly they combine to form a tissue type. When a number of tissue types combine, they form an organ. The most common and important cells with the human body are detailed in Table 2.1. It is important for midwives to understand the normal structure and function of the cell; this will help them understand the health impact if the structure or function changes and how they can identify and treat this in the clinical setting. This chapter considers the structure and function of the cell and how the body's adaptations to pregnancy can impact its normal function (Coad et al. 2019).

The Cell and Organelles

A typical cell will contain a nucleus, cytoplasm and a cell membrane. The cytoplasm is made up of water, electrolytes, carbohydrates, proteins and lipids and they all play a key role in the structure and function of the cell and its organelles. The organelles of the cell include the cell membrane, nucleus, peroxisomes, the endoplasmic reticulum, Golgi apparatus, mitochondria, lysosomes and cytoskeleton (Figure 2.1).

The Nucleus

The nucleus is the largest organelle and is the control centre for the cell. It is bound by a membrane: the nuclear membrane, which allows substances to move into and out of the nucleus via nuclear pores (Figure 2.1). The nucleus contains nucleoplasm, deoxyribonucleic acid (DNA) as chromatin threads, and nucleoli where ribosomal ribonucleic acid (rRNA) is produced. The DNA contains the genetic instructions for the organism and the nucleus helps to store and protect the genetic information of the cell. The nucleus supports with the regulation of cell division through mitosis and meiosis (discussed later in the chapter). The nucleus is also responsible for gene expression, allowing the cell to adapt and respond to signals it receives (Evans and Manson 2008).

Endoplasmic Reticulum

The endoplasmic reticulum is a multifunctional organelle that plays a crucial role in the synthesis, modification and transport of proteins and lipids within the cell (Figure 2.1). It is a complex network of membranous tubules and sacs connected to the nuclear membrane. There are two main types: rough and smooth, each having distinct functions.

Rough endoplasmic reticulum (RER) contains ribosomes on its surface, which gives a rough appearance. The ribosomes are responsible for the synthesis of proteins that are used in the cell membrane or elsewhere in the body. These proteins are modified in the lumen of the RER to give them their distinct structure and transported to the Golgi apparatus.

Smooth endoplasmic reticulum (SER) does not have ribosomes on its surface, giving it a smooth appearance. It is enriched in cells that are involved in lipid metabolism and detoxification of drugs and harmful substances. It is responsible for the regulation of calcium levels within the cell and plays a crucial role in the synthesis of lipids, including phospholipids and cholesterol, which are essential components of the cell membrane (Peate and Evans 2020).

TABLE 2.1 Common types of cells in the human body.

Cell groups in the body	Types of cells
Stem cells	Embryonic stem cells
	Adult stem cells
Red blood cells	Erythrocytes
White blood cells	Granulocytes (neutrophils, eosinophils, basophils)
	Agranulocytes (monocytes, lymphocytes)
Platelets	Fragments of megakaryocytes
Nerve cells	Neurons
	Neuroglial cells
Muscle cells	Skeletal
	Cardiac
	Smooth
Cartilage	Chondrocytes
Bone cells	Osteoblasts
	Osteoclasts
	Osteocytes
	Lining cells
Skin cells	Keratinocytes
	Melanocytes
	Merkel cells
	Langerhans cells
Endothelium	Lining of blood vessels
Epithelium	Lining of body cavities
Fat cells	White adipocytes
	Brown adipocytes
Sex cells	Ova
	Spermatozoa

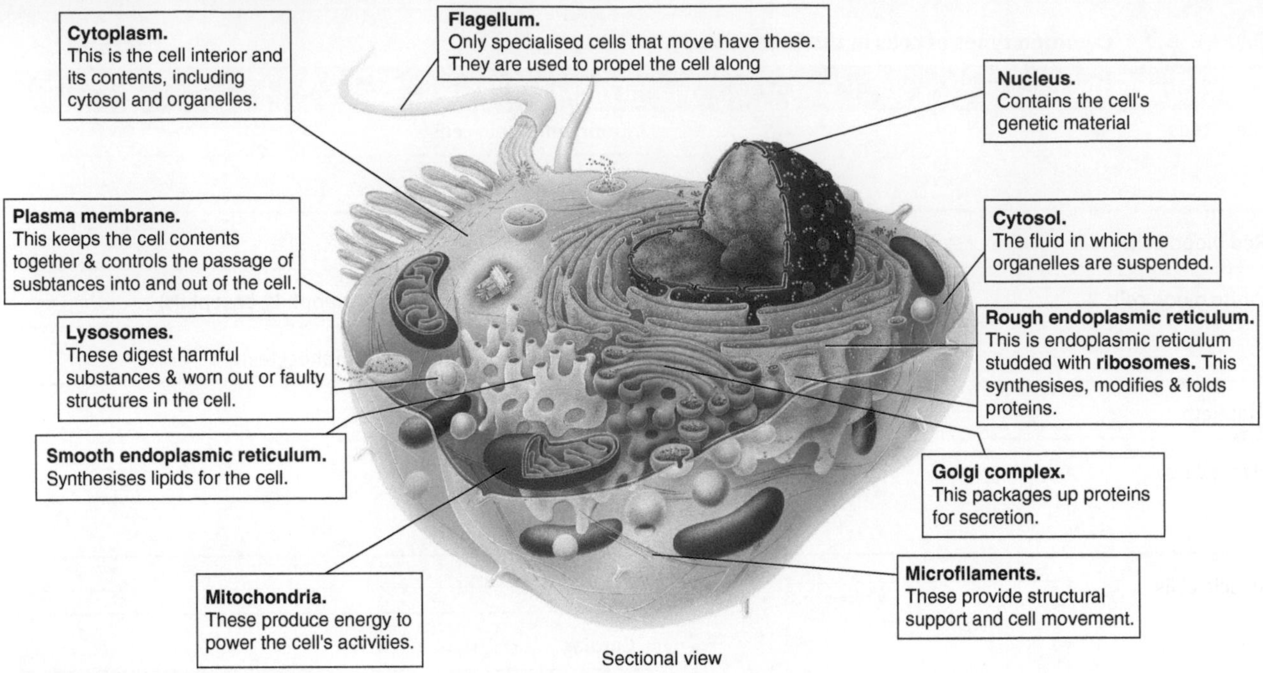

Cytoplasm.
This is the cell interior and its contents, including cytosol and organelles.

Flagellum.
Only specialised cells that move have these. They are used to propel the cell along

Nucleus.
Contains the cell's genetic material

Plasma membrane.
This keeps the cell contents together & controls the passage of susbtances into and out of the cell.

Cytosol.
The fluid in which the organelles are suspended.

Lysosomes.
These digest harmful substances & worn out or faulty structures in the cell.

Rough endoplasmic reticulum.
This is endoplasmic reticulum studded with **ribosomes.** This synthesises, modifies & folds proteins.

Smooth endoplasmic reticulum.
Synthesises lipids for the cell.

Golgi complex.
This packages up proteins for secretion.

Mitochondria.
These produce energy to power the cell's activities.

Microfilaments.
These provide structural support and cell movement.

Sectional view

FIGURE 2.1   Structure of a cell. Source: Nair and Peate (2009)/John Wiley & Sons.

Golgi Apparatus

The Golgi apparatus is a series of membrane-bound sacs arranged in parallel rows, stacked on top of each other. They are responsible for processing, sorting and packaging proteins and lipids for transport to their destination inside or outside the cell. Proteins that are synthesised in the RER move through the Golgi apparatus and are modified in ways that will affect their structure, function and stability. The Golgi apparatus plays a key role in assembling complex lipids, including glycolipids, which are important for the cell membrane, and secretes these proteins from the cell by the process of exocytosis (explained later in the chapter). It also develops lysosomes needed for the breakdown of waste products and foreign substances found within the cell (Alberts et al. 2018).

Mitochondria

The mitochondria are responsible for producing adenosine triphosphate (ATP), the energy needed for a cell to carry out its function. A mitochondrion comprises an inner and outer membrane. The outer membrane consists of a phospholipid bilayer, similar to cell membrane, of transport proteins, which help with the transport of ions and metabolites. The inner membrane consists of lots of folds called cristae, and is the site of ATP production. For cells that use a lot of energy, such as muscles and the liver, the inner membrane includes more folds to increase the capacity to produce ATP (Orchard and Nation 2015).

The Cell Membrane

The cell membrane, also known as the plasma membrane, is a semipermeable membrane surrounding the cell (Figure 2.1). The cell membrane defines the border of the cell and determines how it interacts with the environment around it. It must be adaptable to all the different types of movement of cells, such as red and white blood cells moving through narrow arteries and veins. The membrane needs to have markers that allow similar cells to recognise each other and form tissues and organs. The cell membrane has a function is the transmission of signals to receive and activate vital processes (Evans and Manson 2008).

The cell membrane is made up of a phospholipid bilayer containing molecules such as proteins and lipids, which are involved in the processes of cellular transportation and communication. Phospholipids are molecules with a hydrophilic (water loving) head and two hydrophobic (water hating) tails. In the cell membrane, phospholipids arrange themselves with their hydrophilic heads facing outwards towards the aqueous environments both intracellular and extracellular. The hydrophobic tails are oriented inwards, away from the water, creating a stable, flexible barrier that isolates the cytoplasm from the surrounding medium (Peate and Evans 2020). The proteins contained in the phospholipid bilayer serve various functions, including transport of molecules, enzymatic activity, cell signalling and structural support. Some proteins also act as receptors, allowing the cell to detect and respond to external signals (Alberts et al. 2018).

The cell membrane can be described as a fluid mosaic model, which reflects the dynamic nature of the cell membrane. The components of the cell membrane are not static but rather move laterally within the lipid bilayer. This dynamic behaviour allows the cell membrane to be selectively permeable, controlling the passage of ions, nutrients and other molecules into and out of the cell, which is essential for maintaining cellular homeostasis and regulating cellular activities.

Transport of Substances Across the Cell Membrane

The processes in which substances move through the cell membrane can be split into active and passive processes. The active processes require energy from the cell and are known as active transport, endocytosis and exocytosis. When energy is not required, the processes are passive and consist of osmosis, simple diffusion and facilitated diffusion.

Osmosis

Osmosis is the movement of water across a semipermeable membrane from an area of low solute concentration and high water concentration to an area of high solute concentration and low water concentration. A solute is something that is dissolved in water (e.g. sodium). The process of osmosis continues until there is an equilibrium on each side. It is important in maintaining structure and osmotic pressure within a cell (Lopez and Hall 2020). An example of osmosis in the body is in the kidneys, as water is absorbed into the body for use. This process is regulated by antidiuretic hormone (ADH), which is produced in the pituitary gland. This hormone is released based on a feedback mechanism where there is a reduction in blood pressure or decreased renal perfusion. During pregnancy, the effect of hormones on the blood vessels causes vasodilation, which can cause an increase in ADH and a decrease in plasma osmolarity and sodium levels (Diaz-Perez and Davis 2018).

Clinical Investigations: Fluid Input and Output

A woman who has pre-eclampsia may have a non-osmotic release of ADH, resulting in increased absorption of water, which leads to oedema and circulatory overload. When caring for a woman with pre-eclampsia, it is important to record fluid input and output accurately on a fluid balance chart to minimise the risk of fluid overload. The woman will also be on a fluid-restricted regimen (Hsu et al. 2021; Powell et al. 2020).

Simple Diffusion

Simple diffusion, a form of passive transport, is the process in which molecules move across a cell membrane from an area of high concentration to an area of low concentration along the concentration gradient. This movement occurs without the need for energy from the cell, as it relies on the natural movement of molecules. The movement continues until a balance is reached, with molecules evenly distributed on both sides of the plasma membrane. An example of simple diffusion within the body is the exchange of the gases oxygen and carbon dioxide within the lungs. Oxygen in the lungs moves into the bloodstream because the concentration is lower and, in reverse, carbon dioxide moves from the bloodstream into the lungs. This process is essential for maintaining the proper balance of molecules inside and outside the cell. While simple diffusion is efficient for certain molecules, more complex transport mechanisms are required for larger, charged or polar molecules to move across the cell membrane (Figure 2.2).

Facilitated Diffusion

Facilitated diffusion is the process of molecules moving from an area of high concentration to low concentration using proteins within the cell membrane to transport them. The proteins within the cell membrane help molecules that cannot move easily across the phospholipid bilayer to enter the cells. While the cell uses proteins and protein channels, the process is still passive, as it is moving from an area of high to low concentration and therefore does not require energy. This is useful for essential maintenance of the cell, as it does not require energy. Facilitated diffusion is a selective process, with proteins and protein channels only transporting specific molecules (e.g. ion channels only move sodium, potassium and calcium across the cell membrane). Figure 2.3 shows the different types of passive transport mechanisms.

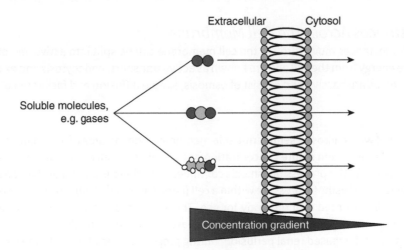

FIGURE 2.2   Diagram showing simple diffusion. Source: Nair and Peate (2009)/John Wiley & Sons.

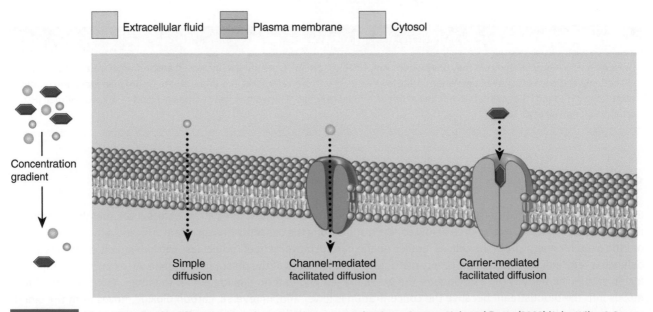

FIGURE 2.3   Figure showing the different types of passive transport mechanisms. Source: Nair and Peate (2009)/John Wiley & Sons.

Active Transport

Active transport is the process in which molecules move across the cell membrane from an area of low concentration to high concentration. As they are moving against the concentration gradient, energy is required to facilitate the process. The energy for this process comes from the breakdown of ATP to adenosine diphosphate (ADP). ATP consists of a base, sugar and three phosphate groups held together by high-energy bonds. During the process of hydrolysis, water is added and the ATP breaks down to ADP and a free phosphate, releasing the energy bonds that are used in the active transport process. The free phosphate is used in the process of creating ATP, which can be used again. Active transport is important for muscle contraction and nerve stimulus. In the sodium–potassium pump, concentration gradients generate electrical energy within the cell. In calcium pumps, calcium ions are transported into the cell to help with muscle contraction (Alberts et al. 2018). Proton pumps can also be found in the lining on the stomach to create acid, which helps with the breakdown of food.

Exocytosis

Exocytosis is a process by which cells release substances from the inside of the cell to the outside of the cell. It is an important process in cell communication and secretion of hormones and neurotransmitters. Previously in the chapter, the role of the Golgi apparatus was discussed in relation to the formation of proteins and hormones. These substances are released from the Golgi apparatus by exocytosis when the body receives a signal for their use. The secretory vesicle fuses with the cell membrane and releases the contents to outside the cell. The secretory vesicle briefly becomes part of the cell membrane, increasing its surface area; however, this process is regulated by endocytosis, which returns the unused proteins and lipids from the vesicle to the Golgi apparatus (Orchard and Nation 2015). Oxytocin is an example of a hormone that is secreted via exocytosis. It is produced in the hypothalamus and released from the pituitary gland when signals are received due to pressure on mechanoreceptors in the cervix and vaginal wall during labour or from suckling during breastfeeding (Walter et al. 2021).

Endocytosis

Endocytosis plays a role in the regulation of the internal environment of a cell. It allows the cell to take in nutrients and other molecules without using the channels and carrier proteins of the plasma membrane by using the plasma membrane itself to engulf the molecule. Once the molecule has been engulfed inwards by the plasma membrane, it is pinched off, forming a vesicle that contains the molecule. There are two types of endocytosis: phagocytosis and pinocytosis (Orchard and Nation 2015).

Pinocytosis occurs in many cells and is also known as 'cellular drinking'. The process involves fluid and dissolved solutes being surrounded by the cell membrane forming a vesicle known as a pinosome; these are used by the cell to regulate the intake of fluids and solutes.

Phagocytosis is a specialised form of endocytosis, known as 'cellular eating'. It has two main functions in the body: breakdown of nutrients from food or defence against bacteria. When large food particles are taken into the cell via endocytosis, they are sent to lysosomes for digestion. It is at this point that the food particles are broken down and the metabolites are used within the cell. The body also has several specialised cells, phagocytic cells, which defend the body against bacteria; examples are macrophages and neutrophils (Alberts et al. 2018). Figure 2.4 shows the types of endocytosis.

Macrophages play a role in tissue remodelling and repair and the formation of new blood vessels via angiogenesis. They are found in the decidua of the uterus, where they are thought to play a role in the maintenance of a healthy pregnancy by helping with trophoblast invasion and the formation of the spiral arteries. However, if this normal process becomes disrupted, an inflammatory event can occur, releasing cytokines, which disrupts the formation of the spiral arteries and can lead to complications such as pre-eclampsia and fetal growth restriction (Ning et al. 2016).

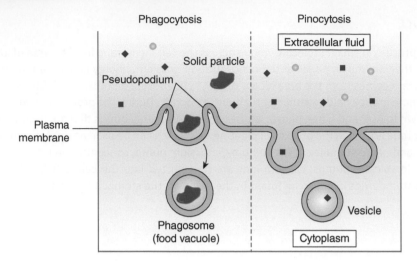

Phagocytosis   Pinocytosis

FIGURE 2.4   Showing the types of endocytosis.

Links to Clinical Practice: The Placenta

The placenta is a temporary organ which develops during pregnancy to support the growth and development of the fetus. The role of the placenta is:

- Gas exchange, providing nutrients and removal of waste between the mother and the fetus.
- Transfer of immunoglobulins from mother to baby.
- Secretion of hormones.

These processes happen via passive and active transport processes.

Water crosses the placenta through osmosis working with the concentration gradient. Simple diffusion allows the exchange of gases in the placenta. Oxygen from the maternal blood is diffused into the fetal circulation for use, while carbon dioxide is removed as a waste product back into the maternal circulation for elimination. Facilitated diffusion is responsible for the delivery of glucose to the fetus as it requires the use of carrier proteins in the placenta membrane.

Amnio acids needed by the fetus for protein synthesis are transferred across the placenta by active transport. Maternal immunoglobulin G antibodies can cross the placenta via pinocytosis to provide passive immunity.

It is important to remember that while the placenta has a protective and supportive role in maintaining a healthy pregnancy, it is not selective, so substances from drugs and their metabolites can cross from the mother to the fetus. The availability of the drug in the fetal circulation depends on the function of the placenta, the transport mechanism, and the type of drug (Griffiths and Campbell 2015; Macnab 2022).

Medications Management: Drugs in Pregnancy

There will be times during pregnancy when drugs are given with the aim of transferring them across the placenta for a therapeutic benefit (e.g. steroids for lung maturation in premature infants). Unfortunately, there are occasions when drugs have been given that have caused devastating adverse effects, most notably thalidomide (Griffiths and Campbell 2015; Macnab 2022).

- Midwives need to consider what is known about a drug in pregnancy before they prescribe or administer and consider alternative options if needed.
- Where there is a known teratogenic effect of a drug, they should be avoided, when possible, in women who want to conceive. For example, sodium valporate is used for the treatment of epilepsy, but because of its teratogenic effects, it should be avoided as a treatment option in women of childbearing potential (MHRA 2021).

Homeostasis

Homeostasis is the ability of the human body to maintain and regulate its internal environment, adjusting to external factors, to protect its function. In the body, it is important that blood glucose levels, blood pressure, electrolyte levels and body temperature are all kept with a certain range to maintain normal body functions (McEwan 2016). Homeostasis is achieved by feedback mechanisms within the body; these can be positive, which encourages a response, or negative, which acts to inhibit a response. The process happens with receptors on cells in the body that are activated. Activation sends a message to a control centre, which sends signals that produce a response. Homeostasis is regulated in many areas in the body; this process discussed in later chapters (Peate and Evans 2020).

During pregnancy, the effect of hormones on the blood vessels causes vasodilation, leading to a reduction in blood pressure. To regulate this reduction, there are increased levels of aldosterone released from the adrenal glands during pregnancy. This hormone increases the absorption of water and sodium back into the system, increasing plasma volume to maintain blood pressure (Scaife and Mohaupt 2017). This increase in blood plasma volume also has a protective function in preparation for delivery to help the body if there is a loss of plasma volume from postpartum haemorrhage (Vricella, 2017).

Clinical Management: Hyperemesis Gravidarum

Hyperemesis gravidarum is a condition of severe nausea and vomiting in pregnancy. Women experiencing hyperemesis have weight loss, nutritional deficiency and fluid and electrolyte imbalance. Symptoms can start from five weeks of gestation and, for some women, the symptoms do not stop until the birth of the baby. It is the most common reason for admission to hospital in early pregnancy.

Women present with signs of dehydration including tachycardia, hypotension and ketonuria. Blood results will show electrolyte imbalance. The treatment of hyperemesis gravidarum is oral or intramuscular antiemetics, vitamins and intravenous (IV) fluids (RCOG 2016; Lee et al. 2011). IV fluids are needed to replace the fluid volume and treat the electrolyte imbalance. The most common IV fluids used to treat dehydration are sodium chloride 0.9% or Hartmann's solution.

Osmoregulation in Cases of Dehydration

The fluid within the human body consists of water, electrolytes, gases, enzymes and hormones. It plays an important role in providing the appropriate environment for cells to perform effectively to carry out their normal function. The body works hard to maintain each of these within a normal range to maintain homeostasis. In cases of severe dehydration, such as hyperemesis gravidarum, the body will release ADH to signal to the kidney to increase water absorption to try to maintain levels. Aldosterone is produced in the adrenal glands and released to help maintain electrolyte balance. Its role is to increase the absorption of water and sodium from the kidneys and also signal for the kidneys to release potassium. However, there are times when fluid and electrolyte replacement is needed to treat the dehydration.

Medications Management: Intravenous Fluids

It is important to remember that IV fluids need an appropriate prescription before they are administered for treatment of dehydration. The fluid requirements will be individual to each woman who needs them. It is important to look at the results of her blood tests to understand what needs to be replaced and to carefully monitor her bloods throughout. Accurate fluid balance charts should be maintained to prevent fluid overload and the IV access site must be monitored to ensure that there is no infection and that the IV line is patent (Macdonald and Johnson 2023).

Cell Division

There are two types of cell division: mitosis and meiosis. Mitosis is the process of making new, identical cells, while meiosis is the process of producing sperm and egg (each containing half the genetic information) for reproduction.

Mitosis

During mitosis, the parent cell, containing 23 chromosome pairs, replicates to produce two daughter cells. These daughter cells contain exactly the same genetic information as the parent. Mitosis is seen in the human body during cell renewal, such as skin renewal, and during repair from tissue damage (e.g. surgery). During pregnancy, the rate of mitosis is amplified because of the increased demands of growth of the fetus and changes in the female body. The stages of mitosis are prophase, metaphase, anaphase and telophase.

- Before mitosis begins, the cells are prepared for cell division by growing and replicating its DNA to produce two identical strands known as chromatids; this phase is known as the *interphase*.
- *Prophase* – this is the first stage of mitosis. The DNA in the nucleus of the cell condenses and chromosomes become visible; the chromatids are held together at the centromere (Figure 2.5). The mitotic apparatus forms, consisting of two centrioles separated by a mitotic spindle, whose role is to separate the chromosome. The centrioles move to opposite ends of the cell and the membrane around the nucleus disappears.
- *Metaphase* – the chromatids start to align in a single plane on each side of the mitotic spindle, in preparation for division (Figure 2.6).
- *Anaphase* – the centromeres divide and the chromatids start to separate, forming separate daughter chromosomes (Figure 2.7).
- *Telophase* – the final stage sees the arrival of the chromosomes at their pole (Figure 2.8). A new nuclear membrane is formed and the content of the cell cytoplasm is split between the sister cells leaving two cell identical to the parent cell.

Once this is process is complete, the whole process starts again (Rankin 2017; Gardner and Davis 2009)

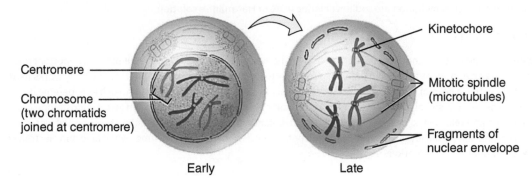

Centromere

Chromosome
(two chromatids
joined at centromere)

Kinetochore

Mitotic spindle
(microtubules)

Fragments of
nuclear envelope

Early   Late

FIGURE 2.5   Prophase.

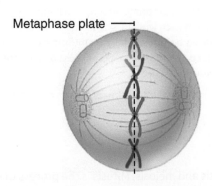

Metaphase plate

FIGURE 2.6   Metaphase.

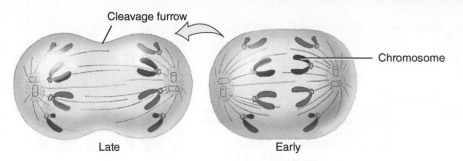

FIGURE 2.7 Anaphase.

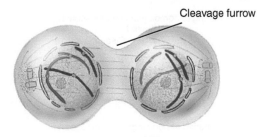

FIGURE 2.8 Telophase.

Meiosis

Meiosis is a specialised type of cell division that occurs to produce gametes – sperm and egg (Figure 2.9). All human cells are diploid, meaning that they contain two sets of chromosomes: one from the maternal egg and one from the paternal sperm. Meiosis is the process whereby the cells split to form haploid cells – gametes, containing only half the genetic information. The process is split into two parts – meiosis 1 and meiosis 2, leading to four genetically different daughter cells (which in turn leads to the diversity we see in the population). Before this process starts, the cells go through interphase, just as in mitosis, to replicate the genetic information (Rankin 2017).

Meiosis 1 consists of prophase 1, metaphase 1, anaphase 1 and telophase 1. Similarly, to mitosis, in prophase 1, the chromosomes condense, the nuclear membrane starts to break down and the chromatids become aligned to become pairs. During this alignment, the chromatids pair with their match (e.g. chromosome 9 pairs with chromosome 9). It is at this point that some of the genetic material is exchanged leading to diversity in humans.

During metaphase 1, the homologue pairs line up at the metaphase plate for separation. A microtubule from one pole attaches to one chromosome of a homologous pair and a microtubule from another pole attaches to the other chromosome of the homologous pair. Moving into anaphase 1, the homologous chromosome separate but the sister chromatids remain together.

When the chromosomes arrive at their separate poles, the cells split and the cellular material is divided; this is known as telophase 1. Quickly, the cells enter meiosis 2.

Meiosis 2 is different to meiosis 1 and mitosis, as it does not start with the replication of DNA. The cells entering meiosis 2 are haploid but there are still two sister chromatids. During prophase 2, the chromosomes recondense, the spindle is reformed and the nuclear membrane breaks up. In metaphase 2, the chromosomes align along the metaphase plate. In anaphase 2, the sister chromatids separate, moving to the opposite poles, becoming separate chromosomes. In the final stage, telophase 2, the chromosomes arrive at their poles, the nuclear membrane is formed and there are four haploid cells containing unique genetic material (Marcus 2010).

There are times when the process of meiosis does not work as planned, resulting in an abnormal number of chromosomes in the daughter cells. Meiotic non-disjunction errors are a result of homologous chromosomes failing to

33

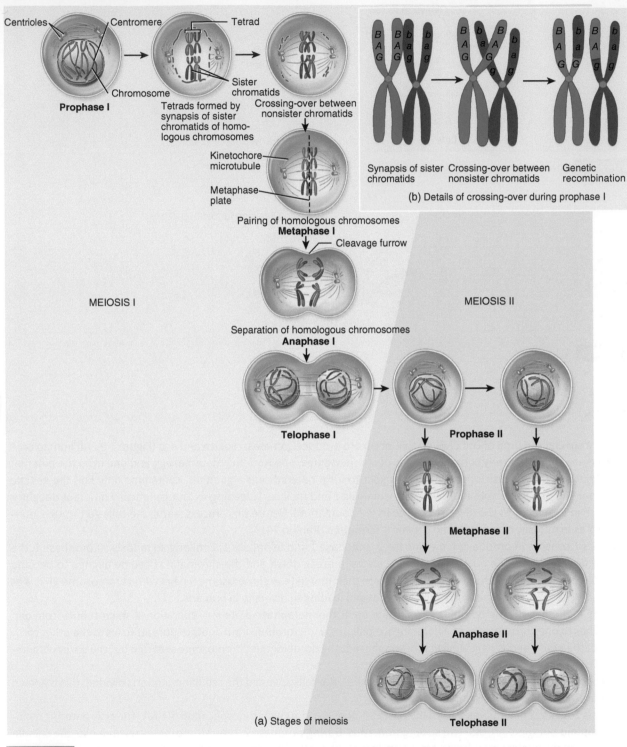

Synapsis of sister chromatids

Crossing-over between nonsister chromatids

Genetic recombination

(b) Details of crossing-over during prophase I

MEIOSIS I

MEIOSIS II

(a) Stages of meiosis

FIGURE 2.9   A diagrammatic representation of meiosis, reproductive cell division.

split during anaphase, meaning that both chromosomes of the pair pass to the daughter cell; this is known as aneuploidy. Aneuploidy usually involves a single chromosome and leads to a trisomy condition such as trisomy 21 (Down syndrome). However, there are times when all the chromosomes are involved, leading to a condition known as triploidy (Strauss et al. 2023).

Clinical Investigations: Screening Tests

During the antenatal period, women are offered screening tests for trisomy 21 (T21), trisomy 18 (T18; Edwards syndrome) and trisomy 13 (T13; Patau syndrome) as part of the NHS fetal anomaly screening programme. These tests are not compulsory, and women can opt out of testing. This screening involves an ultrasound scan and blood test, and take place between 11^{+2} and 14^{+1} weeks of gestation. Maternal age, biochemical markers from blood tests and nuchal translucency, and crown–rump length from the ultrasound scan are combined to determine the chance of the fetus having one of these conditions.

Women who have a screening result which gives them a higher chance of having a fetus with T21, T18 or T13 will be offered further testing to determine whether the fetus is affected by the condition. The options available to them are non-invasive prenatal testing (NIPT) or prenatal diagnostic (PND) tests – chorionic villi sampling or amniocentesis. If a woman selects NIPT and the result is a higher chance, she will be offered PND to confirm the result. If the results from PND confirm that the fetus has the condition, the woman will be offered support to continue with the pregnancy or will be supported and signposted to the appropriate services to end the pregnancy (NHS 2021).

Genomics and Midwifery

Genomics is the study of complex and multifactorial diseases resulting from the interactions of genes and the person's environment. It is an area of research that has expanded over the past 30 years, with the aims of developing new diagnostic tests, and brings with it the potential for novel treatments. Midwives need to understand genomics and how it relates to midwifery practice. This will allow them to present the most up to date evidence-based options to the women they see in clinical practice. Women who may need further investigation would be identified during the booking appointment or from the results of screening tests. Most common next generation sequencing tests offered within the NHS are Non Invasive Prenatal Testing (NIPT) which is a screening test, or Non Invasive Prenatal Diagnosis (NIPD) which is a diagnostic test. Both involve taking a blood sample, which is used to extract cell-free fetal DNA in the maternal blood. This DNA is sequenced and the chromosomes are counted to determine whether there is an abnormal number.

NIPD is used within maternity services to determine the rhesus genotype of a fetus carried by a rhesus negative mother. If the fetus is rhesus positive, the women will receive prophylactic anti D to reduce the risk of rhesus disease. If the fetus is rhesus negative then the mother does not need to receive this treatment (Macdonald and Johnson 2023).

Cell Division and Multiple Pregnancy

In human reproduction, the egg and sperm (haploid gametes) join together to produce a diploid zygote. While meiosis is the cell division cycle responsible for the creation of gametes, mitosis is responsible for the cell division in embryonic development (Gilbert 2000). In the majority of cases, the joining of a single sperm and single egg will result in a singleton pregnancy. However, there is a chance that after fertilization, the zygote will split into two or more, leading to a multiple pregnancy such as twins or triplets.

There are a number of types of twin pregnancies. Dizygotic twins occur when two eggs are fertilised by two different sperm, resulting in two singleton pregnancies. Dizygotic twins are not the results of cell division. These fetuses are not genetically the same and can be different sexes. Each fetus has its own placenta and amniotic sac and the babies are referred to as dichorionic diamniotic (DCDA) twins.

Monozygotic twins occur when the zygote splits following fertilisation. They are genetically identical and will be the same sex. The zygote splits very early in the developmental process, although the cause for this split is unknown. The timing of the split can determine whether the twins will have a separate or shared placenta and amniotic sac (Table 2.2).

Monochorionic diamniotic and monochorionic monoamniotic twin pregnancies are high risk because of the risk of twin-to-twin transfusion and cord entanglements, which can lead to intrauterine growth restriction or intrauterine death (Marshall and Raynor 2020).

Multiple pregnancies of triplets or more fetuses are most probably the results of three single zygote conceptions, or a mixture of twins and singleton zygotes; however, in rare cases, monozygotic triplets are born (Tal et al. 2012).

TABLE 2.2   **The timing of the split.**

Timing of split (days)	Placenta, amnion and chorion	Type of twin
0–3	Separate amnion and chorion but two placentas can be fused or completely separate	DCDA monozygotic
4–8	Sharing of chorion. Separate amnion. 1 placenta	MCDA monozygotic
>8	Sharing of amnion and chorion. 1 placenta	MCMA monozygotic

Reflective Learning Activity

The following is a list of conditions that are associated with the cell. Take some time and write notes about each of the conditions. Think about the conditions and how they might impact individuals and their families. Outline your role and function related to each condition, remember to include aspects of woman-centred care. If you are making notes about people to whom you have offered care and support, you must ensure that you have adhered to the rules of confidentiality.

- Down syndrome
- Edward syndrome
- Hyperemesis gravidarum
- Patau syndrome
- Turner syndrome

Take Home Points

- The cell's unique structure allows it to adapt to carry out its different functions within the body. Cells combine together based on function to form different tissue types. A combination of different tissues leads to organ formation.
- The cell membrane is a made of a phospholipid bilayer, which contains proteins and lipids that are responsible for cellular transportation and communication.
- Active and passive processes are responsible for transportation across the cell membrane. Active processes require energy, which is produced by the cell, while passive processes move along concentration gradients and do not require energy.
- There are two methods of cell division – meiosis and mitosis. Meiosis is the process of producing gametes, which contain half the genetic material of the parent cell. Meiosis produces genetically identical cells to the parent cell and it is responsible for the replication and renewal of cells.
- The cells and their functions adapt to the needs of the body during pregnancy to maintain normal homeostasis and function in the maternal system while also supporting the placenta with gaseous exchange and nutrient transport.

Summary

This chapter has provided an overview of the structure and function of the cell and its organelles. It demonstrates the complex processes and the interactions that happen at cellular level to support normal function of the human body and the adaptations made during pregnancy to maintain homeostasis. It has highlighted the processes of cell division used for growth and repair, as well as the process of gamete formation and how this contributes to genetic diversity in the population. The information in this chapter provides fundamental understanding of cell biology and how it can be applied to clinical practice.

References

Alberts, B., Hopkin, K., Johnson, A.D. et al. (2018). *Essential Cell Biology*, 5th International Student Edition.

Coad, J., Pedley, K., and Dunstall, M. (2019). *Anatomy and Physiology for Midwives e-Book*. Elsevier Health Sciences.

Diaz-Perez, R. and Davis, J.E. (2018). Pathophysiological mechanisms for the development of gestational diabetes insipidus. *Journal of Clinical Investigation and Studies* 1 (2): 1–3.

Evans, J. and Manson, A.L. (2008). *Cell Biology and Genetics*. Elsevier Health Sciences.

Gardner, A. and Davis, T. (2009). *Human Genetics*, 2e. Bristol: Scion.

Gilbert, S.F. (2000). An introduction to early developmental processes. In: *Developmental Biology*, 6e. Massachusetts: Sinauer Associates.

Griffiths, S.K. and Campbell, J.P. (2015). Placental structure, function, and drug transfer. *Continuing Education in Anaesthesia, Critical Care & Pain* 15 (2): 84–89.

Hsu, R., Tong, A., and Hsu, C.D. (2021). Hypervolemic hyponatremia as a reversible cause of cardiopulmonary arrest in a postpartum patient with preeclampsia. *Case Reports in Obstetrics and Gynaecology* 2021.

Lee, N.M. and Saha, S. (2011). Nausea and vomiting of pregnancy. *Gastroenterology Clinics* 40 (2): 309–334.

Lopez, M.J. and Hall, C.A. (2020). *Physiology, Osmosis*. StatPearls Publishing LLC.

Macdonald, S. and Johnson, G. (2023). *Mayes' Midwifery E-Book: Mayes' Midwifery E-Book*, 16e. Elsevier Health Sciences.

Macnab, W.R. (2022). Functions of the placenta. *Anaesthesia & Intensive Care Medicine* 23 (6): 344–346.

Marcus, A. (2010). *Human Genetics: An Overview*. Oxford: Alpha Science International Ltd.

Marshall, J.E. and Raynor, M.D. (2020). *Myles' Textbook for Midwives E-Book*, 17e. Elsevier Health Sciences.

McEwen, B.S. (2016). Central role of the brain in stress and adaptation: allostasis, biological embedding, and cumulative change. In: *Stress: Concepts, Cognition, Emotion, and Behavior*, 39–55. Academic Press.

MHRA (2021). Safer Medicines in Pregnancy and Breastfeeding Consortium A major initiative to ensure pregnant and breastfeeding women can make informed decisions about their healthcare. https://www.gov.uk/government/publications/safer-medicines-in-pregnancy-and-breastfeeding-consortium (accessed 29-November 2023).

N.H.S (2021). *Screening for Down's Syndrome, Edwards' Syndrome and Patau's Syndrome: NIPT*. London: NHS England.

Nair, M. and Peate, I. (ed.) (2009). *Fundamentals of Applied Pathophysiology: An essential guide for nursing students*. John Wiley & Sons.

Ning, F., Liu, H., and Lash, G.E. (2016). The role of decidual macrophages during normal and pathological pregnancy. *American Journal of Reproductive Immunology* 75 (3): 298–309.

Orchard, G. and Nation, B. (ed.) (2015). Cell structure & function. In: *Fundamentals of Biomedical Science*. Oxford: Oxford University Press.

Peate, I. and Evans, S. (ed.) (2020). *Fundamentals of Anatomy and Physiology for Student Nurses*, 3e. Oxford: Wiley.

Powel, J.E., Rosenthal, E., Roman, A. et al. (2020). Preeclampsia and low sodium (PALS): a case and systematic review. *European Journal of Obstetrics & Gynecology and Reproductive Biology* 249: 14–20.

Rankin, J. (2017). *Physiology in Childbearing E-Book: With Anatomy and Related Biosciences*. Elsevier Health Sciences.

RCOG No, 69 G.T.G. (2016). The management of nausea and vomiting of pregnancy and hyperemesis gravidarum.

Scaife, P.J. and Mohaupt, M.G. (2017). Salt, aldosterone and extrarenal Na^+-sensitive responses in pregnancy. *Placenta* 56: 53–58.

Tal, R., Fridman, D., and Grazi, R.V. (2012). Monozygotic triplets and dizygotic twins following transfer of three poor-quality cleavage stage embryos. *Case Reports in Obstetrics and Gynecology* 2012.

Vricella, L.K. (2017). Emerging understanding and measurement of plasma volume expansion in pregnancy. *The American Journal of Clinical Nutrition* 106 (suppl_6): 1620S–1625S.

Walter, M.H., Abele, H., and Plappert, C.F. (2021 Oct). The role of oxytocin and the effect of stress during childbirth: neurobiological basics and implications for mother and child. *Front Endocrinol (Lausanne)*. 27 (12): 742236.

Strauss, J.F., Barbieri, R.L., Dokras, A. et al. (ed.) (2023). *Yen & Jaffe's Reproductive Endocrinology-E-Book: Physiology, Pathophysiology, and Clinical Management*. Elsevier Health Sciences.

Further Reading

Ali, R.A.R., Hassan, J., and Egan, L.J. (2022). Review of recent evidence on the management of heartburn in pregnant and breastfeeding women. *BMC Gastroenterology* 22: 219. https://doi.org/10.1186/s12876-022-02287-w.

Stubbs, M. and Suleyman, N. (2015). *Crash Course Cell Biology and Genetics Updated Edition-E-Book*. Elsevier Health Sciences.

Online Resources

Gene People
The genetic conditions support network
Home - Gene People - For Everyone Affected
HM Government
Genome UK: The future of Healthcare
Genome UK: the future of healthcare (publishing.service.gov.uk)
HM Government
Screening Programmes Across the UK
Screening programmes across the UK - GOV.UK (www.gov.uk)
NHS England
Genomics in Midwifery: Genomics Education Programme
Genomics in Midwifery - Genomics Education Programme (hee.nhs.uk)
NHS England. E-learning for Health Care
About the NHS Screening Programmes
NHS Screening Programmes - elearning for healthcare (e-lfh.org.uk)

Glossary

Active transport	The movement of substances across cell membranes against the concentration gradient, therefore requiring energy in the form of ATP
Adenosine triphosphate (ATP)	A molecule that serves as the primary energy source for cellular activities
Cell	The smallest living part of the human body, makes up all living organisms and tissues
Cell membrane	A semi-permeable, phospholipid bilayer surrounding the cell, separating its internal contents from the external environment, responsible for regulating the movement of substances in and out of the cell
Chromosome	A structure within the nucleus carrying genetic information in the form of DNA.
Endocytosis	The process by which cells engulf external materials (such as nutrients or particles) by forming vesicles from the cell membrane
Endoplasmic reticulum (ER)	A network of membranes involved in protein synthesis and lipid metabolism. There are two types – rough ER (with ribosomes) and smooth ER (lacking ribosomes).
Exocytosis	The process by which cells release substances from the inside of the cell to outside of the cell
Golgi apparatus	A stack of membrane-bound vesicles that processes, sorts and packages proteins and lipids for transport within or outside the cell
Meiosis	A specialised form of cell division that occurs in reproductive cells (gametes), resulting in the production of haploid cells with half the number of chromosomes which has genetic variations.
Mitochondria	Often referred to as the 'powerhouses' of the cell, responsible for producing energy (ATP)
Mitosis	The process of cell division that results in two identical daughter cells, each with the same genetic information as the parent cell.
Organelles	Specialised structures within the cell performing specific functions

Passive transport	The movement of substances across cell membranes along the concentration gradient not requiring cellular energy
Teratogenic	Causing birth defects or abnormalities in a developing fetus.
Triploidy	A genetic condition where cells have three full sets of chromosomes instead of two.
Trisomy	A genetic condition where a chromosome has three copies instead of two.

Multiple Choice Questions

1. Which cellular organelle is responsible for protein synthesis?
   a. Golgi apparatus
   b. Mitochondria
   c. Endoplasmic reticulum
   d. Nucleus

2. The primary function of the mitochondria is to:
   a. Synthesise proteins
   b. Store genetic information
   c. Produce energy (ATP)
   d. Detoxify harmful substances

3. The cell membrane is primarily composed of:
   a. Proteins
   b. Carbohydrates
   c. Nucleic acids
   d. Lipids

4. The genetic material of a cell is located in the:
   a. Mitochondria
   b. Golgi apparatus
   c. Nucleus
   d. Endoplasmic reticulum

5. The process by which a cell engulfs large particles or other cells is called:
   a. Osmosis
   b. Endocytosis
   c. Exocytosis
   d. Diffusion

6. The organelle that packages and modifies proteins for transportation is called the:
   a. Golgi apparatus
   b. Endoplasmic reticulum
   c. Nucleus
   d. Lysosome

7. The process by which water moves across a semipermeable membrane from an area of lower solute concentration to an area of higher solute concentration is called:
   a. Active transport
   b. Facilitated diffusion
   c. Endocytosis
   d. Osmosis

8. Which of the following is responsible for providing energy for active cellular processes?
   a. Mitochondria
   b. Golgi apparatus
   c. Nucleus
   d. Endoplasmic reticulum

9. The process by which a cell takes in substances from the external environment through the cell membrane is called:
   a. Exocytosis
   b. Pinocytosis
   c. Phagocytosis
   d. Endocytosis

10. The process by which a cell divides to form two identical daughter cells is called:
    a. Meiosis
    b. Mitosis
    c. Transcription
    d. Translation

CHAPTER 3

The Female Reproductive System and Associated Disorders

Claire Ford

AIM

This chapter aims to support midwifery students in their practice by providing them with information about the anatomy and physiology of the reproductive system. It aims to support safe and holistic practice by using evidence-based practice and aligning this with women-centred approaches to care.

LEARNING OUTCOMES

After reading this chapter you will be able to:

- Describe the internal and external organs associated with the female reproductive system.
- Understand the structure and function of these organs in relation to fertility, pregnancy and birth.
- Have an awareness of some of the red flags associated with these organs, to provide safe and effective care to women.
- Gain an appreciation of the role of pharmacology in relation to managing and treating some conditions affecting the reproductive organs.

Test Your Prior Knowledge

1. Can you name five of the external structures associated with the female reproductive system?
2. What is the most superior section of the uterus called?
3. How long is the endocervical canal?
4. How many muscle layers can be found in the uterus?

Fundamentals of Maternal Anatomy and Physiology, First Edition. Edited by Ian Peate and Claire Leader.
© 2024 John Wiley & Sons Ltd. Published 2024 by John Wiley & Sons Ltd.

Introduction

The female reproductive system is composed of internal and external organs (Figure 3.1). These organs are designed to adapt and change to produce female gametes, transport the ovum, assist fertilisation, protect the growing fetus and birth and feed a baby (Boore et al. 2021). The reproductive organs are explored in greater depth and reference is made to some adaptations required to undertake the above roles in the reproductive process.

The External Genitalia

The Vulva

The vulva has several functions including protection of the urethra, lubrication of the vagina and, due to an extensive nervous supply, also produces feelings of sensual intensity upon stimulation. However, until recently, the importance of the vulva in sexual pleasure has largely been underplayed and, in some cultures, female pleasure is not encouraged or even discussed.

Arterial blood supply is provided to the vulva by the external and internal pudendal arteries, which branch from the femoral and iliac arteries, respectively. Venous and lymphatic draining occurs via the internal iliac veins and superficial inguinal nodes and the nerves branch from the pudendal nerves (Waugh and Grant 2018).

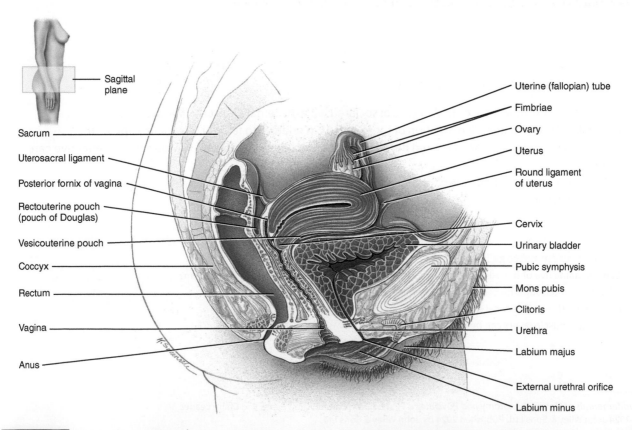

FIGURE 3.1   The female reproductive organs (sagittal plane view). Source: Peate and Evans (2020)/John Wiley & Sons.

Reflective Learning Activity

Take some time to reflect on discussions you have heard, or not heard, on female sexual pleasure.

- What have you read in the media?
- How has this been depicted in movies and television programmes?
- In what ways do you think some cultural and religious beliefs have repressed attitudes towards female sexual pleasure?

Additionally, if the vulva has an increased number of nerves and sensory nerve endings, pain can also be experienced in this region. Vulvodynia is often experienced by women, and can affect not only the vulva but also the inner thighs and perineum. It is often exacerbated by sexual intercourse, tight clothing, the insertion of a tampon or even sitting (Schlaeger et al. 2019).

- Consider how you would care for woman who presented with vulvodynia during and after pregnancy.
- What alternative pain management strategies could you use in the event of perineal trauma during delivery?

The vulva (Figure 3.2) consists of the vaginal orifice, clitoris, mons pubis, labia majora, labia minora, urethral orifice, vulval vestibule and vulval glands.

Mons Pubis

In females, the mons pubis is described as a prominent mound of adipose tissue that is located directly anterior to the pubic bone. It is sometimes referred to as the pubic mound. Its main functions are to ease and facilitate sexual intercourse by cushioning and protecting the pubic bone and secreting pheromones, via the sebaceous glands, to induce sexual attraction. During puberty, hair growth can be seen in this region, which also acts as a protective buffer, reducing friction and acting as a dry lubricant.

Labia Majora and Minora

The words 'labia majora' mean larger lips; these two large prominences form the lateral longitudinal outer boundary of the vulva (Nguyen and Duong 2022). They are created from rounded folds of skin, adipose and fibrous tissue. They join anteriorly and superiorly to the vaginal opening to form the anterior labial commissure at the pudendal cleft, in front of the symphysis pubis, and posteriorly and inferiorly to the vaginal opening to form the posterior labial commissure as it joins with the skin of the perineum (Waugh and Grant 2018). The labia majora contain sebaceous and eccrine sweat glands and hair growth only occurs on the lateral surfaces, leaving the inner surfaces smooth. The hair acts as a protective barrier, reducing friction, and the inner smooth surface acts like a mucous membrane, preventing dryness.

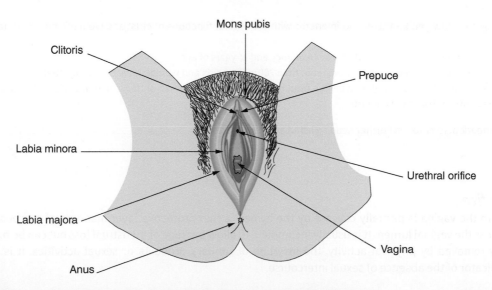

FIGURE 3.2 The vulva (external genitalia). Source: Peate and Evans (2020)/John Wiley & Sons.

The words 'labia minora' mean smaller lips, which are also folds of skin with sebaceous and eccrine sweats glands but, as the name suggests, are smaller in size and completely hairless. They are found between the labia majora, and their main function is the protection of the vestibular, urethra, vagina and clitoris. The anterior folds of the labia minora encircle the clitoris, which creates the clitoral hood and the frenulum of the clitoris (Nguyen and Duong 2022). These folds then descend obliquely and downwards to the posterior ends, encompassing the vulva vestibule, before terminating as they are linked together by a skin fold called the frenulum. It is suggested to have a significantly greater nerve supply than the labia majora, possibly as the outer labia are more exposed to surface irritants. It is also not unusual for both the labia minora and majora to appear swollen with or without sexual arousal, due to the increased blood flow, and darker in colour as a result of the hormonal changes associated with pregnancy.

Clitoris

The main function of this organ is for sexual pleasure; consequently, it is constructed largely of sensory nerve endings and erectile tissue. It is approximately 2 cm in diameter and consists of a shaft (body) and a glans (tips), which is the part of the clitoris that is visible. The glans clitoris is highly innervated by nerves and is estimated to contain over 8000 nerve endings. The underlying tissue that makes the clitoris is the corpus cavernous and erectile tissue, which is perfused by many blood vessels and responds to arousal by enlarging and becoming firm (Peate 2017). A fold of skin derived from an extension of the labia minora, known as the clitoral hood, protects this very sensitive organ.

Urethral Orifice

This is often referred to as the urinary meatus and is the exit point of urine out of the body, from the bladder, through the urethra. It is located 2.5 cm inferior and posterior to the clitoris and superior and anterior to the vagina (Boore et al. 2021).

Red Flag Alert: Female Genital Mutilation

The World Health Organization (WHO; 2023) recognises female genital mutilation (FGM) as a violation of the human rights of women and girls and suggests that the practice reflects deep-rooted gender inequalities. It is illegal in the UK and constitutes a form of child abuse. It is imperative that midwives and midwifery students observe for signs of FGM and ask women about any possible alterations to the external genitalia, as these may increase the risk of intrapartum complications and neonatal mortality. As it also constitutes an extreme form of discrimination, it may also alert healthcare professionals to possible safeguarding concerns for the woman and female infants.

Some of the main facts regarding FGM published by the WHO (2023) include:

- FGM involves the partial or total removal of external female genitalia or other injury to the female genital organs for non-medical reasons (Table 3.1).
- FGM damages healthy genital tissue and interferes with the natural functions of girls' and women's bodies, it has no health benefits and can result in loss of life.
- FGM is mostly carried out on young girls between infancy and 15 years of age.
- In areas of the world where FGM is practised, more than 200 million girls and women have been subjected to FGM.
- The practice violates a person's rights to be free from torture and cruel, inhuman or degrading treatment and a person's rights to health, security and physical integrity.

For more information, refer to the Further Reading listed after the references.

Vaginal Orifice

The introitus to the vagina is partially covered by the hymen, a thin protective layer made up of mucous membranes stretching across the vaginal lumen. It is usually incomplete to allow passage of menstrual loss but can be broken further or completely removed by physical activity, the insertion of sanitary products or sexual activities. It is therefore an unreliable indicator of the absence of sexual intercourse.

Vestibular Bulbs

The vestibular bulbs are structures formed from corpus spongiosum tissue, a type of erectile tissue (Nguyen and Duong 2022). These bulbs commence close to the inferior side of the body of the clitoris before extending, splitting and surrounding the lateral border of the urethra and vagina. During sexual arousal, they become engorged with blood, which exerts pressure on the clitoris, inducing feelings of pleasure.

TABLE 3.1   Types of female genital mutilation.

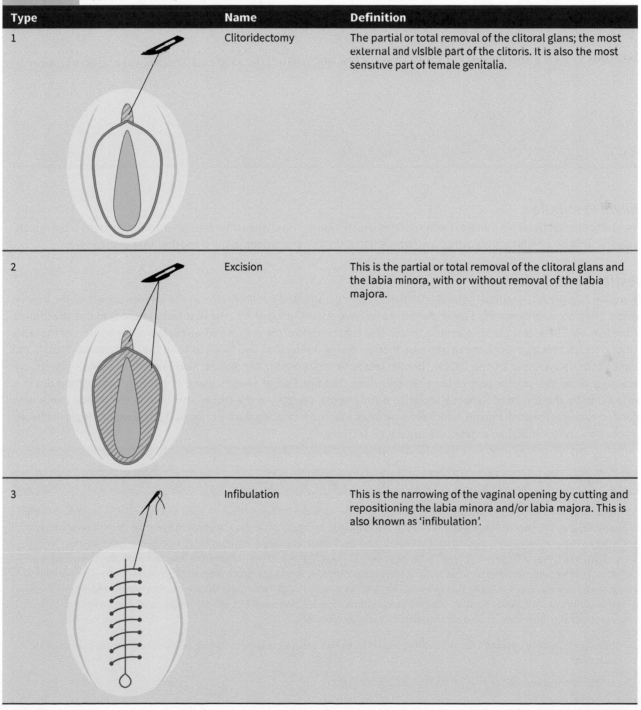

Type		Name	Definition
1		Clitoridectomy	The partial or total removal of the clitoral glans; the most external and visible part of the clitoris. It is also the most sensitive part of female genitalia.
2		Excision	This is the partial or total removal of the clitoral glans and the labia minora, with or without removal of the labia majora.
3		Infibulation	This is the narrowing of the vaginal opening by cutting and repositioning the labia minora and/or labia majora. This is also known as 'infibulation'.

(Continued)

TABLE 3.1   (Continued)

Type	Name	Definition
4	Other (e.g. stretched labia)	This includes all other harmful procedures to the female genitalia for non-medical purposes including: • pricking • piercing • incising • scraping • cauterising

Vulval Vestibule

The cleft between the labia minora is referred to as the vestibule. The change from the vulva vestibule to the labia minora is clearly defined by Hart's lines, which are formed when the skin transitions to the smoother skin of the vulva.

Vestibular Glands

There are two greater vestibular glands (Bartholin's glands) situated on either side of the inferior aspect of the vaginal orifice. They are approximately 1 cm in diameter and have ducts that open into the vestibule, laterally to the attachment of the hymen. These two glands secrete a mucus-like substance into the vagina and within the outer borders of the labia minora, which acts as a lubricant to decrease friction during intercourse and helps to keep the vulva moist (Waugh and Grant 2018; Nguyen and Duong 2022). The two lesser or minor vestibular glands, also known as Skene's glands, are located around the inferior part of the urethral orifice. The function of Skene's gland is not fully understood but it is believed to be the source of female ejaculation during sexual arousal, as the tissue surrounding the glands swells with blood, creating force on the gland, which then secretes a fluid, particularly during orgasm. The substance is also believed to act as an antimicrobial, to prevent urinary tract infections.

Medications Management: Bartholin's Cyst

If the ducts of the Bartholin's gland become blocked, usually because of a bacterial infection, such as *Escherichia coli*, gonorrhoea or chlamydia, they can become engorged with fluid, expanding to form a cyst. Some may be small and resolve on their own; however, others can become very large, causing significant pain and discomfort, and may become infected resulting in an abscess.

Suspected infected cysts will need to be swabbed to identify the bacteria responsible and to target the treatment more effectively. Generally, narrow-spectrum antibacterials are preferred to broad-spectrum antibacterials unless there is a clear clinical indication for their use. Antibiotic therapies for infected cysts include ceftriaxone, ciprofloxacin, doxycycline and azithromycin. Topical or local anaesthetics such as lidocaine and bupivacaine are also used to treat abscesses, and oral analgesics such as paracetamol and ibuprofen are also recommended to manage the pain.

• Ciprofloxacin: dose by mouth for an adult initially 500 mg twice daily, increasing to 750 mg twice daily in severe or deep-seated infections.

For further information, see Lee et al. (2015), BNF (2022a), NHS (2022).

Perineum

The perineum is a triangular structure extending from the labia minora to the anal canal. Its main function as the central tendon of the perineum to act as the main attachment mechanism for the muscles of the pelvic floor (Figure 3.3). It consists of connective tissue, muscle and adipose tissue, and tearing of these structures can often occur during childbirth. The Royal College of Obstetricians and Gynaecologists (2023a) states that almost 9 of 10 first-time mothers who have a vaginal birth will experience some trauma to the perineum. This trauma can occur inside the vagina or other parts of the vulva, including the labia. For most women, the tears are minor and heal on their own. However, for approximately 3.5 in 100 women, the tear may be deeper, resulting in significant damage to the anal sphincter, leading to complications such as anal incontinence, infections, fistulas and weakened pelvic floor (Table 3.2).

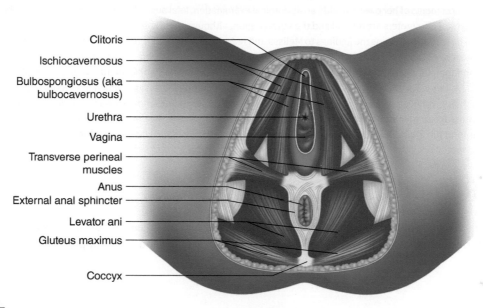

Clitoris
Ischiocavernosus
Bulbospongiosus (aka bulbocavernosus)
Urethra
Vagina
Transverse perineal muscles
Anus
External anal sphincter
Levator ani
Gluteus maximus
Coccyx

FIGURE 3.3 Muscles of the pelvic floor.

TABLE 3.2 Classifications of peritoneal trauma.

Grade	Description
1	Damage to the perineal skin and/or vaginal mucosa; will normally heal quickly and requires no intervention
2	Damage to the perineal muscles and skin but not anal sphincter; usually requires sutures to close the skin and muscle layers; can be performed by a trained midwife or a student nurse
3	Damage to the skin, muscles and anal sphincter. Three subgroups: 3a) damage to external anal sphincter (EAS) <50% thickness 3b) damage to EAS >50% thickness 3c) internal sphincter also torn Surgical repair will be performed by obstetric medical staff in theatre
4	Injury to both the external and internal anal sphincter as well as the anal epithelium. Again, repair will be carried out in theatre, under local, regional or general anaesthetic by a member of the obstetric medical team

Source: Adapted from Royal College of Obstetricians and Gynaecologists (2015, 2023a)

Snapshot 3.1   Perineal Trauma

Melissa Gilbert is 27-year-old woman expecting her first child. At 34 weeks of gestation, she contacted her midwife as she was experiencing some swelling and discomfort in her vulval region, particularly towards her perineum. She has several friends who have already experienced birth and she is extremely worried about the delivery, and trauma to her vulva and perineal area. She is worried how this will impact her recovery, lifestyle and sexual relationship with her partner. She has read several blogs on the internet and is worried she will get a third- or fourth-degree tear and incontinence.

The midwife first reassures Melissa that feelings of anxiety about the delivery are to be expected and that she has done the right thing by making the appointment to see her. She gains consent to obtain a more thorough gynaecological history and asks questions about Melissa's presenting symptoms, such as when she noticed the changes to her vulva, how this is impacting on her lifestyle and wellbeing, and any changes to the colour and consistency of her vaginal discharge or episodes of pain. She also asks her about her sexual health and undertakes physical assessments of her overall health, an abdominal examination, fetal auscultations and examination of her vulva.

All maternal and fetal parameters are normal and the vulval region, although slightly swollen and discoloured, shows no signs of infection or trauma. The midwife explains the findings to Melissa and reassures her that the changes to her vulva are often experienced during pregnancy because of the increased blood flow and release of hormones. She provides her with the latest information on rates of perineal trauma and that, for most women, the trauma is often mild and will need no significant intervention. She also explains that she can start to prepare her vulva and perineum for delivery with the use of perineal massage, which may reduce the risk of tearing. She includes tips such as involving partners, using warm baths to loosen the muscles around the perineum, ensuring that the nails on the hands used for massage remain short, ensuring that each partner is comfortable with adequate back support and using lubricants like vitamin E oil, almond oil or olive oil to reduce friction (Royal College of Obstetricians and Gynaecologists 2023a).

Internal Reproductive Organs

The internal organs of the reproductive system sit within the pelvic cavity and consist of the vagina, the uterus, two ovaries and two uterine tubes (Figures 3.1 and 3.4). Each organ has its own blood and nerve supply (Waugh and Grant 2018).

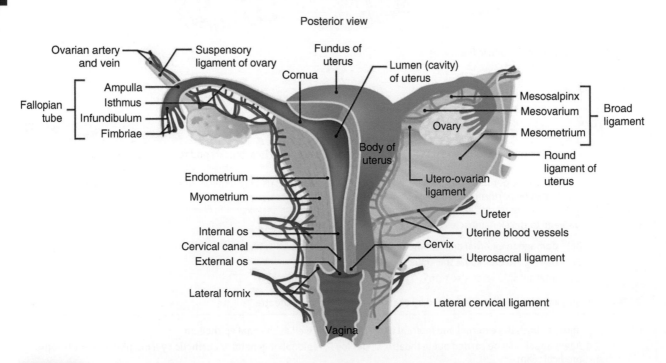

FIGURE 3.4   Vagina, uterus, ovaries and supporting structures. Source: Lecturio GmbH/https://www.lecturio.com/concepts/uterus-cervix-and-fallopian-tubes.

The Vagina

This is a fibromuscular tube which acts as a passageway for menstrual fluid and the birth of a baby. It connects with the vestibule at one end and the uterine cervix at the other (Peate 2017). The arterial and venous blood supply to the vagina is via the internal iliac arteries and veins and lymphatic draining is through the deep and superficial iliac glands. The nerve supply is more complex, with a mixture of sympathetic fibres from the lumbar outflow, somatic sensory fibres from the pudendal nerves and parasympathetic fibres from the sacral outflow (Boore et al. 2021). The vagina is also not completely vertical, but rather at an upward, inverted angle of about 45 degrees, anterior to the rectum and posterior to the bladder and urethra. Hence, it has a longer posterior wall, around 9 cm, and a shorter anterior wall of approximately 7.5 cm. While. the vagina itself has no secretory glands, it is kept moist by the cervical secretions With the assistance of oestrogen and lactic acid-secreting friendly bacteria, the vagina maintains an acidic bacteriostatic environment, inhibiting the growth of other microorganisms (Peate 2017).

The Uterus

The uterus is a pear-shaped organ situated in the pelvic cavity posterior and superior to the bladder and anterior to the rectum. For most women, it leans forward (anteverted), unlike the vagina, and is approximately 7.5 cm long, 5 cm wide, and weighs between 30 and 40 g (Waugh and Grant 2018). It is divided into several sections, the largest of which is the body, occupying two-thirds of the uterus. The fundus is the rounded superior section commencing after the openings of the uterine tubes; the narrow inferior portion is referred to as the isthmus, which attaches to the cervix (discussed later). It is held in place within the pelvic cavity by the mesometrium ligaments, which attach to the pelvic floor, and the round ligaments, which anchor the anterior wall of the uterus to the pelvic cavity. The mesovarium (and the mesometrium), otherwise referred to as the broad ligaments, also help to preserve the position of the uterus within the pelvic cavity and maintain the relationship of the uterine tubes to the ovaries and the uterus.

The uterus is an extremely muscular organ, about 2.5 cm thick, with walls constructed from three varying muscle layers: the perimetrium, the myometrium and the endometrium.

- *Perimetrium*: this is the outer serous and protective layer of the uterus which merges with the peritoneum.
- *Myometrium*: this is the central and thickest part of the uterus, which contains several smooth muscle layers, running in various directions, and interlaced with blood vessels and nerves. This structural design aids contraction during labour and menstruation, and enables the uterus to grow and expand up to 20 times its normal size during pregnancy (Peate 2017).
- *Endometrium*: this is the inner layer of the uterus, constructed from a basal and functional layer of mucosa. The basal layer, which is permanent and closest to the myometrium, plays a role in the replication and regeneration of the uterine lining during the menstrual cycle. The functional layer is the section of the mucosa which sheds during menstruation if the ovum released by the ovaries is not fertilised or implanted.

The uterus is extremely vascular and significant amounts of blood can be delivered to the uterus via the uterine arteries, which branch from the internal iliac arteries. There are two uterine arteries on either side of the uterus supplying the endometrium, splitting further into straight radial arteries that feed the basal layer and the spiral radial arteries that supply the functional layer. The myometrium is fed via the arcuate arteries.

49

Medications Management: Uterine Contraction

After successful delivery of the baby and the placenta, it is vital to palpate the uterus for signs of continued contraction as this action is essential to prevent blood loss during the postpartum period. If the uterine tone is soft and weak (uterine atony), the uterine muscles will be prevented from clamping the large placental blood vessels shut and the woman could be at risk of postpartum haemorrhage (PPH).

Obstetric haemorrhage remains one of the major causes of maternal death in both developed and developing countries. Primary PPH, commonly defined as a blood loss of 500 ml or more within 24 hours after birth, affects about 6% of all women giving birth. To minimise the risk of bleeding, pharmacological intervention in the form of prophylactic uterotonics are often used in maternity and obstetric practice to stimulate and encourage uterine contraction. Several uterotonics have been developed, including prostaglandin analogues (misoprostol, sulprostone, carboprost) and ergot alkaloids (ergometrine/methylergometrine). However, the most popular and widely used are the oxytocin receptor agonists (oxytocin or carbetocin), with oxytocin 10 iu by intramuscular injection being recommended following the birth of the baby for the prevention of PPH for all births.

For further information about PPH, see Mavrides et al. (2022), Vogel et al. (2019), BNF (2022b).

The Cervix

The cervix, the narrowest part of the uterus, is a thickened ring of muscle and fibrous tissue which changes during pregnancy and, in particular, labour. The external os of the cervix can be found protruding into the fornix of the vagina and the internal os opens into the uterus. The endocervical canal between these openings is approximately 2.5 cm long and is the only pathway between the uterus and the vagina. It is held in place by the lateral cervical ligaments, which attach the cervix and the vagina to the lateral pelvic walls.

Reflective Learning Activity

The cervix is the gatekeeper of the uterus. It not only acts to restrict the invasion of microorganisms into the uterus, but is also integral to maintaining the safe closure of the uterus so it can remain a safe home for the growing fetus. Towards the due date and during labour, the cervix must soften, shorten and dilate to enable the baby to move out of the uterus; however, if this cervix has a weakness, its function is compromised, which could increase the risk of preterm birth (Nott et al. 2016).

- What is your current understanding of preterm birth?
- Have you read evidence making links between some preterm births and cervical weaknesses?

Reflective Learning Activity

During midwifery education, students will have the opportunity to physically examine cervixes as part of a vaginal examination. However, this is an invasive procedure and it is therefore important to consider the following in relation to this clinical skill:

- What is your understanding of informed consent regarding vaginal examination and what would you do if consent was not provided?
- Have you seen chaperones being used in practice?
- How have you seen respect and dignity being maintained when observing this skill in practice?
- If you have undertaken this skill under supervision in practice, how did you feel? Did you find it difficult to feel the cervix and identify the external os?
- Were you able to feel the difference when examining a cervix during the effacement and ripening stages of change?

The Ovaries

Within females, gametes are produced in the ovaries, which are also responsible for the production of several sex hormones (Table 3.3). There are usually two flat, almond-shaped ovaries, 2.5–3.5 cm long, 2 cm wide and 1 cm thick, situated in a shallow fossa, flanking both the right and left side of the uterus, inferior to the uterine tubes (Waugh and Grant 2018). The ovaries are suspended in place within the peritoneal cavity by the suspensory ligaments, which attach the ovary to the pelvic floor, the ovarian ligament, which anchors the ovary to the uterus, and the mesovarium,

TABLE 3.3   **Female reproductive hormones.**

Hormone	Description
Oestrogen	Main function is to mature and maintain the reproductive system
	Responsible for maturation and release of the ovum
	Aids the thickening of the lining of the uterus
	High levels have been linked to acne, constipation, reduced sex drive, depression, cancer and cardiovascular disease
	Reduced levels associated with osteoporosis and mood swings
Progesterone	Secreted by the corpus luteum
	Triggers thickening of the uterine lining
	Prohibits uterine muscle contractions
	Low levels can result in abnormal menstrual cycles or difficulties with conception
	High levels have been linked to anxiety and agitation, breast swelling and tenderness and swelling, depression, fatigue and weight gain
Relaxin	Secreted in the ovary by the corpus luteum
	Relaxes the wall of the uterus and prepares it for pregnancy
	Aids in implantation and placenta growth
	Prevents uterine contractions to prevent early labour
	During labour, helps to relax the ligaments in the pelvis
Testosterone	Produced in small quantities
	Essential for the development of new blood cells, enhancing libido and influencing follicle-stimulating hormones
	Low levels are associated with fatigue, muscle weakness and mood changes
Anti-Müllerian	Helps in the early development of follicles, which hold and support eggs before fertilisation
	Measuring levels can indicate remaining egg supply
	Levels are highest during puberty and decline after menopause

Source: Adapted from Davidge-Pitts and Burt Solorzano (2022).

which acts as the main suspension ligament. Blood is supplied to the ovaries via the ovarian and uterine artery (Figure 3.4) and the ovaries are supplied with parasympathetic and sympathetic nerves from the sacral and lumber outflow, respectively. Although the primordial ova (eggs) are present within the ovaries at birth, they are held in stasis and are only activated at puberty. Ova are then released during menstruation, and slowly reduce in number as the woman ages.

Menstrual Cycle

For most women, the menstrual cycle (consisting of menses, follicular/proliferation, ovulation and luteinising/secretion phases) occurs around every 28 days (Figure 3.5). It is associated with changes in the uterus, ovaries, breast and vagina and aligned with hormonal fluctuations (Figure 3.6). Regulation and control of the menstrual cycle are highly dependent on the anterior pituitary gland and the release of follicular stimulating hormones (FSH) and luteinising hormones (LH). FSH, as the name suggests, simulates several immature ovarian follicles to grow and secrete oestrogen, and LH causes at least one follicle to mature, rupture and eject an ovum and stimulates the development of the corpus luteum (Huether and McCance 2016).

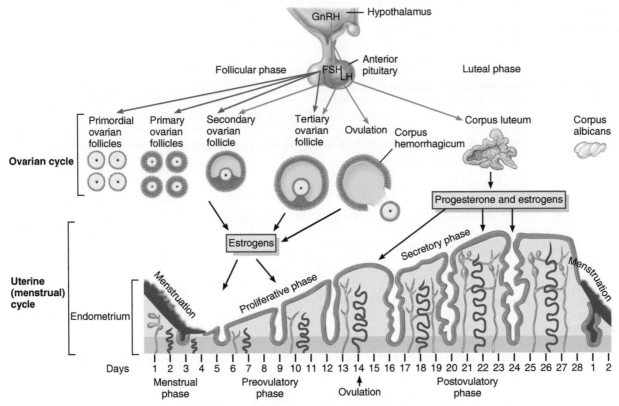

Hormonal regulation of changes in the ovary and uterus

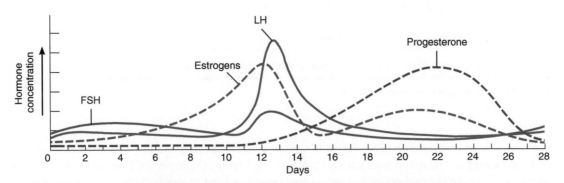

Changes in concentration of anterior pituitary and ovarian hormones

FIGURE 3.5   Phases of the menstrual cycle. Sources: Huether and McCance (2016); Patton et al. (2018).

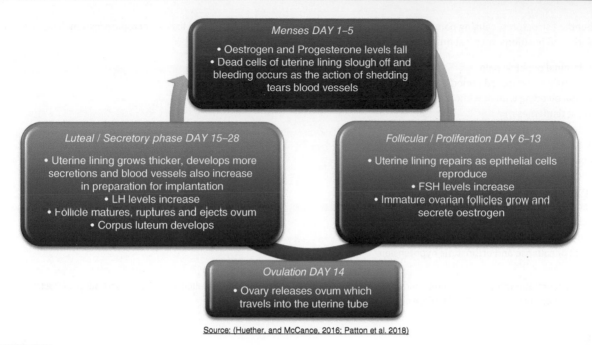

Source: (Huether, and McCance, 2016; Patton et al. 2018)

FIGURE 3.6 A typical 28-day menstrual cycle.

One of the most crucial periods of the menstrual cycle is ovulation. The fertilisation of the oocyte by sperm can only occur within a limited time frame, as most sperm's fertilising abilities diminish after 72 hours post-ejaculation and most ejected oocytes are no longer viable after 48 hours (Patton et al. 2018). The window for possible fertilisation is therefore very small and restricted to three to six days in every menstrual cycle.

The Uterine (Fallopian) Tubes

The ovum released from the ovaries is directed towards the uterine tubes (otherwise referred to as the fallopian tubes or salpinges) by the action of the fimbriae, which are tentacle-like ciliated protections situated at the funnel end (infundibulum) of the uterine tube, the longest of which is the ovarian fimbria. Due to peristaltic and kinetic movement of the ciliated inner wall lining, the ovum moves towards the uterus for implantation, through the uterine tube, which is approximately 10 cm long (the largest part being the ampulla, and the narrowest and final section the isthmus; Peate 2017). The uterine tubes are suspended and held in place by the mesosalpinx.

Red Flag Alert: Ectopic Pregnancy

An ectopic pregnancy occurs when the fertilised ovum implants outside of the uterus. The Royal College of Obstetricians and Gynaecologists (2023b) states that in the United Kingdom, 1 in 90 pregnancies results in an ectopic pregnancy; women are at higher risk if they have previously had an ectopic pregnancy. Most ectopic pregnancies develop in the uterine tubes, but in 3–5% they can occur in the cervix, ovary and abdominal cavity. An ectopic pregnancy is life threatening and, if suspected, should be managed quickly via surgical, pharmacological or conservative interventions. As the fetus grows, trauma can occur to the surrounding structures, causing pain, and ruptured vessels can result in significant blood loss. As ectopic pregnancies can occur in a variety of positions, atypical presentation is common, but symptoms can include:

- abdominal or pelvic pain
- amenorrhoea or missed period
- vaginal bleeding with or without clots
- breast tenderness
- gastrointestinal symptoms
- dizziness, fainting or syncope and pallor
- shoulder tip pain
- urinary symptoms
- passage of tissue per vagina
- rectal pressure or pain on defaecation
- abdominal distension and enlarged uterus
- tachycardia or hypotension
- shock or collapse and orthostatic hypotension.

For further information about ectopic pregnancy, see National Institute for Health and Care Excellence (2023a), Royal College of Obstetricians and Gynaecologists (2016) and Royal College of Obstetricians and Gynaecologists (2023b).

The Breasts

The female breasts contain the mammary glands and are considered external accessory sexual organs and part of the reproductive system, as they play a pivotal role in the nurturing and feeding of newborns (Peate 2017; Figure 3.7). They are not located within proximity to the other reproductive organs already mentioned within this chapter; instead, they are located on the upper chest, between the third and seventh rib, and are supported in place by the pectoral muscles. The breasts are made of adipose tissue, fibrous connective tissue and glandular tissue, which provides support and structure to the breast and is further divided into 15–25 lobes. These lobes are comprised of alveolar glands 'lobules', which produce milk, and are connect to the nipple via small lactiferous ducts. During the last two-thirds of pregnancy, the breasts enlarge due to the proliferation of additional glandular tissue, and milk is stored in the lactiferous sinuses. Blood supply to the breasts is provided via the thoracic branches of the axillary arteries and the internal mammary and intercostal arteries (Waugh and Grant 2018). Lymphatic draining is carried out via the superficial axillary lymph vessel and nodes and the breast is supplied with many nerves branching from the fourth, fifth and sixth thoracic nerves. There are also several sensory nerve endings in the breast, especially around the nipple, which when stimulated by sucking, pass impulses to the hypothalamus to increase the secretion of oxytocin, a hormone needed for milk production.

Snapshot 3.2   Mastitis

Blessing Adhio is a 32-year-old mother of a newborn boy. With the support of her family and midwife, she is successfully breastfeeding her son, who is thriving. At the last visit before handing over care to the health visiting team, the midwife notices that Blessing is having some trouble holding the baby and seemed to wince when her breasts are touched. Blessing admits when asked that her breasts have been very tender for the past two days and she found it difficult to feed her son this morning and needed to use some of her saved breast milk and bottles.

The midwife suspected mastitis and therefore needed to ask further questions to ascertain the severity of the condition and whether an immediate referral was needed. She gains consent to obtain a more thorough history and asks questions about her presenting symptoms, such as when she noticed the pain and discomfort, what makes the pain worse, what makes it better, and whether there are any other changes to her breasts, such as discoloration, swelling, discharge. She also asks Blessing about breastfeeding, and if she thinks it is still going well, if her son was latching on correctly and so forth. She also gains consent from Blessing to physically examine her breasts and undertakes some vital observations.

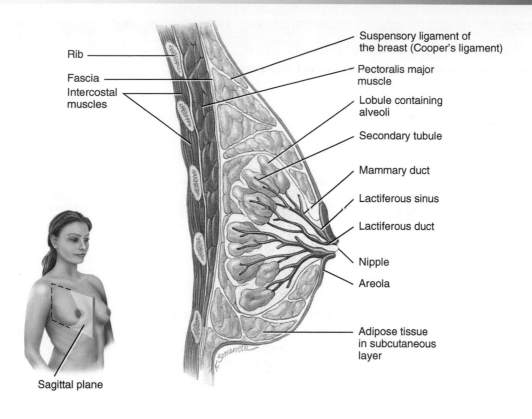

Sagittal plane

Sagittal section

FIGURE 3.7 Sagittal view of the breast. Source: Peate and Evans (2020)/John Wiley & Sons.

Blessing's observations were within normal parameters, but she described the pain as throbbing and scored it a 6 out of 10 using the numerical rating scale. There were no signs of an abscess but both breasts were swollen and there were signs of erythema. The midwife did not think that admission was required but did suspect that both breasts were inflamed and affected by mastitis. She reassured Blessing that this happens in around 30% of breastfeeding mothers, especially during the first few weeks, and that mastitis should resolve, and her breasts should return to normal size, shape and function after treatment.

She suggested the use of warm compresses, or for Blessings to bathe or shower in warm water, to relieve pain and help the milk to flow. She also advised the use of analgesics such as paracetamol and ibuprofen and advocated continued breastfeeding, with additional expressing if the breast were not emptied, ensuring that her baby was latching correctly (National Institute for Health and Care Excellence 2023b). The midwife should observe a feed if possible and check the baby's latch, as the most common reason for mastitis/engorgement is poor latching technique.

Take Home Points

- When caring for any woman, it is important to have a sound understanding of the anatomy and physiology of the reproductive system and how it adapts and changes during pregnancy and birth.
- This understanding enables midwives to carry out procedures safely but also to recognise disease and reproductive disorders that may negatively impact the perinatal journey.
- It is essential to include women and their partners in their care and not to make a decision for women, but with women.
- Any decisions made must be tailored to the individual needs of the woman and need to take into consideration their holistic picture.

Reflective Learning Activity

The following is a list of conditions that are associated with the reproductive system:

- Symphysis pubis dysfunction
- Molar pregnancy
- Polycystic vary syndrome
- Uterine fibroids
- Endometriosis

Take some time and write notes about each of the conditions. Think about the anatomy and physiology involved. Remember to include aspects of patient care. Remember that if you are making notes about people you have offered care and support to you must ensure that you have adhered to the rules of confidentiality.

Summary

The reproductive organs play an essential role in the repopulation of the human race and as the midwife's primary role is to 'be with woman', before, during and after birth, midwifery students must understand the anatomy and physiology to practice safely and effectively. The female body goes through a series of adaptations to develop and deliver life, but these processes do not always change in the way that they should; thus, this chapter has also provided additional information on some of the complications that can occur and some alternative strategies that midwives may need to employ.

References

BNF (2022a). Ciprofloxacin. In: *British National Formulary*. London: BMJ and Parmaceutical Press https://bnf.nice.org.uk/drugs/ciprofloxacin.

BNF (2022b). Oxytocin. In: *British National Formulary*. London: BMJ and Parmaceutical Press https://bnf.nice.org.uk/drugs/oxytocin.

Boore, J., Cook, N., and Shepherd, A. (2021). *Essentials of Anatomy and Physiology for Nursing Practice*, 2e. London: Sage.

Davidge-Pitts, C. and Solorzano, C, B. (2022). Reproductive hormones, patient resources. *Endocrine Library* (24 January). https://www.endocrine.org/patient-engagement/endocrine-library/hormones-and-endocrine-function/reproductive-hormones (accessed 23 October 2023).

Huether, S.E. and McCance, K.L. (2016). *Understanding Pathophysiology*, 6e. St Louis, MO: Elsevier Mosby.

Lee, M.Y., Dalpiaz, A., Schwamb, R. et al. (2015). Clinical pathology of Bartholin's glands: a review of the literature. *Current Urology* 8 (1): 22–25.

Mavrides, E., Allard, S., Chandraharan, E. et al. (2022). Prevention and management of postpartum haemorrhage. *BJOG* 24: e106–e149.

National Institute for Health and Care Excellence (2023a). Ectopic Pregnancy and Miscarriage: Diagnosis and initial management. NICE Guideline NG126. London: National Institute for Health and Care Excellence. https://www.nice.org.uk/guidance/ng126 (accessed 23 October 2023).

National Institute for Health and Care Excellence (2023b). *Mastitis and Breast Abscess*. Clinical Knowledge Summary. London: National Institute for Health and Care Excellence. https://cks.nice.org.uk/topics/mastitis-breast-abscess (accessed 23 October 2023).

Nguyen, J.D. and Duong, H. (2022). *Anatomy, Abdomen and Pelvis, Female External Genitalia*. Treasure Island (FL): StatPearls Publishing.

NHS (2022). Treatment: Bartholin's cyst. https://www.nhs.uk/conditions/bartholins-cyst/treatment (accessed 23 October 2023).

Nott, J.P., Bonney, E.A., Pickering, J.D., and Simpson, N.A.J. (2016). The structure and function of the cervix during pregnancy. *Translational Research in Anatomy* 2: 1–7.

Patton, K.T., Thibodeau, G.A., and Hutton, A. (2018). *Anatomy and Physiology*. St Louis, MO: Elsevier.

Peate, I. (2017). The reproductive system. In: *Fundamentals of Anatomy and Physiology for Nursing and Healthcare Students*, 2e (ed. I. Peate and M. Nair), 371–402. Chichester: Wiley.

Peate, I. and Evans, S. (2020). *Fundamentals of Anatomy and Physiology for Nursing and Healthcare Students*, 3e. Chichester: Wiley.

Royal College of Obstetricians and Gynaecologists (2015). *The Management of Third- and Fourth-Degree Perineal Tears*. Green-top Guideline No. 29. London: Royal College of Obstetricians and Gynaecologists.

Royal College of Obstetricians and Gynaecologists (2016). Diagnosis and management of ectopic pregnancy. Green-top Guideline No. 21. *BJOG* 123 (13): e15–e55.

Royal College of Obstetricians and Gynaecologists (2023a). Perineal tears and episiotomies in childbirth. www.rcog.org.uk/for-the-public/perineal-tears-and-episiotomies-in-childbirth (accessed 23 October 2023).

Royal College of Obstetricians and Gynaecologists. (2023b). *Ectopic Pregnancy*. Information for You. London: Royal College of Obstetricians and Gynaecologists. www.rcog.org.uk/for-the-public/browse-all-patient-information-leaflets/ectopic-pregnancy-patient-information-leaflet (accessed 23 October 2023).

Schlaeger, J.M., Patil, C.L., Steffen, A.D. et al. (2019). Sensory pain characteristics of vulvodynia and their association with nociceptive and neuropathic pain: an online survey pilot study. *Pain Reports* 4 (2): e713.

Vogel, J.P., Williams, M., Gallos, I. et al. (2019). WHO recommendations on uterotonics for postpartum haemorrhage prevention: what works, and which one? *BMJ Global Health* 4 (2).

Waugh, A. and Grant, A. (2018). *Ross and Wilson Anatomy and Physiology in Health and Illness*, 13e. London: Elsevier.

World Health Organization (2023). Female genital mutilation. Key facts. https://www.who.int/news-room/fact-sheets/detail/female-genital-mutilation (accessed 23 October 2023).

Online Resources

Dahlia Project: https://www.dahliaproject.org

Ectopic Pregnancy Trust: www.ectopic.org.uk

FGM National Clinical Group: http://www.fgmnationalgroup.org

Tommy's. Ectopic pregnancy: signs, treatment and support: http://www.tommys.org/pregnancy-information/pregnancy-complications/ectopic-pregnancy

NCT. Breastfeeding support from NCT: www.nct.org.uk/baby-toddler/feeding/early-days/breastfeeding-support-nct

Glossary

Adipose tissue	Connective tissue consisting mainly of fat cells.
Amenorrhea	The absence of menstruation.
Anterior	Near to the front.
Anteverted	Tilted forward.
Cleft	A hollow between ridges or protuberances.
Commissure	A point or line of union between two anatomical parts.
Effacement	The thinning of tissue.
Fistula	An abnormal passage that leads from one hollow organ or part to another.
Frenulum	A connecting fold of membrane serving to support a part of the body.
Fundus	The large upper end of the uterus.
Gamete	Sex cell.
Glans clitoris	The conical, highly innervated body forming the external extremity of the clitoris.
Inferior	Situated lower down.
Infibulation	The complete excision of the clitoris, labia minora and most of the labia majora followed by stitching to close up most of the vagina; illegal in the UK.
Introitus	The orifice of a body cavity.
Isthmus	A narrow anatomical part or passage connecting two larger structures or cavities.

Lateral	Of or relating to the side.
Lumen	The cavity of a tubular organ or part.
Osteoporosis	A condition that is characterised by a decrease in bone mass with decreased density and enlargement of bone spaces.
Ovum	A female gamete.
Pheromones	A chemical substance produced to serve as a stimulus to other individuals of the same species.
Posterior	Situated behind.
Superior	Situated higher up.
Vulvodynia	Chronic discomfort of the vulva.

Multiple Choice Questions

1. Arterial blood supply is provided to the vulva by which arteries?
   a. Pudendal arteries
   b. Labial arteries
   c. Uterine arteries
   d. Inguinal arteries

2. The endocervical canal is how long?
   a. 1.5 cm
   b. 2.0 cm
   c. 2.5 cm
   d. 3.0 cm

3. What is the name of the thin protective layer which is made up of mucous membranes stretching across the vaginal lumen?
   a. Hymale
   b. Hymen
   c. Hymate
   d. Hyman

4. What part of the clitoris is visible?
   a. Isthmus
   b. Fundus
   c. Shaft
   d. Glans

5. What is the diameter of the clitoris?
   a. 1 cm
   b. 2 cm
   c. 3 cm
   d. 4 cm

6. The urethral orifice is situated directly?
   a. Inferior and posterior to the clitoris
   b. Inferior and anterior to the clitoris
   c. Inferior and posterior to the labia
   d. Inferior and anterior to the labia

7. FGM is mostly carried out on females of what age?
   a. Infancy to 15 years
   b. 15–18 years
   c. 18–21 years
   d. 21–24 years

8. Damage to the skin, muscles and > 50% thickness of external anal sphincter is which classification of perineal trauma?
   a. 3a
   b. 3b
   c. 3c
   d. 3d

9. The uterus weighs how many grams?
   a. 20–30 g
   b. 25–35 g
   c. 30–40 g
   d. 35–45 g

10. The spiral radial arteries supply which part of the uterus?
    a. Endometrium – basal layer
    b. Endometrium – functional layer
    c. Myometrium – basal layer
    d. Myometrium – functional layer

CHAPTER **4**

Embryology and Fetal Development

Jenny Brewster

AIM

The aim of this chapter is to introduce the reader to the development of the embryo/fetus from fertilisation until birth. This chapter focuses on the embryo/fetus. Cell division and metabolism can be reviewed in Chapter 2, and the development of the placenta is considered in Chapter 7.

LEARNING OUTCOMES

After reading this chapter you will be able to:

- Understand the terminology related to embryology and the development of the fetus.
- Consider the stages of development of the embryo for the eight-week period starting at the point of fertilisation.
- Be aware of the further development and growth that takes place in the fetus from this point until birth.
- Have an awareness of how this knowledge relates to the care provided by midwives during pregnancy, intrapartum and postnatal periods.

Test Your Prior Knowledge

1. What is the name given to the oocyte following fertilisation by the spermatozoa?
2. From eight weeks following fertilisation of the ovum until term, what name is used?
3. What does the term 'organogenesis' refer to?
4. The blastocyst has an outer layer of trophoblast cells and an inner cell mass. What does the inner cell mass develop into?

Introduction

From the moment that the spermatozoon penetrates the oocyte in the uterine tube, the growth of a new human being starts. During the embryological period, cells multiply, diversify into the approximately 350 different cell types within the body (Rankin and Matthews 2017) and migrate in a specific direction to their final destination, controlled by a genetic

Fundamentals of Maternal Anatomy and Physiology, First Edition. Edited by Ian Peate and Claire Leader.
© 2024 John Wiley & Sons Ltd. Published 2024 by John Wiley & Sons Ltd.

signalling system. Cells also recognise and attach themselves to each other. Another process involved in embryology is *apoptosis* or programmed cell death. An example of this is the removal of webbing between fingers and toes.

This development of the new human being from fertilisation until birth is divided into different time periods. The *pre-embryonic* period is the first three weeks from the time of fertilisation when the zygote travels along the uterine tube and includes embedding in the endometrium. This is followed by the *embryonic* period, which lasts until the completion of eight weeks, during which time most of the major structures are formed, and finally, the *fetal* period lasting until birth, during which the fetus matures and grows in size. Figure 4.1 indicates the time periods and stages of development of the organ systems.

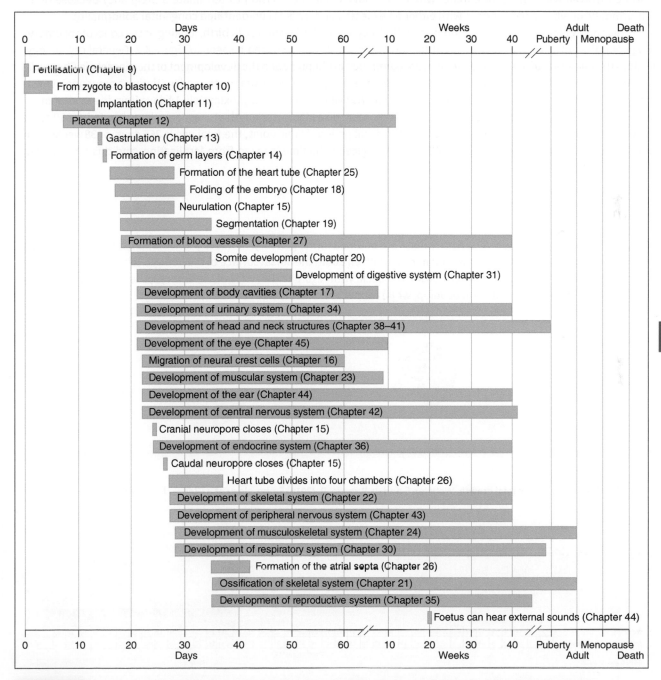

FIGURE 4.1 The time periods and stages of development of the fetal organ systems. Webster, S and de Wreede, R. (2016) Embryology at a Glance/John Wiley & Sons.

An understanding of the basics of embryology can help the midwife in supporting parents in the decisions they make about screening, as the development process is prone to error at any of the stages. This can result in either spontaneous miscarriage or the birth of a baby with a congenital abnormality, which may be related to structure, function or metabolic activity (Moore et al. 2015). Congenital abnormalities can be the result of a failure in the developmental process. They may be caused by teratogens, such as certain drugs or viruses, or they may be genetic. It is thought that more than half of all fertilised oocytes have some form of malformation and are spontaneously miscarried, and that 6% of live births have a congenital malformation that is either identified at birth or during the first year of life (Moore et al. 2015). Midwives may also be involved with caring for parents where they have made the decision to terminate a pregnancy because of an abnormality, or when a baby is born with either an expected or previously unidentified congenital abnormality.

This chapter focuses on the development of the oocyte from fertilisation until birth, looking at the concepts of embryology and the growth and development of the fetus. The stages of growth can be seen in Figure 4.2. General cell biology, such as the processes of mitosis and meiosis, are considered in Chapter 2 and the development of the placenta in Chapter 7.

When considering embryology and fetal growth, the timings used vary from those used for timing a pregnancy, which is taken from the first day of the last menstrual period. As ovulation occurs approximately 14 days from the start of menstruation, there is a period of 2 weeks before fertilisation can take place. The length of pregnancy is seen as being 280 days, which is 40 weeks from the first day of the last menstrual period. At this point, the fetal age is 266 days, or 38 weeks. The link between timings is shown in Table 4.1. Embryologically, the time is taken from fertilisation, and this time is used throughout this chapter.

Terminology

Many of the words associated with embryology are outlined in the glossary. However, to aid understanding, the terms used with relation to direction are outlined here. As with an adult, the dorsal surface of the embryo relates to the back and the ventral surface is the front, or that opposite the back. With regard to the poles of the embryo, the cranial end refers to the area in which the head and brain develop, while caudal refers to the tail.

    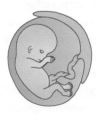 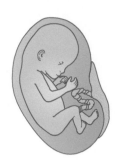

FIGURE 4.2   The stages of fetal growth. Webster, S and de Wreede, R. (2016) Embryology at a Glance/John Wiley & Sons.

TABLE 4.1   **Timings of clinical gestation related to embryological timings.**

	Last menstruation																																								
		Fertilisation																								Antenatal period															
				First Trimester												Second Trimester									Third Trimester															
				Embryogenesis									Fetal Development and growth																											
Week no	1	2	3	4	5	6	7	8	9	10	11	12	13	14	15	16	17	18	19	20	21	22	23	24	25	26	27	28	29	30	31	32	33	34	35	36	37	38	39	40	41
Embryological week no			1	2	3	4	5	6	7	8	9	10	11	12	13	14	15	16	17	18	19	20	21	22	23	24	25	26	27	28	29	30	31	32	33	34	35	36	37	38	39
																						50% survival chance																		
Birth Classification																												Preterm											Term		Post

Source: Adapted from Webster and de Wreede (2016).

Fertilisation of the Oocyte

Once ovulation occurs, the oocyte is wafted into the uterine tube by the fimbriae and starts to travel along the tube. Fertilisation needs to occur within the next 24 hours. The spermatozoa are released into the vagina during ejaculation, where they become hyperactive as they move through the cervix to the uterus and then into the uterine tubes. Once the spermatozoa reach the oocyte, there are two barriers to overcome. First, the cumulus cells on the outer surface have to be broken through, and then the zona pellucida. This is achieved by the breakdown of the acrosomal cap, which forms the head of the spermatozoon, releasing enzymes that dissolve the zona pellucida. Once a spermatozoon has reached the membrane of the oocyte, both membranes fuse and the zona pellucida alters so that no other spermatozoa are able to enter.

The oocyte and spermatozoon each contain 23 chromosomes in their individual pronucleus; that is, half of the normal cell number of 46. As the spermatozoon and the oocyte fuse together, the pronuclei come together to form the nucleus of the new cell. This then contains a unique genetic pattern, having half the genetic material from the mother and half from the father (Bailey 2020a). Whereas the oocyte carries the x chromosome, the spermatozoa contains either an x or y chromosome, which determines the sex of the embryo, x for a female or y for a male.

The Pre-embryonic Period

The process of cell division and differentiation is controlled by a genetic cell to cell signalling system. At about 18 hours following fertilisation, the zygote undergoes cleavage, the first of what will be many cell divisions, where the single cell of the zygote divides into two cells, or blastomeres, by mitosis (Figure 4.3). The cell reproduction continues, so that there are 4 cells by 2 days after fertilisation, 8 cells at 2.5 days, and 16 cells by day 3. This stage is called the morula, as it resembles a mulberry. At this stage, the cells are identical but have the ability to differentiate into any of the cells within the body. This is known as *totipotency*.

Despite the increase in the number of cells, the embryo does not increase in size in the initial stages. Instead, the cells become smaller as they pack together within the boundaries of the zona pellucida, to enable easy passage along the uterine tubes to the uterus (Coad et al. 2020). The cells are already beginning to communicate with each other.

On day 4, the morula enters the uterine cavity and develops into the blastocyst. A cavity develops in the morula, the blastocoele, with the outer layer of cells becoming the trophoblast, which will develop into the placenta and chorion, and the inner cell mass or embryoblast, which will become the embryo and amnion, moves towards one end of the blastocyst. The move from morula to blastocyst is shown in Figure 4.4.

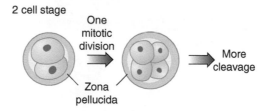

FIGURE 4.3　Cleavage; the single cell of the zygote divides into two blastomeres by mitosis. Webster, S and de Wreede, R. (2016) Embryology at a Glance/John Wiley & Sons.

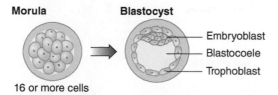

FIGURE 4.4　The change from morula to blastocyst. Webster, S and de Wreede, R. (2016) Embryology at a Glance/John Wiley & Sons.

Once in the uterine cavity, the secretions within the uterus start to dissolve the zona pellucida, allowing the blastocyst to start to increase in size. This is known as hatching. After around two days, the blastocyst will then embed in the endometrial lining of the uterus, where the placenta will start to grow and develop. This development is covered in Chapter 7.

Twins

A twin pregnancy may either be dizygotic or monozygotic. Dizygotic twins occur as multiple ova are released at ovulation, become fertilised and embed in the uterine lining (Figure 4.5). These twins have individual placentas, although they may fuse together and appear to be one large placenta. Monozygotic twins are the result of one fertilised zygote dividing into two. This is most likely to happen during the blastocyst stage. If this occurs between days 4 and 9, then the twins will have individual amniotic sacs but a shared placenta. Where the division happens at a later stage, the twins may share an amniotic sac, and divisions occurring after 12 days may be incomplete, resulting in conjoined twins (Webster and de Wreede 2016).

Week 2

As the blastocyst embeds in the endometrium and the development of the placenta commences, the embryoblast also starts to undergo changes as the cells differentiate into a bilaminar disc consisting of the epiblast layer and the hypoblast layer. These layers will go on to form the structures of the embryo. A cavity in the epiblast layer also appears, which will develop into the amniotic cavity. This is soon surrounded by cells that have separated from the epiblast to form a thin membrane, the amnion. The cells from the hypoblast also extend to form a membrane lining the blastocyst cavity, the exocoelomic mesoderm, from which the primary umbilical vesicle forms. Previously, this was known as the yolk sac, but the name has been changed to reflect the fact that there is no yolk present (Moore et al. 2015).

Towards the end of the second week following fertilisation, the bilaminar disc develops into an ovoid shape, with the cranial end thickening to form the site of the mouth of the embryo, the prechordal plate. The buccopharyngeal membrane covers the plate initially, and the cloacal membrane covers the end that will become the anus. This is an early sign indicating the organisation of the embryo.

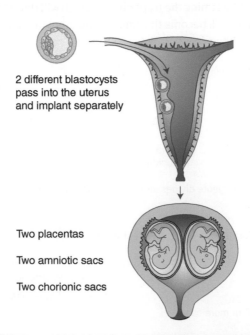

2 different blastocysts pass into the uterus and implant separately

Two placentas

Two amniotic sacs

Two chorionic sacs

FIGURE 4.5 Development of twins. Webster, S and de Wreede, R. (2016) Embryology at a Glance/John Wiley & Sons.

Week 3

During week 3, several changes take place within the blastocyst, which are the precursors for the organs and systems of the body that will develop in the following weeks. Early in week 3, the process of *gastrulation* takes place, converting the bilaminar embryonic disc into the trilaminar disc. The first process is the formation of the primitive streak, with cells from the epiblast migrating to the dorsal aspect of the caudal end of the embryonic disc. The cranial end of the streak develops a rounded mound, the primitive node and a groove appears along the length of the primitive streak, ending in a depression in the primitive node, the primitive pit.

The migration of epiblast cells leads to the development of the trilaminar disc, with the first cells to migrate slipping under the primitive streak to form the mesoderm, connective tissue which provides support for the embryo. This is known as mesenchyme. Further migration of epiblast cells through the primitive groove leads to the endodermal layer, which replaces the hypoblast, and the epiblast becomes the ectodermal layer. The contribution of these layers to the body systems can be seen in Table 4.1. As the ectoderm and endoderm meet at the mouth and the anus, the epithelial linings are formed from both layers.

Cavities also appear in the embryo from around day 2. Initially, there are two cavities, the thoracic and abdominal cavities, then membranes develop, resulting in a pericardial cavity surrounding the primitive heart, two pleural cavities and a peritoneal cavity. The diaphragm also develops from these membranes, the main one being the septum transversum.

With the germ layers in place, the cells within them, further cell movement and differentiation continues as the organs of the body now start to develop. This starts with neurulation, the formation of the rudimentary nervous system.

Days 18–28

The notochordal process is formed as mesenchyme cells continue to migrate from the primitive node and primitive pit, forming a cord shape. The notochordal process continues to grow towards the prechordal plate, and gradually develops a lumen so that is becomes the notochordal canal. The notochordal process and the underlying endoderm fuse together around day 20 forming the notochordal plate. These cells continue to multiply and lift from the endoderm to form the notochord, a rod-like structure that gives structure to the embryo (Figure 4.6).

The main function of the notochord is to act as a signalling centre for the cells of the ectoderm, where there is thickening to develop the neural plate, which will become the brain and spinal cord. The cells in this area are now neuroectoderm cells and are also involved in the development of the retina. Once formed, the neural plate starts to dip along its length and then to fold over to form a neural groove (Figure 4.7). The sides of the groove are the neural folds and the top points that will come together are the neural crests. As the neural crests come together, a tube of neuroectoderm from the cranial to the caudal end is formed, which is the neural tube as seen in (Figure 4.8). Initially, the ends of the tube are open, the neuropores, the cranial end closing on day 24 and the caudal end on day 26 (Webster and de Wreede 2016). From this point, the brain and central nervous system will continue to develop. At the cranial end, the neural tube will dilate and fold to become the brain, while the remainder develops into the spinal cord.

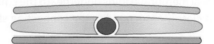

FIGURE 4.6 Formation of the notochord. Webster, S and de Wreede, R. (2016) Embryology at a Glance/John Wiley & Sons.

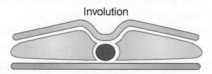

FIGURE 4.7 Formation of the neural groove. Webster, S and de Wreede, R. (2016) Embryology at a Glance/John Wiley & Sons.

65

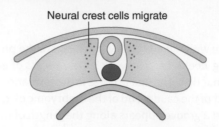

FIGURE 4.8 Formation of the neural tube. Webster, S and de Wreede, R. (2016) Embryology at a Glance/John Wiley & Sons.

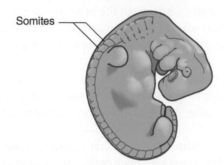

FIGURE 4.9 Somites develop during weeks 4 and 5. Webster, S and de Wreede, R. (2016) Embryology at a Glance/John Wiley & Sons.

In the neural crests, specialist cells develop, the neural crest cells. These cells migrate throughout the embryo, differentiating to become part of several organs and structures. This migration starts before the neuropores close, with the cells having specific destinations. Should this process be interrupted so that the cells do not reach their intended destination, this can result in congenital abnormalities, such as a cleft lip and palate, if there are insufficient cells in the face to form the mesenchyme structure that is required.

The mesoderm of the trilaminar layer itself has three individual layers, the paraxial mesoderm, the intermediate mesoderm and the lateral mesoderm, which is involved with the development of different structures in the body. Late in the third week from fertilisation, the paraxial mesoderm on either side of the neural tube thickens and divides to form pairs of somites. Pairs of somites develop at a recognised rate during the fourth and fifth weeks and are also prominent on the surface of the embryo, so can be used as a means of dating the pregnancy(Figure 4.9). The first somites form at the cranial end of the embryo as a result of complex genetic signalling. By the end if week 5, there will be 3 pairs of occipital somites, 8 cervical, 12 thoracic, 5 lumbar, 5 sacral and 3–5 coccygeal.

As the cells of the trilaminar discs multiply and grow at different rates, the embryo starts to fold and curl, changing from the flat layers of the discs to a more recognisable embryo shape. Neurogenesis is the start of the folding process, and this continues as the cranial end of the embryo folds over, so that the early neural tube is above the buccopharyngeal membrane and, at the caudal end, the cloacal membrane folds underneath the embryo. The remaining part of the umbilical vesicle will develop into the gut, and is closely associated to the connecting stalk, the link between the embryo and the placenta.

As well as folding longitudinally, lateral folds also develop, so that the ectoderm on each side comes together to form the external surface of the embryo. The mesoderm and endoderm also meet, with the endoderm forming the lining of the gastrointestinal tract. This is complete by the end of week 4. Should this process fail, the result is gastroschisis, where the intestines herniate through the abdominal wall.

The development of the cardiovascular system also begins in week 3, as the embryo needs to acquire oxygen and nutrients from the developing placental circulation. Blood vessels begin to form in the umbilical vesicle and the connecting stalk and blood cells initially develop from specialised cells within the vessels so that there is an early uteroplacental circulation in place by the end of the third week (Moore et al. 2016).

The Embryonic Period

From week 4 onwards, the process of organogenesis takes place, with the establishment of all the major organs and systems in the body. This is the time of greatest risk to the fetus, when exposure to teratogens, such as certain drugs, viruses or bacteria, could interrupt the development of one or more organs resulting in congenital abnormalities. The growth and development of the organs can occur in three ways. Growth occurs through mitosis, normal cell division and multiplication. The development of the shape and size of the organs and features occurs through morphogenesis, which is controlled by specific genes. Here, the cells change their size, shape and location, as well as interacting with other genes. Finally, the cells differentiate to form tissues and organs with specific functions. This is mediated by various signalling centres (Coad et al. 2020).

Week 4

The structure of the embryo changes during week 4, with the continuation of the folding started in week 3, and the somites are seen as small protuberances on the dorsal surface. Many of the systems and organs of the body start to form during this week. The forebrain starts to develop, showing as the cranial end of the embryo extends upwards. Limb buds become visible during week 4, the oric pits, early ears, develop and the site where the eyes will grow are seen as the lens placodes.

Week 5

There are fewer changes in week 5, but there is noticeable growth of the head as the brain develops. The site of the early kidneys, the mesomorphic kidneys, starts to develop in this week.

Week 6

During week 6, the embryo first starts to move, although this is not felt until much later by the mother. There are signs of fingers developing on the hand plates, with the toes starting to show towards the end of this week. Development of the eyes and ears continue, with the early earlobe now being present. At this stage, the abdominal cavity is too small for the intestines, and these herniate into the umbilical vesicle.

Week 7

Week 7 sees the beginning of ossification of the bones of the arms, where the digits have become more pronounced.

Week 8

By the end of week 8, the embryo is taking on the appearance of human, with the disappearance of the tail-like eminence at the caudal end by the end of the week, although the head is still much larger in relation to the rest of the body. The development of the digits of the hand continues so that they are now separated, but still maintain the webbing between the fingers, and there is ossification in the long bones of the legs.

Overview of the Development of Body Systems and Organs

Cardiovascular System: Days 16–28

Initially, angioblasts in the mesoderm clump together to form islands of blood, and the process of vasculogenesis sees the development of new blood vessels. At the cranial end of the embryo, the blood islands merge together and start to fold to form a horseshoe shaped tube. This and the great vessels develop from mesenchymal cells that diversify into myoblasts. Neural crest cells also migrate to contribute to the development of the early heart. This primitive heart will start beating around day 22 and will continue to fold and change shape between days 23 and 27. Initially, two bulges appear, the bulbus cordis at the cranial end and the primitive ventricles at the caudal end (Figure 4.10). The folding continues in week 4 (Figure 4.11) in preparation for the establishment of the four chambers of the heart. Septa start to appear in week 5, with the atrioventricular canal separating the tube into two by the end of week 6. The atrial septum develops but maintains a flap between the two atrium, the foramen ovale, one of the temporary structures in the fetal circulation to by-pass the fetal lungs (Figure 4.12). The septum between the ventricles is completed during week 7.

Blood vessels also develop from about 17 days, with angioblast cells leading to the formation of the early blood vessels. This is vasculogenesis. Further new vessels branch off from these vessels in the process of angiogenesis. Early blood cells develop from multipotent stem cells, which are found in the mesoderm layer of the umbilical vesicle. As the embryo grows, blood cells are then produced in the aorta, and later, the liver, spleen and bone marrow. The embryonic circulatory system can be seen in Figure 4.13.

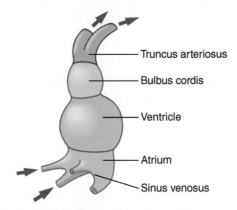

FIGURE 4.10 Development of the primitive heart; the bulbus cordis at the cranial end and the primitive ventricles at the caudal end. Webster, S and de Wreede, R. (2016) Embryology at a Glance/John Wiley & Sons.

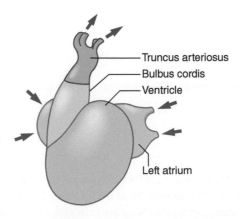

FIGURE 4.11 Folding in preparation for the establishment of the four chambers of the heart. Webster, S and de Wreede, R. (2016) Embryology at a Glance/John Wiley & Sons.

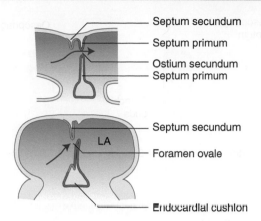

FIGURE 4.12 The atrial septum develops but maintains a flap between the two atrium, the foramen ovale, one of the temporary structures in the fetal circulation to by-pass the fetal lungs. Webster, S and de Wreede, R. (2016) Embryology at a Glance/John Wiley & Sons.

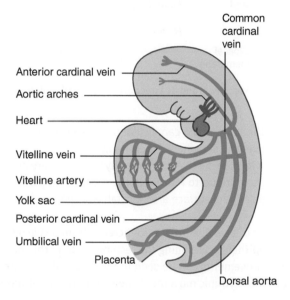

FIGURE 4.13 The embryonic circulatory system. Webster, S and de Wreede, R. (2016) Embryology at a Glance/John Wiley & Sons.

Structural development of the heart is one of the most common areas of congenital abnormality, with 6 in 1000 children being born with heart defects (Webster and de Wreede 2016). The most common of these is a ventricular septal defect (VSD) where the ventricular septum does not fuse completely. Should the foramen ovals fail to close at birth, this results in an atrial septal defect.

Respiratory System: Day 28 Onwards

The beginning of the respiratory system can be seen during week 4 when a bud branches from the tube of the gut, which then divides again during the fifth week. These buds then continue to branch out and divide, forming three lobes on the right hand side and only two on the left (Figure 4.14). This is seen as the embryonic stage of development of the lungs. The second stage is the pseudoglandular stage, from about 6–17 weeks, where with continual growth results in the structures of the respiratory system being in place, except those specifically involved in the exchange of gases. The lung type II alveolar cells, which later produce surfactant, also develop during this period.

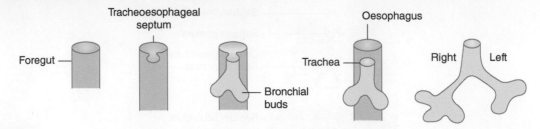

FIGURE 4.14   The beginnings of the respiratory system. Webster, S and de Wreede, R. (2016) Embryology at a Glance/John Wiley & Sons.

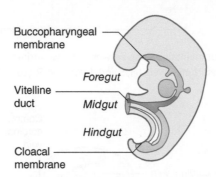

FIGURE 4.15   The three sections of the gut. Webster, S and de Wreede, R. (2016) Embryology at a Glance/John Wiley & Sons.

The next stage of development of the lungs is the canalicular stage from 16 to 25 weeks, when the primitive alveoli develop, flatten and become the type I alveolar cells where the exchange of gas takes place. Towards the end of this period, the lungs are sufficiently developed for a fetus to survive supported by intensive care as the system is very immature.

From 25 weeks until birth, the lungs continue to mature in the saccular stage. Surfactant is now produced, which helps to prevent the alveoli from collapsing; the surface area available for gas exchange and the blood–air barrier also develop.

The alveolar stage sees the number of alveoli continue to increase from 36 weeks and throughout childhood. The alveoli also mature in this stage as the epithelial cells lining the respiratory tract thin out.

From about 12 weeks, respiratory movements can be seen in the fetus, which increases from about 24 weeks. The fetus is not able to breath as such, but the rhythmic movements help with the maturation of the respiratory system.

Gastrointestinal Tract: Days 21–50

As described earlier in this chapter, the tube which will develop into the gut forms with the initial folding of the embryonic plates. The lining is endodermal in origin, except for the caudal end where the endoderm and ectoderm layers meet. The buccopharyngeal membrane covering the orifice that will form the mouth opens during the fourth week, so that the mouth is then open to the amniotic cavity, and the cloacal membrane covering what will become the anus ruptures in the seventh week.

There are three sections to the gut, indicated in Figure 4.15. the foregut goes on to form the pharynx, oesophagus, stomach and the initial part of the duodenum. The midgut develops into the remainder of the duodenum as well as the small and part of the large intestine, while the hindgut forms the remainder of the large intestine from the transverse colon to the start of the anal canal.

As the embryo grows, so does the foregut, with an area beginning to dilate in week 4, which will form the stomach. Further buds form, which will become the liver, gallbladder and pancreas. The liver grows rapidly, being about 10% of the total weight of the embryo by week 10, although this reduces to 5% by the time of birth. As mentioned previously, one of the functions of the liver at this stage is the production of red blood cells. The pancreas, by week 7, has a system of ducts

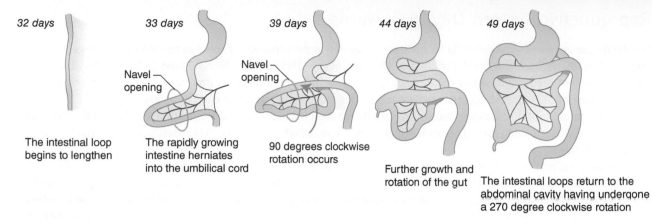

FIGURE 4.16 The growth and development of the midgut. Webster, S and de Wreede, R. (2016) Embryology at a Glance/ John Wiley & Sons.

which fuse together to form the main pancreatic duct. In the third month, the islets of Langerhans are formed, which are secreting insulin within a few weeks.

The growth of the midgut is also rapid, especially during the sixth week. The growth is so considerable that it herniates into the umbilical cord to have sufficient room, returning to the abdominal cavity around week 10, as well as undergoing several twists and turns (Figure 4.16). The development of the hindgut is completed during the seventh week. The urorectal septum forms from mesoderm in the cloacal area, forming the anorectal canal and a urogenital sinus from which the bladder and urogenital tract will develop.

The spleen is also slinked to the gastrointestinal tract, developing around week 5. From the second trimester until birth, red and white blood cells are produced here.

The Urogenital System

The urinary and genital systems develop independently, but from both arise from the intermediate mesoderm. Initially, a collection of cells gather in the abdomen, and these divide into the nephrogenic cord and the gonadal ridge.

The Renal System: Day 21 to Birth

During the development of the renal system, there are three sets of kidneys. The pronephroses is a non-functioning kidney, developing around week 3 and disappearing soon afterwards, which triggers the subsequent processes that result in the development of the full kidney. In week 4, the mesonephric ducts develop as tubes in the mesoderm and extend to the cloaca in the area where the bladder will develop. Small amounts of urine are produced here from about week 6 until they degenerate between weeks 7 and 10.

The permanent kidneys are the metanephros, which start to develop from the fifth week from the mesonephric duct, taking on the form of the adult kidney with the renal pelvis, calyces, collecting tubules, nephrons and the ureter. The kidneys continue to develop until birth. Urine is produced from around week 12, mainly as part of the amniotic fluid as excretion is via the placenta.

The urogenital sinus from the cloaca has three parts to it, with the largest section at the top developing into the bladder, the middle section is the urethra in the female, and the upper part of the urethra in the male, while the lowest section is the vestibule in the female and the lower part of the urethra in the male.

Reproductive System: Day 35 Onwards

For the first seven weeks, the genitalia for both sexes develop in the same way, known as the indifferent stage, from the mesonephric ducts from the renal system and the paramesonephric ducts which lie next to them. The changes in the development are influenced by the inheritance of either the x or y chromosome from the spermatozoon. In the male, the mesonephric ducts become the efferent ductules, the epididymis and the vas deferens.

The paramesonephric ducts are involved in the development of the uterus and uterine tubes in the female. The ducts meet in the pelvic region and form the uterovaginal primordium, which later becomes the uterus, while the ducts become the uterine tubes.

The external genitalia start to develop from around week 9 from the cloacal membrane but are not easily identified on ultrasound until week 11. The changes that then occur are mediated in the female by oestrogens from the placenta and fetal ovaries stimulating the growth of the clitoris and vestibule, containing the vaginal and urethral openings. The development of the penis in the male is stimulated by androgens from the testes. Figure 4.17 shows the development of the female external genitalia and the development of the male external genitalia is demonstrated in Figure 4.18.

The gonads develop from day 30 onwards from the mesoderm of the urogenital ridge and germ cells, which originate in the umbilical vesicle. These migrate to the urogenital ridge during week 6, leading to an indifferent gonad. In the female, from the fourth month, the germ cells are surrounded by epithelia to form the primary follicle. Each of the germ cells becomes an oogonium, which undergoes cell division prior to birth.

The male produces testosterone by week 8 from Leydig cells developed from the gonadal ridge. By the fourth month, the primitive germ cells that will produce spermatozoa are found in the seminiferous tubules.

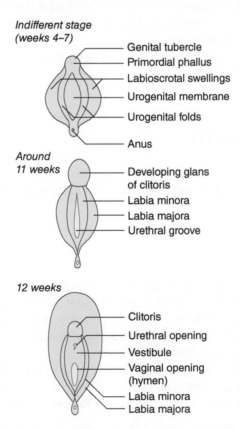

FIGURE 4.17   Development of the female external genitalia. Webster, S and de Wreede, R. (2016) Embryology at a Glance/ John Wiley & Sons.

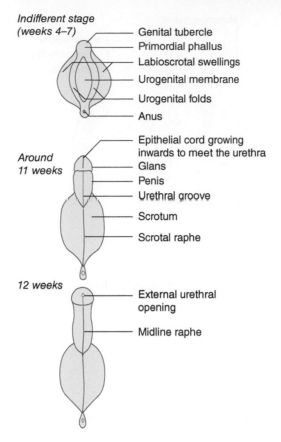

Indifferent stage (weeks 4–7)

- Genital tubercle
- Primordial phallus
- Labioscrotal swellings
- Urogenital membrane
- Urogenital folds
- Anus

Around 11 weeks

- Epithelial cord growing inwards to meet the urethra
- Glans
- Penis
- Urethral groove
- Scrotum
- Scrotal raphe

12 weeks

- External urethral opening
- Midline raphe

FIGURE 4.18 Development of the male external genitalia. Webster, S and de Wreede, R. (2016) Embryology at a Glance/John Wiley & Sons.

Central Nervous System: Day 22 Onwards

The early development of the nervous system, neurulation, is described earlier in this chapter with the formation of the neural tube from neuroectoderm.

The brain develops at the cranial end of the neural tube with the formation of three vesicles, the prosencephalon, or forebrain, the mesencephalon, or midbrain and the rhombencephalon, or hindbrain. With continued growth, the neural tube folds, and the forebrain and hindbrain each divide into two during the fifth week. These divisions are demonstrated in Figure 4.19. The telencephalon area of the forebrain becomes the cerebral cortex posteriorly and the basal ganglia towards the front, while the diencephalon area develops into the optic cup and stalk, the pituitary gland, thalamus, hypothalamus and pineal body.

The myelencephalon is the caudal part of the hindbrain, and this becomes the medulla oblongata, while the other area, the metacephalon, forms the pons and cerebellum. These, plus the midbrain, form the brainstem. The ventricles all contain cerebrospinal fluid.

At the caudal end, the neural tube lengthens to form the spinal cord, with the neurocoel, a canal in the centre of the tube, forming by week 9. This is lined by neuroepithelial cells, which differentiate to become neuroblasts, the eventual neurons that form the grey matter. The white matter surrounds the neurocoel and contains the axons leading from the neurons.

During the embryonic period, the spinal cord is the length of the vertebral column. However, at the end of this period, the number of coccygeal vertebrae reduces and there is lengthening of the vertebral column so that the end of the spinal cord reaches the third lumbar vertebra by term, and the first or second lumbar vertebrae in adults.

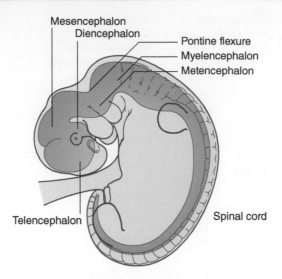

FIGURE 4.19 Division of the neural tube folds, and the forebrain and hindbrain in week 5. Webster, S and de Wreede, R. (2016) Embryology at a Glance/John Wiley & Sons.

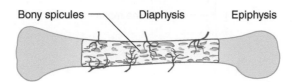

FIGURE 4.20 The beginning of ossification of the long bones. Webster, S and de Wreede, R. (2016) Embryology at a Glance/John Wiley & Sons.

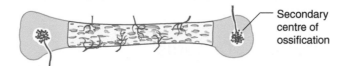

FIGURE 4.21 Secondary ossification. Webster, S and de Wreede, R. (2016) Embryology at a Glance/John Wiley & Sons.

Skeletal System: Week 5 to Adulthood

There are two main areas to the development of the skeletal system, these being the axial skeleton, formed of the cranium, vertebral column, ribs and sternum and then the limbs which form the appendicular skeleton.

The precursors of the skeletal system are the mesodermal cells, which form connective tissue in the embryo and go on to form both the bones and joints. The long bones of the appendicular skeleton develop through endochondral ossification. Tightly packed mesodermal cells form the shape of the future bone, and this differentiates to become cartilage. Ossification begins in the shaft, or diaphysis, of the bone where the cartilage cells enlarge and become calcified, with the ossification of the limb bones starting at 56 days after fertilisation, towards the end of the embryonic period. This process continues after birth in the ends of the bones, the epiphysis. Bone also forms around the edges of the diaphysis, where the layer of cells surrounding this, the periosteum, differentiate to become osteoblasts. These stages can be seen in Figures 4.20–4.22. The precursor cells for the bone marrow are bought to the long bones through developing blood vessels.

Flat bones, such as those of the skull, ossify through intermembranous ossification. The mesenchyme forms a hollow shape that contains precursor cells that will form the osteoblasts. Calcium deposits aid the process of the formation of the bone, with the cells maturing from osteoblasts to osteocytes. In intermembranous ossification, the formation of the bone starts towards the centre of the preformed mesenchyme membranous shape and then radiates outwards.

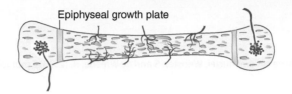

Epiphyseal growth plate

FIGURE 4.22 Position of the growth plates in the ossified bone. Webster, S and de Wreede, R. (2016) Embryology at a Glance/ John Wiley & Sons.

The axial skeleton is mainly formed from the somites, as discussed earlier in the chapter. Cells from the somites differentiate further to form the sclerotome and dermomyotome. The sclerotome cells differentiate into the vertebrae as well as the intervertebral discs, ribs and connective tissues. Ossification of the vertebrae begins during week 7 from fertilisation, continuing until the age of 25 years. Initially, the ribs are formed of cartilage, with ossification developing during the fetal period.

Snapshot 4.1 Spina Bifida

Following the birth of baby Simon, the midwife notices a hairy patch of skin on the back of the baby, overlying the vertebrae. On discussing with the parents, they ask what this might be and what may have caused it.

- The midwife can explain that this may be an occult spina bifida, seen when the two halves of the vertebrae do not fuse together. This leaves a small gap in the vertebral column (Figure 4.23).
- A referral to the neonatologist is required, and an x-ray will be arranged to confirm the diagnosis.
- This is the least severe form of spina bifida, generally leading to very minor or even no symptoms.

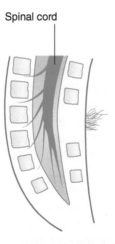

Spinal cord

FIGURE 4.23 Occult spina bifida. Webster, S and de Wreede, R. (2016) Embryology at a Glance/John Wiley & Sons.

The dermomyotome layer of the somites splits again into myotome, which differentiate to form the skeletal muscles and the muscles of the limbs, and the dermatome cells, which become part of the dermal and subcutaneous tissues of the skin. Skeletal muscle is formed from myoblasts, which are the precursors to the muscle cells. Initially, they form long myotubes followed by long muscle fibres, which have several nuclei (Figure 4.24). Early skeletal muscle is visible from the end of 12 weeks as microfibres that have strands of actin and myosin.

The limb buds appear around day 26, with muscle precursor cells migrating into the limbs. These cells join together to form muscle masses, then split into the individual muscles of the relative limbs. This process is mostly completed by nine weeks. On ultrasound, limb movement can be detected by 7 weeks but this is clearer from around week 10.

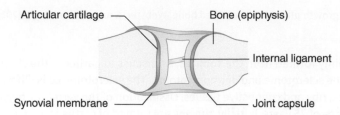

FIGURE 4.24   Long muscle fibres have several nuclei. Webster, S and de Wreede, R. (2016) Embryology at a Glance/John Wiley & Sons.

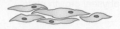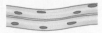

Articular cartilage — Bone (epiphysis)

— Internal ligament

Synovial membrane — Joint capsule

FIGURE 4.25   A synovial joint. Webster, S and de Wreede, R. (2016) Embryology at a Glance/John Wiley & Sons.

The various joints of the skeletal system also develop from the mesenchyme starting in the sixth week from fertilisation and look like the adult joint by the end of week eight. Where there is a cartilaginous joint, such as in the ribs and sternum, the mesenchyme differentiates to form the fibrous supporting tissue. The symphysis pubis is formed from fibrocartilage.

Synovial joints, such as the knee joint, comprise different tissue types (Figure 4.25). The mesenchyme differentiates into the joint capsule, with the tissue in the centre disappearing to form the synovial cavity of the joint. The synovial membrane forms from the mesenchyme lining the capsule, and this secretes the synovial fluid. Supporting ligaments also develop from the mesenchyme.

The Skull and Face

The skull is divided into the neurocranium covering the brain and the viscerocranium, forming the face. Cells from the occipital somites, together with neural crest cells, form the neurocranium from plates of cartilage, which ossify through endochondral ossification to form the frontal, parietal and occipital bones as well as part of the temporal bone. This process is incomplete at birth, leaving membranous gaps, suture lines, between the bones with larger areas, the fontanelles, where two or more bones meet. During labour, this allows for slight overlapping of the bones, known as moulding, to help facilitate progress through the pelvis. The process of ossification is not complete until about 18 months of age (Coad et al. 2020).

The viscerocranium also originates from cartilage and membrane. During week 4, six pairs of pharyngeal arches, clefts and pouches into which neural crest cells migrate appear in the sides of the cranial end of the embryo. These structures go on to form the bones of the face, as well as the mouth, nasal cavity, larynx, pharynx and neck and the associated muscles and nerves that are involved with chewing and swallowing, facial expression and speech. Although six pairs of arches form, the fifth pair disappears soon after development and has no role to play. The centre of the pharyngeal arches consists of mesoderm and they are covered in ectoderm on the outside, which forms the pharyngeal grooves separating the arches and endoderm on the inside, forming pharyngeal pouches.

The early mouth can be seen as an indentation in the surface of the embryo, the stomodeum, from week 4, and is continuous with the gut. This is covered with the oropharyngeal membrane until day 26 when the early pharynx and foregut comes into contact with the amniotic fluid (Moore et al. 2016). Figure 4.26 shows the embryo at four weeks demonstrating the position of the pharyngeal arches and the stomodeum.

The first pharyngeal arches divide to from the maxillary and mandibular prominences, while the ectoderm and endoderm layers contribute to the formation of the mucous membrane and glands of the tongue. During week 5, the maxillary prominences grow towards the centre of what will be the face and the development of the nose commences with the formation of the nasal placodes. Mesenchyme accumulates around the nasal placodes to become the nasal prominences,

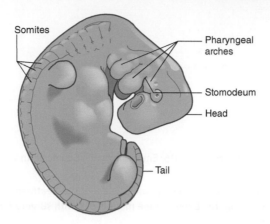

FIGURE 4.26 The embryo at four weeks, demonstrating the position of the pharyngeal arches and the stomodeum. Webster, S and de Wreede, R. (2016) Embryology at a Glance/John Wiley & Sons.

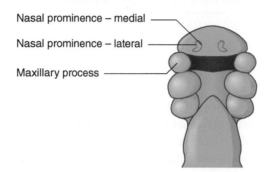

FIGURE 4.27 Formation of the nose. Webster, S and de Wreede, R. (2016) Embryology at a Glance/John Wiley & Sons.

which move together and merge in the midline before fusing with the maxillary prominence forming the upper lip (Mitchell and Sharma 2009). This early development can be seen in Figure 4.27. The nasal placodes also turn inwards to form nasal pits, which then appear on the face as the nostrils. The septum between the nostrils develops during week 9.

The palate also develops from the maxillary prominences, initially growing along the side of the tongue and moving to their horizontal position by the end of week 9, when they fuse together. Failure of this process results in a cleft palate. The muscles of the tongue will start to work during this time.

Some of the pharyngeal structures, such as the hyoid bone, originate from the third pair of pharyngeal arches, while arches four and six eventually fuse together to form structures within the neck, such as the muscles of the larynx and pharynx. The fifth pair of arches forms, but soon disappears and has no function in development.

Snapshot 4.2   Cleft Lip

At the 20 week ultrasound scan, the sonographer identified and pointed out to Aisha and Mohammed that she could identify a cleft lip on the fetus. They are now with the midwife and have asked a number of questions about what this means and how it may have occurred.

- A cleft lip is where the fusion of the nasal prominence with the maxillary prominence has not been completed. This can either affect just the lip, which is known as being incomplete (Figure 4.28) or can extend to the nose, which is complete, and may also occur on just one side of the mouth or both sides.
- Although it can be seen on ultrasound, a cleft lip may be accompanied by a cleft palate, where the palate has failed to fuse as it develops from the maxillary process. This is not diagnosed until after birth.

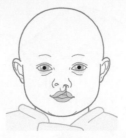

FIGURE 4.28 Cleft lip. Webster, S and de Wreede, R. (2016) Embryology at a Glance/John Wiley & Sons.

- Aisha and Mohammed will have discussions with the neonatologists about the treatment for the baby following birth. For the cleft lip, surgery should be carried out before the baby is three months old, with surgery for a cleft palate, if diagnosed, being required before the baby's first birthday.
- Generally, surgery is effective and it is often difficult to see where the defect was. There may be initial difficulties with feeding, for which support will be needed, and possible speech therapy.
- Prevention of these defects can be promoted by taking folic acid prior to pregnancy.

Ears and Eyes

The ear consists of the outer, middle and inner ear, with the outer and middle ear developing from the first and second pharyngeal arches, cleft and pouch. The inner ear develops first, starting around day 22 with a thickening of the ectoderm on either side of the cranial end of the embryo, the otic placode. This folds inwards to become the otic vesicle, which modifies its shape to develop into the semicircular canals and the cochlea. During week 6, the cochlea spirals into the surrounding mesenchyme, completing two and a half spirals by the end of week 8, and being fully developed by 24 weeks.

The first pharyngeal arch contributes to the formation of the middle ear in the form of the incus and malleus bones, the stapes bone being formed from the second pharyngeal arch. The bones of the middle ear can be seen in Figure 4.29. The tubotympanic recess becomes the middle ear cavity and the Eustachian or auditory tube is developed from the related pouch. The tympanic membrane, or eardrum, is the beginning of the external ear at the point where the internal tympanic cavity meets the ectoderm of the external auditory meatus, which is formed from the cleft of the pharyngeal arch. By week 20, The ear is developed sufficiently for the fetus to hear sounds from outside the uterus.

The eyes also originate from the thickened ectodermal placodes, with the optic vesicle developing at the beginning of the fourth week from fertilisation, which leads to the formation of the lens placode from the ectoderm. The optic vesicle folds inwards to form the optic cup, and the lens placode replicates this movement to lie in the optic cup as the lens vesicle (Figure 4.30). Primary lens fibres form over the next two weeks, with secondary lens fibres developing from the epithelial cells at the centre of the lens. This process continues throughout life.

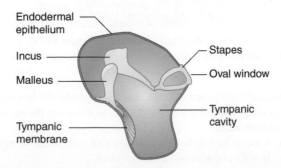

FIGURE 4.29 The bones of the middle ear. Webster, S and de Wreede, R. (2016) Embryology at a Glance/John Wiley & Sons.

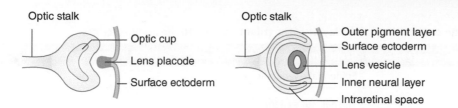

FIGURE 4.30 The optic vesicle folds inwards to form the optic cup, and the lens placode replicates this movement to lie in the optic cup as the lens vesicle. Webster, S and de Wreede, R. (2016) Embryology at a Glance/John Wiley & Sons.

The retina develops from the optic cup, with the outside layer becoming the pigmented layer and the inner layer the rods and cones, as well as neural cells, which differentiate to become the optic nerve by the end of week 9. Anteriorly, the layers of the retina become the iris and ciliary body, with the ciliary muscles developing from mesenchyme in this area. Formation of the eye is complete by 20 weeks, with rapid eye movements being observed from 21 weeks; the eyes are sensitive to light from 30 weeks. The eyelids, however, which develop from folds of ectoderm, are fused until around 24 weeks of gestation.

Integumentary System

In the early embryonic stages, the skin of the embryo develops from the ectoderm and mesoderm layers of the trilaminar disc (Table 4.2). The ectoderm starts as a single layer, to which others are added to form the epidermis, and the mesoderm forms the dermal layer of the skin, giving a thin covering to the embryo by the end of the fourth week with development continuing to the 24th week following fertilisation. The pigmentation of the skin is from melanocytes, which originate as neural crest cells.

Hair, which also originates from the ectoderm, develops on the fetus from 9 weeks, with the body being covered with lanugo, fine downy hair, by 20 weeks. Most of this hair has been shed by term. The nails also develop from the ectoderm, with fingernails appearing from about 10 weeks and toenails much later, at 18 weeks (Bailey, 2020b).

The Fetal Period

As discussed above, the tissues and organs of the body are formed during the embryonic period, but further differentiation and overall growth continues from the end of the eighth week until birth, the fetal period. During this time, there is both an increase in cell numbers, hyperplasia and an increase in cell size, hypertrophy. The process of apoptosis is also involved in the growth and development of the fetus. For the first 16 weeks, the growth is mainly due to hyperplasia. At this point, hyperplasia growth slows and much of the growth is due to hypertrophy until 32 weeks, when hypertrophy is the main reason for growth.

At four weeks, the length of the embryo from the crown to the rump is 4 mm, with the embryo growing by 1 mm a day until it reaches 30 mm. Weeks 8–28 see the most rapid period of growth, with an increase of 1.5 mm a day. Until 16 weeks, embryos are all a similar size, which allows for early dating of the pregnancy by ultrasound measurements, as there is little variation. The crown–rump length is generally used in the first trimester. However, if this length is over 84 mm, the head circumference is the measurement that is used; the biparietal diameter or femur length is used in the second trimester.

From this point, the rates of growth vary from embryo to embryo due to the influence of genetic and environmental factors, such as the availability of oxygen and nutrients from the mother (Coad et al. 2020). Not only does maternal nutrition have an effect on the rate of growth, as the stores of fat depend on the nutrition that is available to the fetus, but it is thought that maternal height also has an influence, as smaller women tend to have smaller babies (Patrick 2017). The levels of insulin in the fetus also contribute to the birth weight.

Where there is a lack of oxygen and nutrition available for the fetus, adaptations are made to the metabolism, and blood flow is redirected to protect the major organs, especially the brain. About 10% of pregnancies are affected by fetal growth restriction, which can lead to perinatal morbidity and mortality.

TABLE 4.2 **The contribution of the layers of the trilaminar disc to the body systems.**

Layer	Structures
Ectoderm	Epidermal layer of the skin
	The nervous system
	Neural crest cells (vital to the development of several structures)
Mesoderm	Dermal layer of skin
	Skeletal system
	Striated skeletal muscle
	Smooth muscle
	Cardiovascular and lymphatic systems
	Reproductive system
	Kidneys and ureters
	Linings of body cavities
	Cells of the cardiovascular system and immune system formed in the bone marrow
Endoderm	Epithelial lining of the digestive, respiratory and urinary systems
	Pancreas
	Liver
	Epithelia of the urethra and bladder
	Tonsils
	Thyroid gland

The rates of growth of different areas of the fetus vary, with the growth of the head circumference, abdominal circumference and femur peaking at 16–17 weeks (Ohuma et al. 2021). Towards term, the rates of growth of the head circumference, biparietal diameter and femur length slow, while the growth of the abdominal circumference is maintained throughout the pregnancy. Sex also affects the rate of growth, with males generally being larger than females (Coad et al. 2020), which is thought to be because testosterone is produced in fetal life, giving the effect of anabolic steroids.

Snapshot 4.3   Gastroschisis

Susan and Tom have just returned from their 20 week scan, where they were told that the baby had gastroschisis. They have come to see you for further explanations of what this is and what the future holds for them and the baby.

Gastroschisis is where the intestines herniate through a defect in the abdominal wall where the peritoneum and skin layers have failed to completely join together as the abdominal wall forms during the embryonic period. The prognosis is generally very good, with surgery being required soon after birth to repair the defect.

Snapshot 4.4   Ventricular Septal Defect

Baby Niram has just had the newborn and infant physical examination at 24 hours of age. The paediatrician detected a heart murmur and has explained that further investigations will be needed to provide a diagnosis. However, he suspects a VSD. The parents have asked for more information on this condition.

A VSD is one of the most common of heart abnormalities, accounting for about 40% (McEwan 2017) and can vary in severity. The septum dividing the ventricles has failed to form completely, allowing the deoxygenated blood from the right ventricle to mix with the oxygenated blood in the left ventricle. The defect ranges from leaving a very small hole, which may heal spontaneously, to a large defect that would require surgical repair, although this is not carried out in the immediate neonatal period. Generally, these defects are not noted during the pregnancy and allow the fetus to develop normally as the lungs are not used for oxygenation.

Take Home Points

- Embryology is an extensive and complex subject. The changes that take place through cell multiplication and differentiation from the moment of fertilisation are immense, as can be seen when reading through this chapter.
- As a midwife, it is important to have a basic understanding of the stages of development so that you can discuss the stages of development with parents as needed and, as mentioned previously, provide explanations and advice related to any abnormalities that are detected.
- A background knowledge is also useful for preconceptual guidance for those who may be on medication for an underlying condition.

References

Bailey, J. (2020a). Hormonal cycles: fertilisation and early development. In: *Myles Textbook for Midwives*, 17e (ed. J. Marshall and M. Raynor). Edinburgh: Elsevier.

Bailey, J. (2020b). The fetus. In: *Myles Textbook for Midwives*, 17e (ed. J. Marshall and M. Raynor). Edinburgh: Elsevier.

Coad, J., Pedley, K., and Dunstall, M. (2020). *Anatomy and Physiology for Midwives*, 4e. Edinburgh: Elsevier.

McEwan, T. (2017). Developmental anatomy: related cardiovascular and respiratory disorders. In: *Physiology in Childbearing with Anatomy and Related Biosciences* (ed. J. Rankin). Edinburgh: Elsevier.

Mitchell, B. and Sharma, R. (2009). *Embryology: An Illustrated Colour Text*, 2e. Edinburgh: Elsevier.

Moore, K.L., Persaud, T.V.N., and Torchia, M.G. (2015). *The Developing Human: Clinically Oriented Embryology*, 10e. Philadelphia, PA: Elsevier.

Moore, K.L., Persaud, T.V.N., and Torchia, M.G. (2016). *Before We Are Born*, 9e. Philadelphia, PA: Elsevier.

Ohuma, E.O., Villar, J., Feng, Y. et al. (2021). Fetal growth velocity standards from the fetal growth longitudinal study of the INTERGROWTH-21st project. *American Journal of Obstetrics and Gynecology* 224 (2): 208.e1–208.e18.

Patrick, H. (2017). Fetal growth and development. In: *Physiology in Childbearing with Anatomy and Related Biosciences* (ed. J. Rankin). Edinburgh: Elsevier.

Rankin, J. and Matthews, L. (2017). General embryology. In: *Physiology in Childbearing with Anatomy and Related Biosciences*, 4e, Chapter 9 (ed. J. Rankin). Edinburgh: Elsevier.

Webster, S. and de Wreede, R. (2016). *Embryology at a Glance*, 2e. Chichester: Wiley Blackwell.

Further Reading

Britten, S., Soenksen, D.M., Bustillo, M., and Coulam, C.B. (1994). Very early (24–56 days from last menstrual period) embryonic heart rate in normal pregnancies. *Human Reproduction* 9 (12): 2424–2426.

DeRuiter, C (2010). Somites: formation and role in developing the body plan. https://embryo.asu.edu/pages/somites-formation-and-role-developing-body-plan (accessed 15 August 2022).

Donovan, M.F. and Cascella, M. (2021). Embryology, weeks 6–8. https://www.ncbi.nlm.nih.gov/books/NBK563181 (accessed 7 September 2022).

Elshazzly, M., Lopex, M.J., Reddy, V., and Caban, O. (2022). Embryology, central Nervous System. https://www.ncbi.nlm.nih.gov/books/NBK526024 (accessed 7 September 2022).

Khan, Y. S and Ackerman, K. M. (2022) Embryology, week 1. https://www.ncbi.nlm.nih.gov/books/NBK554562 (accessed 7 September 2022).

Moore, K.L., Persaud, T.V.N., and Torchia, M.G. (2016). *Before We Are Born*, 9e. Philadelphia: Elsevier.

Nilsson, L. and Forsell, L. (2020). *A Child Is Born*, 5e. New York: Merloyd Lawrence.

Although originally published over 40 years ago, this book has photographs of the development from fertilisation until birth.

NHS England (2023). *Fetal Anomaly Screening Programme Handbook*. Lodno, NHS England: https://www.gov.uk/government/publications/fetal-anomaly-screening-programme-handbook.

Rehman, B. and Muzio, M.R. (2023). *Embryology, Week 2–3*. Treasure Island, FL: StatPearls Publishing https://www.ncbi.nlm.nih.gov/books/NBK546679.

Schoenwolf, G.C., Bleyl, S.B., Brauer, P.R., and Francis-West, P.H. (2021). *Larsen's Human Embryology*, 6e. Philadelphia, PA: Elsevier.

Wolpert, L., Tickle, C., and Martinez Arais, A. (2019). *Principles of Development*, 6e. Oxford: Oxford University Press.

Online Resources

Imperial College London. (2019). Human Embryo Development. [video 3.34 minutes]. https://www.youtube.com/watch?v=1zpV5rzWXMA (accessed 24 October 2023). This is an animation of the sequence of events from fertilisation until birth.

There are numerous videos available online related to embryology. One series which is clearly explained is Easy Embryology by Dr. Minass:

Dr. Minass. (2016). Introduction to Embryology – Fertilisation to Gastrulation (Easy to Understand). [video 18.41 minutes]. https://www.youtube.com/watch?v=l5gUARhXWTY (accessed October 18th 2022).

Glossary

Apoptosis	Programmed cell death important for the final layout of the cells and for the formation of body cavities.
Bilaminar disc	Early differentiation of cells to form the epiblast and hypoblast layers of the embryo.
Blastocyst	A fluid-filled cavity appearing in the morula, with the trophoblast cells around the outside and the formation of the inner cell mass.
Blastomere	The cells formed by cleavage in the zygote.
Buccopharyngeal membrane	Where the endoderm and ectoderm meet at the cranial end of the embryo. Goes on to form the mouth.
Cranial end	Superior end of embryo.
Caudal end	Tail end of embryo.
Cleavage	The first cell division that occurs in the zygote.
Cloacal membrane	Goes on to form the anus; this is where the endoderm is in contact with the ectoderm at the caudal end of the embryo.
Conceptus	The resulting products of the fertilisation of the oocyte by the spermatozoon, including the embryo and the tissues needed to support this.
Dermatome	Part of the somite which develops into the dermis.

Differentiation	Cells change to adopt a specific form or function.
Ectoderm	The outer layer of the trilaminar disc, which will develop into the epidermis, nervous tissue and sensory organs.
Embryo	From implantation of the fertilised ovum until the end of the eighth week.
Embryogenesis	Cells migrate through the embryo and differentiate to form the organs and tissues.
Endoderm	The inside layer of the trilaminar disc, which develops into the gastrointestinal tract and the respiratory system.
Fertilisation	The fusion of a spermatozoon with an oocyte leading to the development of the embryo.
Fetus	From the beginning of the ninth week until birth.
Gastrulation	The conversion of the two bilaminar embryonic discs into the three trilaminar embryonic discs This is the beginning of the formation of the nervous system.
Hypertrophy	Overall increase in size caused by the increase in the size of the cells.
Hypoplasia	Increase in size brought about by an increase in the number of cells.
Mesoderm	The middle layer of the trilaminar disc, which develops into connective tissue, muscle, bone, the urogenital and circulatory systems.
Morphogenesis	The development of the organs and tissues of the body through organised movement and diversification of cells.
Morula	(Latin for mulberry.) The zygote has reached the 16-cell stage, usually around three days after fertilisation.
Neural crest cells	Cells originate in the ectoderm before migrating and differentiating into many cell types.
Neurulation	The beginning of the formation of the nervous system.
Notochord	A rod-like structure that forms the basis of the axial skeleton. The vertebral column will form around this structure.
Organogenesis	The period of time from gastrulation until birth when the internal organs of the fetus develop.
Pluripotent	The cells are able to develop into either of the cells of the germ cell layer – endoderm, mesoderm or ectoderm – from the 16-cell stage.
Somite	Groups of paraxial mesoderm cells that develop into the dermis, muscle and vertebrae.
Totipotency	The cells of the zygote are able to differentiate into any of the cells of the organism, and thus become part of any of the body tissue. This can occur prior to the morula stage of development.
Trilaminar disc	Formed during gastrulation to give the ectoderm, mesoderm and endoderm layers of the developing embryo.
Zona pellucida	Outer membrane of the ovum.
Zygote	When the spermatozoa has penetrated the ovum and fertilisation has occurred.

Multiple Choice Questions

1. The first cell division of the zygote is known as what?
   a. Totipotency
   b. Conceptus
   c. Cleavage
   d. Multiplication

2. The developing infant is known as a fetus from how many weeks?
   a. 4 weeks
   b. 6 weeks
   c. 9 weeks
   d. 10 weeks

3. When considering directional terms, the caudal refers to which part of the embryo?
   a. The head end
   b. The tail end
   c. The sides
   d. The back

4. At the 16-cell stage, the zygote is known as what?
   a. The morula
   b. The blastocyst
   c. The embryo
   d. The fetus

5. Which layer of the trilaminar disc develops into the skeletal system?
   a. The ectoderm
   b. The mesoderm
   c. The endoderm

6. Which cells go on to form the vertebra and ribs?
   a. Endoderm
   b. Ectoderm
   c. Somites

7. What are the primitive cells of the heart called?
   a. Myoblasts
   b. Haemoblasts
   c. Cardioblasts
   d. Trophoblasts

8. What type of cells produce surfactant?
   a. Type I alveolar cells
   b. Type II alveola cells
   c. Saccular cells
   d. Epiblast cells

9. All fetuses are of a similar size until how many weeks?
   a. 8 weeks
   b. 10 weeks
   c. 12 weeks
   d. 16 weeks

10. What measurement is used to estimate the gestation of the fetus in the first trimester?
    a. Abdominal circumference
    b. Biparietal diameter
    c. Crown–rump length
    d. Femur length

CHAPTER 5

Genetics

Sarah Malone and James Castleman

AIM

The aim of this chapter is to enable the reader to gain an understanding of the fundamental concepts underpinning genetics.

LEARNING OUTCOMES

On completion of this chapter you will be able to:

- Describe the structure and function of DNA.
- Understand the normal process of DNA replication and how DNA is read.
- Understand the common problems that can occur with chromosome number, arrangement and amount of genetic material on chromosomes.
- Understand what a single gene disorder is and patterns of inheritance and understand other modes of inheritance such as triplet repeats.
- Appreciate the difference between genotype and phenotype and the factors that may affect gene expression.

Test Your Prior Knowledge

1. What is a chromosome?
2. What is a gene?
3. What does DNA stand for?
4. Which base pair does thymine pair with?
5. What is the most common mechanism for trisomy 21?

Introduction

Midwives provide care for pregnant people throughout the perinatal period. An understanding of genetics is essential when discussing screening for common chromosomal conditions such as Down, Edwards and Patau syndromes, as well as assessing risks of genetic conditions such as thalassaemia or sickle cell disease to offspring.

Fundamentals of Maternal Anatomy and Physiology, First Edition. Edited by Ian Peate and Claire Leader.
© 2024 John Wiley & Sons Ltd. Published 2024 by John Wiley & Sons Ltd.

Deoxyribose Nucleic Acid

The very smallest component of every living organism is a cell. Humans are made up of trillions of cells, each one having a particular specialised function. A cell must have three components: a nucleus, cytoplasm and a cell membrane. The cell membrane protects the cell. It consists of a phospholipid bilayer and has various channels and proteins which help to control what can enter and leave the cell. The cytoplasm is a fluid containing components such as glycogen, lipids, ribosomes, filaments and microtubules, all involved with the function of the cell. The nucleus is the main place in the cell where the cell's genetic information is stored and from where the activity of the cell is coordinated. Chapter 2 of this text discusses the cell.

This genetic information exists as deoxyribose nucleic acid (DNA). Most of the cell's DNA resides in the nucleus but a small amount is in the mitochondria. The mitochondria are organelles present in the cytoplasm whose main function relates to the production of energy for the cell (Figure 5.1).

DNA is a double-stranded molecule; each strand is made up of a string of nucleotides. A nucleotide is deoxyribose – a sugar phosphate backbone, with a nucleic acid, (a nitrogenous base) attached. There are four types of nitrogenous bases – adenine (A), guanine (G), cytosine(C) and thymine (T). The nitrogenous base will join only to a complementary base pair – A and T will form a bond, as will C and G. These two strands of DNA are held together by the bond between each complementary base pair (Figure 5.2).

The double strand of DNA twists to form a double helix (Figure 5.3). That DNA double helix wraps itself around protein molecules called histones. This forms a densely packed structure called chromatin. Histones help to form the shape of the DNA structure and influence the way that the genetic material is read and copied to the next cell.

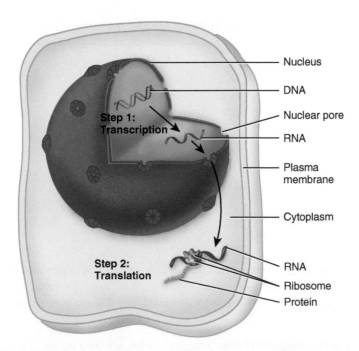

FIGURE 5.1   The cell nucleus. Source: Tortora and Derrickson (2017); reproduced with permission of John Wiley and Sons, Inc.

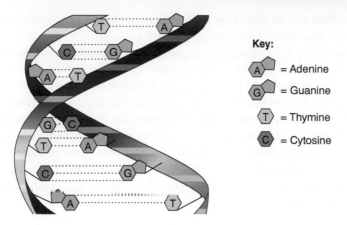

FIGURE 5.2 A portion of the double helix. Source: Tortora and Derrickson (2017); reproduced with permission of John Wiley and Sons, Inc.

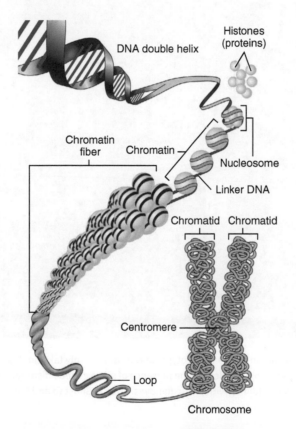

FIGURE 5.3 DNA from a double helix to chromosome. Source: Tortora and Derrickson (2017); reproduced with permission of John Wiley and Sons, Inc.

Chromosomes

When a cell is not dividing, there is no particular pattern as to how the DNA is arranged. When a cell starts to divide, it arranges the DNA, and thus the genetic material, into chromosomes. In a human body cell, there are 23 pairs of chromosomes; 22 of these are known as *autosomes* and the 23rd pair is known as the *sex chromosomes*. In normal circumstances, for the female sex, the 23rd pair is XX and for male sex it is XY. This means that, overall, there are 46 chromosomes. This would be described for a female sex as 46XX and for a male sex as 46XY. The word *karyotype* describes an individual's complete set of chromosomes, which can be seen under a microscope (Figure 5.4).

The chromosomes are arranged in homologous pairs, which means that chromosome 1 inherited from the mother will match up with chromosome 1 from the father, chromosome 2 will do the same, and so on.

A chromosome is pinched in the centre by a centromere. Often, it is not exactly in the centre, which means that one side may be shorter than the other. The shorter end is known as the short arm or 'p' (this comes from the French word *petite*). The longer end is known as the long arm or 'q' (simply because this is the next letter in the alphabet to p). This is important as, when we describe changes in a gene, we can describe where those changes are (otherwise known as the locus) by denoting which chromosome we are talking about and which arm. The tip of each chromosome is known as a telomere (Figure 5.5).

Cells containing 46 chromosomes are known as *diploid*. Not all cells contain 23 pairs (46 in total) of chromosomes. Our sex cells, known as gametes (sperm in males and oocytes in females) have 23 chromosomes only – they do not have pairs. These cells are known as *haploid*.

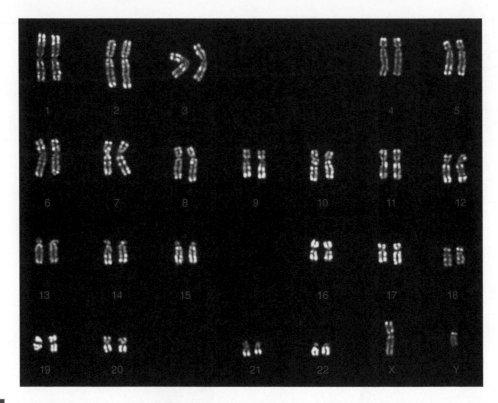

FIGURE 5.4   The chromosomes of a human male – a karyotype. Chromosomes only take on this particular shape during cell division. The assessment of karyotype can be performed to identify the presence of some genetic disorders. Each chromosome is identified by its size and 'banding' pattern following staining with particular dyes. Source: Snustad and Simmons (2012) / with permission of John Wiley & Sons.

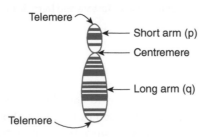

FIGURE 5.5   A telomere.

Mitosis

All living organisms must continue to replicate their cells as old ones die. To do this, the cell must pass on its genetic information to the new cell. The original cell is known as the mother cell. It forms two new cells that should be exact copies of itself. These are called daughter cells. This is achieved by a process known as *mitosis*. A cell has different phases of activity regarding this replication process. This is known as the cell cycle (Figure 5.6):

1. *Interphase*: this is the stage that a cell is resting or in its 'normal' state. Because there are pairs of chromosomes, the amount of genetic material is said to be 2n, where n = a single chromosome. When a cell gets ready to duplicate itself, it replicates its DNA so that there is a second exact set. The cell goes from 2n to 4n and the chromatid now has an identical copy of itself. They are known as sister chromatids. The sister chromatids are joined together by a centromere. Chromatids are only present during cell division.

2. *Prophase*: this is the first real stage of mitosis. In this phase, the chromosomes are now two sister chromatids. The genetic material condenses and becomes visible under a microscope. Two microtubule organisation centres arrange themselves at each side of the cell and attach to the centromeres with tubulin fibres.

3. *Prometaphase*: the outside membrane of the cell dissolves.

4. *Metaphase*: the chromosomes line up in the middle of the cell.

5. *Anaphase*: the sister chromatids separate and move to opposite sides of the cell due to the tension in the tubulin fibres increasing.

6. *Telophase*: the chromatids are now considered to be chromosomes. The cells separate – this is known as cytokinesis. After the separation of the chromosomes, there are now two new cells, the daughter cells. The cells form a surrounding membrane and the chromosomes relax and are no longer lined up in a recognisable form.

Figure 5.7 provides an overview of mitosis.

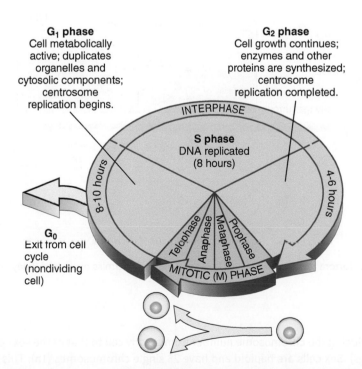

FIGURE 5.6 The cell cycle. Source: Tortora and Derrickson (2017); reproduced with permission of John Wiley and Sons, Inc.

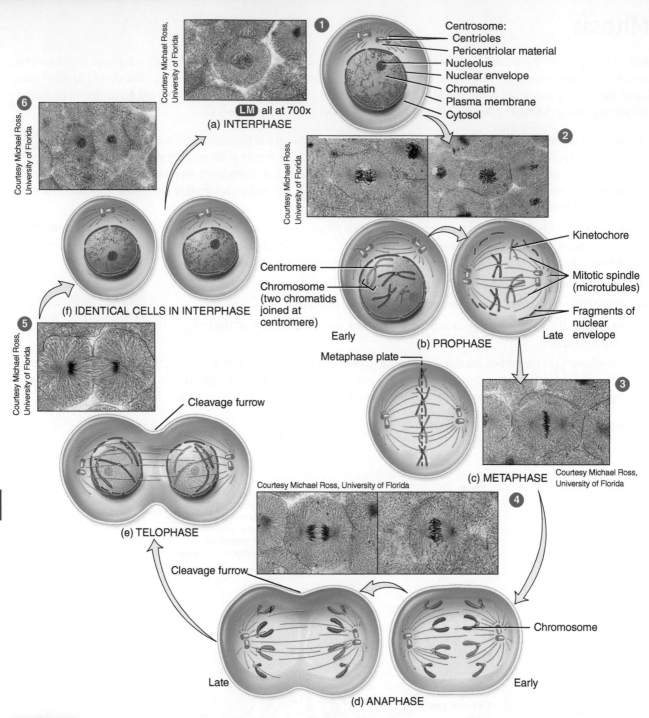

Courtesy Michael Ross, University of Florida

LM all at 700x
(a) INTERPHASE

① Centrosome:
  Centrioles
  Pericentriolar material
Nucleolus
Nuclear envelope
Chromatin
Plasma membrane
Cytosol

②

Kinetochore

Centromere
Chromosome (two chromatids joined at centromere)

Mitotic spindle (microtubules)

Fragments of nuclear envelope

Early   (b) PROPHASE   Late

(f) IDENTICAL CELLS IN INTERPHASE

Metaphase plate

③

Cleavage furrow

(c) METAPHASE   Courtesy Michael Ross, University of Florida

(e) TELOPHASE

④

Courtesy Michael Ross, University of Florida

Cleavage furrow

Chromosome

Late   Early

(d) ANAPHASE

FIGURE 5.7   Mitosis. Source: Tortora and Derrickson (2017); reproduced with permission of John Wiley and Sons, Inc.

Meiosis

Meiosis is the process of reducing the chromosome number from a body cell to that of the sex cells (otherwise known as gametes – i.e. sperm or eggs). Sex cells are haploid and have 23 single chromosomes (1n). This process again begins in interphase, where the cell with 46 chromosomes (2n) duplicates its genetic material to now have 4n. Because we need to end up with 23 chromosomes (n), the phases prophase through to telophase essentially occur twice. There are a few differences however. The beauty of meiosis is that the DNA is recombined so that no two daughter cells will have the same combination of genetic material. This is helpful otherwise we would all be identical to our siblings. This is the process that underpins genetic variation between individuals.

Prophase I

When the cells enter prophase for the first time (prophase I), the DNA condenses into chromatids. They form two sister chromatids, as in mitosis. This time, the two sister chromatids overlap each other, making what is known as a tetrad. Bits of DNA or alleles (an allele is a specific pattern in a gene, e.g. an allele that codes for blue eyes and one for brown) are swapped between themselves. This is known as 'crossing over' (Figure 5.8). This means that there are now uniquely random mixes of both maternally and paternally derived genetic material in the new chromatids. The wall of the nucleus disappears. Centrioles move to opposite ends of the cell and spindle fibres run out from them.

Metaphase I

The homologous pairs of chromosomes line up in the middle of the cell and attach to the spindle fibres at the opposite poles.

Anaphase I

The spindle fibres separate the homologous chromosomes and pull them apart to opposite sides of the cell.

Telophase I

One chromosome from each homologous pair is now at separate poles. The spindle fibres disappear. Each chromosome still consists of sister chromatids but they are no longer identical because of the allele exchange which happened during crossing over. Cytokinesis occurs which describes the division of the cells into two – the result is two separate daughter cells with paired sister chromatids that are genetically different. The cells are diploid.

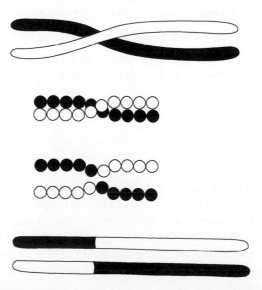

FIGURE 5.8 Gene crossover. Source: Peate and Nair (2016); reproduced with permission of John Wiley and Sons Ltd.

Second Meiotic Division

To become haploid, the cells need to undergo another cell cycle to halve the genetic material. Crossing over does not happen again. There is no DNA replication this time before entering the cell cycle.

Prophase II

The wall of the nucleus disappears and the spindle fibres fan out from the two sets of paired centrioles.

Metaphase II

Sister chromatids line up in the middle of the cell and attach to the spindle fibres from both poles of the centriole.

Anaphase II

Sister chromatids separate and move to opposite sides of the cell. Once they are separated, they are known as chromosomes.

Telophase II

The spindle fibres disappear, the wall of the nucleus reforms and cytokinesis separates both cells resulting in four genetically different daughter cells with one set of chromosomes (Box 5.1).

BOX 5.1	Key Points About Meiosis

- The process begins with a diploid cell.
- The process ends with four genetically different haploid cells (which will be the gametes – for females, oocytes and for males, sperm).
- The cells have to go through the cell cycle twice.
- Genetic recombination happens at prophase I. Each chromatid joins its homologous pair to make a tetrad. Sections of DNA (alleles) switch from one chromatid to another and so new gene combinations are created.

Genes

A gene is a section of DNA which contains the code to make a specific protein. Not all genes code for protein. The gene is therefore an arrangement of nitrogenous base pairs (A,T,C,G) of a certain length.

The human genome project was an international collaborative research project which first sequenced the whole human genome. They identified that humans have about 22 000 genes that make up about three million base pairs.

Genes can vary in size. Our genes determine everything that makes us who we are. They code for everything down to our eye colour, our skin type and even our susceptibility to certain conditions. Our genes code for proteins, which are produced by transcription and translation.

Transcription and Translation

A gene is a section of DNA. That DNA will code for a specific sequence of amino acids which will go on to make a specific protein. As proteins cannot be formed directly from DNA, we have the help of messenger ribonucleic acid (mRNA). Transcription describes the process of DNA code being read and made into mRNA. The DNA strand is zipped open by an enzyme called RNA polymerase. Figure 5.9 shows a DNA double helix separated to make new strands of DNA, with transcription however, that new strand (depicted as green in the figure) is mRNA.

The mRNA reads the code on the DNA and binds a matching nitrogenous base pair to that presented on the DNA. The matching of base pairs is a little different than that we have already seen with DNA; with mRNA, uracil matches with adenine as there is no thymine in RNA (Figure 5.10).

This strand of mRNA is now known as the template strand. Once the template strand has been copied from the DNA in the gene, it moves out of the nucleus to structures within the cytoplasm called ribosomes.

Translation is the part where the mRNA is made into protein. Three base pairs from the mRNA codes for a specific amino acid. These are known as triplets or codons. There are 20 amino acids and 64 codon combinations. The ribosome and the mRNA template strand join, the code of the first three base pairs is read and transfer RNA (tRNA)

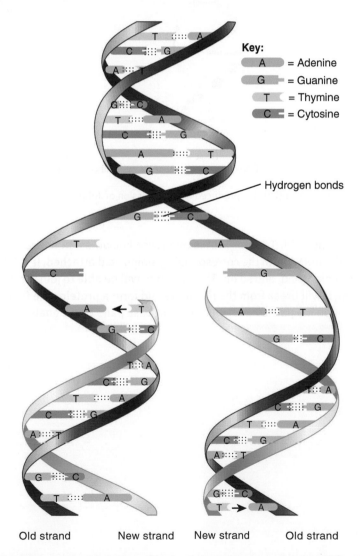

Key:
- A = Adenine
- G = Guanine
- T = Thymine
- C = Cytosine

Hydrogen bonds

Old strand   New strand   New strand   Old strand

FIGURE 5.9 The separation of DNA and the production of further DNA. Source: Tortora and Derrickson (2017); reproduced with permission of John Wiley and Sons, Inc.

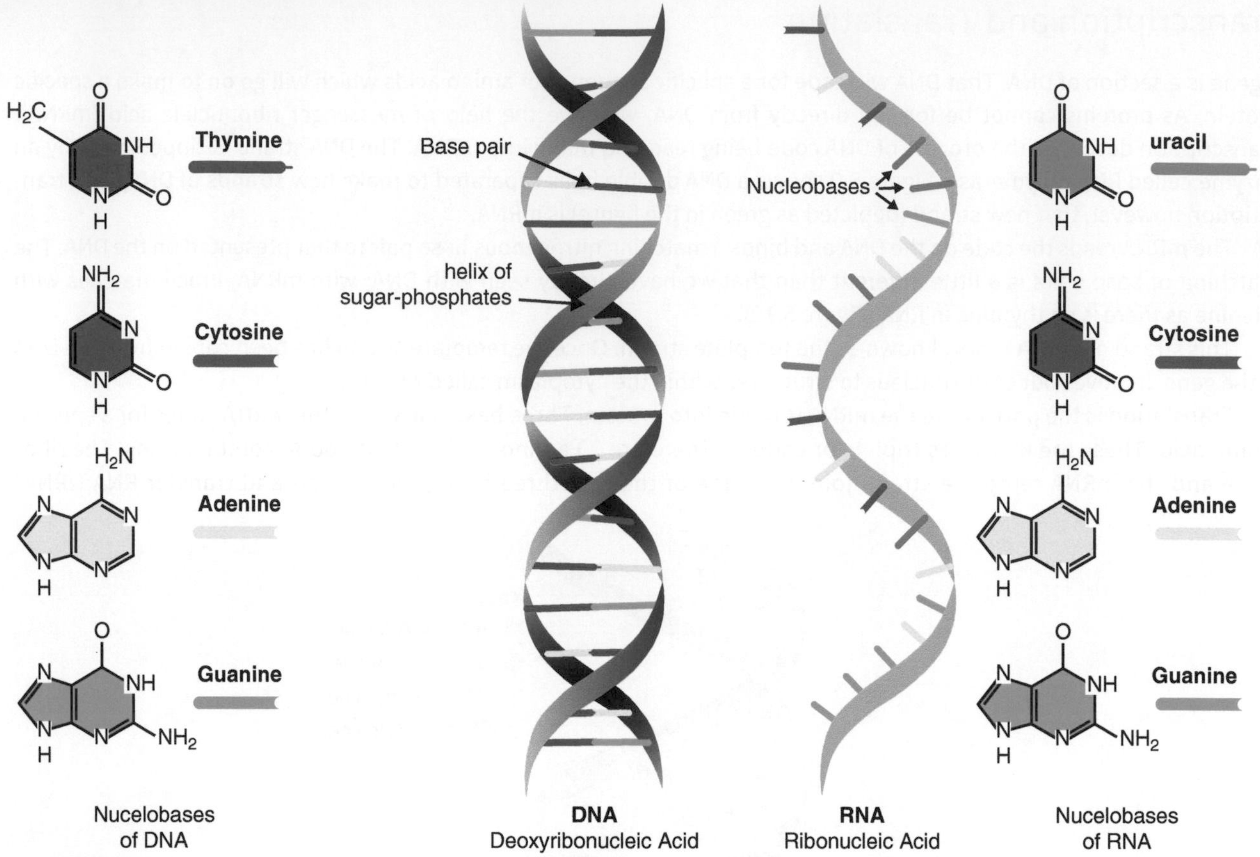

FIGURE 5.10   DNA and RNA. Peate and Nair (2015); reproduced with permission of John Wiley and Sons Ltd.

presents the corresponding amino acid. Transfer RNA is otherwise known as an anticodon – it is a group of three complementary base pairs to the mRNA with the corresponding amino acid attached. It will then go to the next three base pairs and make the next amino acid, and so on. The ribosome will be able to join the amnio acids together and, as the chain continues to form, it will break from the ribosome and form a protein. The final part of the mRNA codes for what is known as a stop codon – a particular combination of base pairs that signals that the amino acid chain is complete (Figure 5.11).

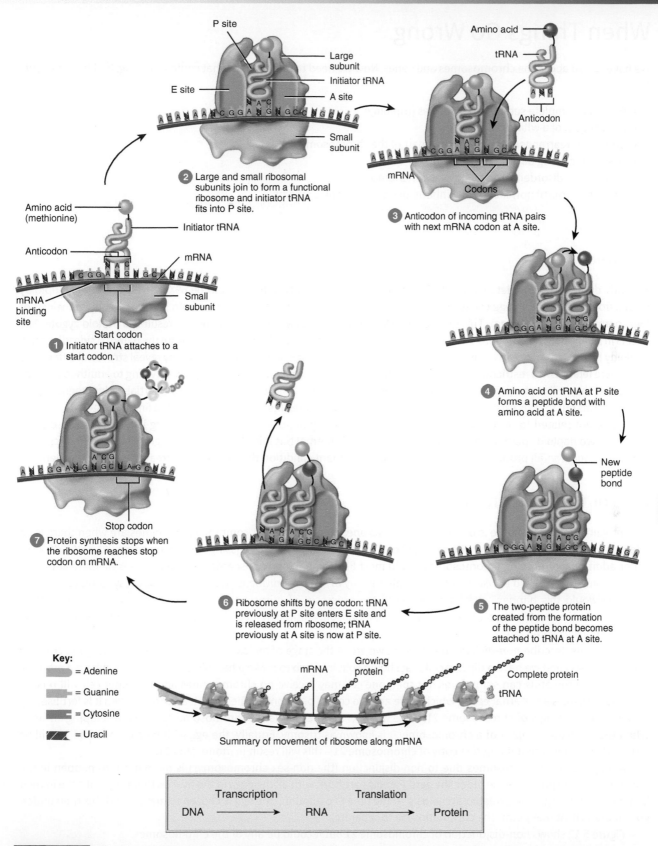

P site

Large subunit

Initiator tRNA

E site

A site

N A C

Small subunit

2 Large and small ribosomal subunits join to form a functional ribosome and initiator tRNA fits into P site.

Amino acid

tRNA

A N G

Anticodon

mRNA

Codons

3 Anticodon of incoming tRNA pairs with next mRNA codon at A site.

Amino acid (methionine)

Initiator tRNA

Anticodon

mRNA

mRNA binding site

Small subunit

Start codon

1 Initiator tRNA attaches to a start codon.

N A C A C G

4 Amino acid on tRNA at P site forms a peptide bond with amino acid at A site.

New peptide bond

N A C A C G

Stop codon

7 Protein synthesis stops when the ribosome reaches stop codon on mRNA.

N A C A C G

6 Ribosome shifts by one codon: tRNA previously at P site enters E site and is released from ribosome; tRNA previously at A site is now at P site.

5 The two-peptide protein created from the formation of the peptide bond becomes attached to tRNA at A site.

95

Key:

= Adenine

= Guanine

= Cytosine

= Uracil

mRNA

Growing protein

Complete protein

tRNA

Summary of movement of ribosome along mRNA

Transcription   Translation

DNA ⟶ RNA ⟶ Protein

FIGURE 5.11 Movement of ribosomes along mRNA and a brief summary of protein synthesis. Source: Tortora and Derrickson (2017); reproduced with permission of John Wiley and Sons, Inc.

When Things Go Wrong

We have talked about the chromosomes and genes. Now we need to understand what could go wrong. In this section, we discuss:

- Gain of a complete set of chromosomes (triploidy)
- Loss or gain of a whole chromosome
- Change or rearrangement to whole or part of the chromosome
- Losing or gaining part of a chromosome
- Single gene disorders (and Mendelian inheritance)
- Other patterns of non-Mendelian inheritance such as triplet repeats.

Triploidy

Triploidy describes a complete extra set of chromosomes. The karyotype here would be 69XXX, 69XXY or 69XYY. Triploidy results from a sperm or an egg cell which had a diploid amount of chromosomes (either from non-disjunction in meiosis or two sperms fertilising one egg). This diploid sex cell fertilises with a haploid sex cell and the result is a triploid zygote. The effects in a baby depend on whether the diploid cell came from the maternal side (digynic) or from the paternal side (diandric). Triploidy has a high chance in ending in miscarriage. Surviving to a later stage of pregnancy may reveal structural differences and severe fetal growth restriction. Most of these babies will die soon after birth, with very few surviving to adulthood; If they do survive, they will have significant health problems. Diandric triploidy is otherwise known as a partial molar pregnancy. An embryo forms but there is excessive placental tissue and this usually results in a miscarriage in the first trimester.

While not related to triploidy, a complete molar pregnancy happens when an empty egg is fertilised by a diploid sperm or two haploid sperms. The chromosomal amount is normal but it is all paternal in origin. These pregnancies are non-viable and a small proportion can transform to a malignant condition that needs to be treated with chemotherapy.

Loss or Gain of a Chromosome

Loss or gain of a chromosome is otherwise known as *aneuploidy*. The most common aneuploidies are when there is an additional chromosome on chromosome 13, 18 or 21 or if there is an extra or missing sex chromosome (X0, XXY, XXX, XYY). Other additional or missing chromosomes would most likely end in early miscarriage. When there is an extra copy of a chromosome this is called a *trisomy* – for example trisomy 21. This condition is also known as Down syndrome.

Why would this happen? We have discussed the processes of mitosis and meiosis earlier in the chapter. Non-disjunction is the most likely cause of aneuploidy of monosomy although it can be more rarely caused by Robertsonian translocations (covered later).

First let us describe *non-disjunction*. Imagine we are at the stage of meiosis II. We have already undergone crossing over in meiosis I and we have a diploid cell that should split into two to make a haploid cell. Now this is where a problem occurs. The chromatids can sometimes not split, one cell may receive no chromosomes and the other cell will receive both. So, if there is a maternal egg in which there are two copies of chromosome 21 instead of one, when it is fertilised by a sperm with one copy of chromosome 21, there will now be three copies of chromosome 21 in the developing embryo. When there are three copies of a chromosome, it is known as trisomy. Equally, the egg with no chromosome 21 will be fertilised by a sperm containing one copy of chromosome 21 – this will result in monosomy 21.

Aneuploidy of the autosomes due to non-disjunction (the non-sex chromosomes) is more likely to happen in the oocytes a woman produces the older she gets. Females are born with all the eggs in the ovaries that they will have in their lifetime. All these eggs are arrested at meiosis. At the time of ovulation, one egg is chosen to mature and this then under-goes meiosis II. At that point, the chromatids fail to separate.

Figure 5.12 shows non-disjunction of chromosome 21 but it could be any of the chromosomes.

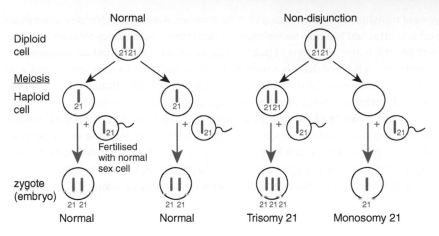

FIGURE 5.12 Non-disjunction of chromosome 21.

Other Rearrangements of Chromosomes

We have discussed rearrangements of entire chromosomes but now we turn to some possible rearrangements of material within the chromosomes.

Inversion

In inversion, the bonds are broken in a particular segment of DNA. This breaks off from the chromosome. The segment of broken DNA reverses its orientation and then reattaches to its original chromosome. There is the same amount of genetic material as before the inversion took place, it is now just arranged differently on the chromosome. As long as there is no extra or missing DNA, inversion would not usually cause problems for an individual.

Deletion

In deletion, a fragment of DNA breaks off from a chromosome. There is no reattachment and now there is less genetic material than there is supposed to be. The effects in an individual would depend on how big the deleted part of DNA was, and which genes were missing within that part of chromosome.

Duplication

Duplication is when there is a duplication of genetic material within a chromosome. The effects depend on the size of the duplication and the genes involved.

Translocations

A *balanced translocation* is when the location of the genetic material has changed but, overall, there is the correct amount of genetic material. When an unequal transfer of genetic material has occurred, this is an *unbalanced translocation* – the exchange of genetic material has led to an incorrect amount of genetic material – some is missing or there is extra material.

Balanced translocations usually cause no problems as the correct amount of genetic material is present, just in a different configuration. An individual with a balanced translocation may be at increased risk of offspring with an unbalanced translocation.

Red Flag Alert: Unbalanced Translocations

Unbalanced translocations can cause differences in the individual which would depend on the size and genes involved. They are also a cause of miscarriage.

There are two types of translocation, reciprocal and Robertsonian. A reciprocal translocation describes a segment of DNA that has broken off and attached to a non-homologous chromosome. Sometimes this can be a direct swap; for example, the same volume of genetic material is present but it is now located on a different chromosome.

A Robertsonian translocation is when there is a translocation but instead of a segment of DNA, a whole chromosome is swapped. This can happen in only some of the chromosomes because of their shape. Remember that we talked about how there are two arms of the chromosome: the short arm (p) and the long arm (q) and the centromere, which is the centre part holding them together. Some of the chromosomes (13, 14, 15, 21 and 22) have such a tiny, short arm that, if a translocation occurs at the level of the centromere, essentially the whole chromosome will have moved. Two long arms of the chromosome will fuse together to form one long chromosome. Robertsonian translocation carriers again may have no loss or gain of genetic material. The rearrangement can lead to problems, however, when meiosis occurs to make sex cells. Figure 5.13 is an example of Robertsonian translocation carrier who has a translocation between chromosome 14 and 21.

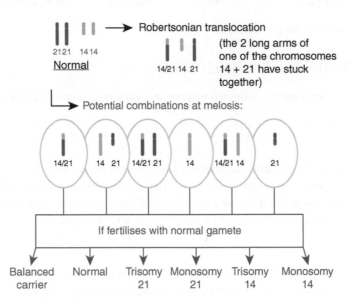

FIGURE 5.13   An example of Robertsonian translocation.

Snapshot 5.1   Trisomy 21

Razia is 42 years old. She has been trying to get pregnant for five years now. She has had three miscarriages in the past at approximately 8–12 weeks of gestation. She has no significant medical or family history. Her partner Leon is also 42 years old with no significant medical or family history. She is currently pregnant at 12 weeks of gestation. She has had an ultrasound showing that the baby has an increased nuchal translucency and a combined risk of trisomy 21 of 1:5 and risk of trisomy 13 and 18 of 1:15. She went on to have chorionic villus sampling, which confirmed trisomy 21.

Reflective Learning Activity

Before you read on, try to answer the following questions:

- What is trisomy 21?
- What is Razia's main risk factor for having a baby with trisomy 21?
- What is the most likely mechanism by which Razia's baby came to be affected with trisomy 21?
- From the history, why would it be important to rule out a Robertsonian translocation in Razia and Leon?

Clinical Investigations

Trisomy means three chromosomes instead of the usual two. Trisomy 21 means that the three chromosomes are where the 21st pair of chromosomes would normally be. Trisomy 21 is also known as Down syndrome and is one of the most common chromosomal differences in humans. Jenny's biggest risk factor for having a baby with trisomy 21 is her age. At the age of 40 years, the background risk of having a baby with trisomy 21 is about 1 in 100.

Non-disjunction is the most likely mechanism in any affected pregnancy but more so because of Jenny's age. This means that at meiosis II, the chromatids did not pull apart and one of Jenny's oocytes had two chromosomes 21 rather than just one. At fertilisation, this met with Leon's sperm, which contained one copy of chromosome 21.

All cases of a trisomy should have a karyotype checked to locate where the extra piece of chromosome is. If it is stuck to a different chromosome entirely then this would fit with a Robertsonian translocation rather than non-disjunction. In this case, either Jenny or Leon may have a piece of their chromosome 21 swapped with another of their chromosomes. They would have no symptoms as they have the right amount of chromosomal material overall. When they came to make sex cells at meiosis, some of the sex cells might have extra or missing parts of chromosome 21. When these cells are fertilised by a normal haploid sex cell, there could be an abnormal amount of chromosome 21 (Figure 5.12). It is important to identify this, as it increases the recurrence risk for future pregnancies having the same trisomy. The other part of the history is that Jenny has had recurrent miscarriages. Having a Robertsonian translocation can be a rare but important cause of recurrent miscarriage. This is usually investigated by either checking the karyotype of the miscarried pregnancy tissue and then checking parental or going straight for karyotype tests for both parents.

Mosaicism

Mosaicism is when there are two cell lines within an individual. For example, one group of cells may be 46XX and the second group of cells may be 45X0. The ratio of cells is variable. This happens after conception during mitosis and is caused by non-disjunction. The effect on an individual will depend on the ratio of affected cells but is generally milder than a full set of chromosomes affected with aneuploidy. This can still be difficult to predict based on the genotype alone.

When Things Go Wrong at the Level of the Gene

As the DNA forms the original template for the formation of mRNA and the subsequent protein, you can see how a single spelling mistake in the DNA could go on to cause some changes in the subsequently formed protein. Take this hypothetical DNA base pairs in a gene:

AAT TCG CGC CCT TCA

Problems occur when there is a mistake in the base pairs, as the amino acid will still be formed in the group of three. If one of the first A's is deleted, it will now look like this:

ATT CGC GCC CTT CA

You can see how one deletion here changed the whole row of base pairs and therefore all the amino acids formed by this gene. If an extra A gets in the line:

AAA TTC GCG CCC TTC A

Again, this changes the amino acids and therefore may affect the protein that is made by this gene. These are known as *frameshift mutations*. The insertion or deletion of a base pair has changed the reading frame.

If one of the amino acids is swapped for a different one, this may affect the protein that is made by the gene. This is a *missense mutation*. In this case, the A is now mistakenly a T:

ATT TCG CGC CCT TCA

A *nonsense mutation* could form a stop codon – this is a triplet repeat which signals that translation stops and therefore there are no further amnio acids produced.

The result of these mutations can be variable. It is possible there will be no effect, as the new change may code for amino acid that was always intended. This is a *silent mutation*. A mutation could cause a change to the resulting protein made. When there is a change in a protein, it may cause a gain or loss of function and it is possible that this could cause disease.

Patterns of Inheritance

Mendelian inheritance was discovered by an Austrian monk called Gregor Mendel, who undertook experiments with pea plants to try to work out how certain traits are passed to the next generation. His work led to the theory of recessive and dominant traits of inheritance. There are two copies of each gene – one that has been passed down from the mother and one from the father. If there is a mistake in one of the genes, as described above, it will depend on whether a gene is dominant or recessive as to whether it will cause a problem in that individual.

A Pedigree

A pedigree is the term used to describe a detailed family tree that explores both maternal and paternal sides of a family. Making a pedigree is helpful for clinicians as this is a graphic representation of the relationships within families and to identify how a condition may have been inherited. As you read the descriptions about patterns of inheritance, you will begin to understand how this may be apparent by using a pedigree.

Autosomal Dominant Conditions

In dominant conditions, if the gene is present, it will mean that the trait or disease will be expressed in the individual. It is an all or nothing situation. Figure 5.14 shows how this happens. The mother on the left of the figure has a condition, which we have marked as A⁺. There is a 50% chance that she will pass on the condition/trait to her offspring. There is also a 50% chance that her offspring will be unaffected. It is not possible to be a silent carrier of the trait or condition. Clinical examples of autosomal dominant conditions include:

- Adult polycystic kidney disease
- Huntington's disease
- Myotonic dystrophy
- Noonan syndrome
- Neurofibromatosis
- Marfan syndrome
- *BRCA1* and *BRCA2* genes
- Achondroplasia.

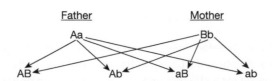

FIGURE 5.14 Autosomal dominant conditions.

Autosomal Recessive Conditions

In autosomal recessive conditions, both parents must be carriers of the same faulty gene change. They have one copy of a faulty gene and one copy of the corresponding normal gene. This is known as being heterozygous. They are asymptomatic.

When two carriers reproduce, there are a few possibilities. In Figure 5.15, A⁺ is the faulty gene from maternal side and A the normal gene; B⁺ is the faulty gene from the paternal side and B the normal paternal gene. The mother may pass on the faulty gene and the father may also do so. There is a one in four chance of that happening. This means that the offspring will be affected, as there will be no normal gene at all. This is known as being homozygous for a condition. There is a one in two chance that either one of the parents' faulty genes will be passed on, but they will have a normal gene from the other parent. This means that the offspring will be carriers of a condition and are heterozygous. They do not have the condition, the fact that they still have a normal gene protects them. It does mean that if they had a baby with someone who was also a carrier for the same faulty gene then they could pass this on, as described in the example in Figure 5.16. There would be a one in four chance that both parents would pass on the normal copy of their gene, which would mean that their child would not be affected with the condition, nor could they pass the gene on to their future offspring.

This pattern of inheritance can happen to anybody, but it is more common in people who are related to each other (consanguineous) and have children. Clinical examples of autosomal recessive conditions include:

- Cystic fibrosis
- Haemochromatosis
- Tay–Sachs disease
- Sickle cell anaemia
- Phenylketonuria
- Wilson's disease
- Bartter syndrome.

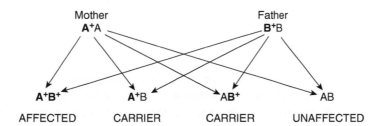

FIGURE 5.15 Autosomal recessive conditions.

X-Linked Dominant Conditions

X-linked dominant conditions are passed to the offspring by genes with a locus on the X chromosome. Remember, those born as female sex have two X sex chromosomes (XX) and those born as males have one X sex chromosome and one Y (XY). Just like in autosomal dominant conditions, only one affected gene is needed to mean that the individual has the condition.

Let us see how someone with a faulty gene on the X chromosome could pass on the condition. We will begin with an affected male (Figure 5.16). In this example, we can see that there is a 50% chance of having female offspring and 50% male. It is always the sperm that determines the sex of the offspring as eggs are derived from female cells (XX) so only X chromosomes are present. In meiosis, when sperm is created, it is from a male cell (XY) and therefore half of the sperm should contain and X and half should contain Y chromosome.

The affected male is only able to pass on an X chromosome that contains the faulty gene. This means that all the daughters of an affected male will have the condition. The son of an affected man in an X-linked condition will always be unaffected. There is a one in two chance of each possibility.

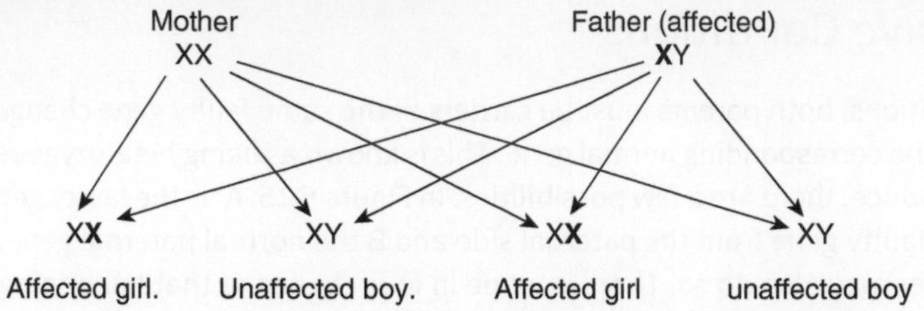

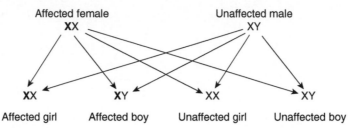

FIGURE 5.16   X linked dominant inheritance: When the faulty X chromosome is derived from the male.

Now let us look at what happens when a female with an X-linked dominant condition reproduces. Remember that, because this is a dominant condition, if she has just one abnormal copy of the gene and the other is normal, she will be affected (Figure 5.17). The affected mother has therefore passed on the faulty gene to half of her sons and half of her daughters. Thus, there is a one in two chance overall of her offspring having the condition, where one in four would be an affected son and one in four an affected daughter.

Fragile X is a condition that is inherited in an X-linked dominant pattern.

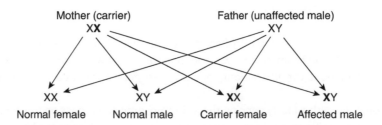

FIGURE 5.17   X linked dominant inheritance: When the faulty X chromosome is derived from the female.

X-Linked Recessive Conditions

For an X-linked recessive condition to cause problems, there must not be another normal copy of the gene on the other X chromosome. For a female to be affected, they must be homozygous for the faulty gene (i.e. both the genes are faulty). If a female is heterozygous for the faulty gene on the X chromosome, she will be a carrier. As males only have one copy of an X chromosome, if they have only one copy of the faulty gene on their X chromosome, they will be affected.

Let us look at the possible child combinations when a mother is a carrier for an X-linked recessive condition (Figure 5.18):

Mother (carrier)
X**X**

Father (unaffected male)
XY

XX
Normal female

XY
Normal male

X**X**
Carrier female

XY
Affected male

FIGURE 5.18   X-linked recessive condition.

- There is a one in four chance of a female who is unaffected and is not a carrier.
- There is a one in four chance of a male who is unaffected.
- There is a one in four chance of a female carrier.
- There is a one in four chance of an affected male.

Examples of X-linked conditions include:

- Dominant:
  - Fragile X
- Recessive:
  - Haemophilia
  - Fabry's disease
  - Duchenne muscular dystrophy.

Snapshot 5.2   Haemophilia

Jess and Harry have attended the booking appointment. Jess is eight weeks pregnant. Her father has haemophilia A (an X-linked recessive condition). This is Jess's first pregnancy. She is well. Her sister's son also has haemophilia A.

Questions and calculations that need to be asked include:

- What is the chance that Jess is a carrier of haemophilia A?
  - 100% – all daughters of an affected man would be obligate carriers.
- What is the chance of Jess's baby having haemophilia A?
  - One in four (50% of Jess's sons would acquire her affected X chromosome).
- What is the chance that Jess has a baby that is not affected and not a carrier?
- The chance would be one in two.
- What is the chance of having a baby that was a carrier of haemophilia A?.
  - The chance would be one in four.

Triplet Repeats

As we have seen earlier in the chapter, amino acids are coded by three base pairs, which are known as a trinucleotide. In some individuals, the trinucleotide can repeat. It can be quite normal to have a small number of trinucleotide repeats, but when they are above a certain threshold, this can cause disease. Some examples of conditions which can cause this are:

- Myotonic dystrophy – expansion of the CTG triplet repeat
- Fragile X syndrome – expansion of the CGG triplet repeat
- Huntington's disease – expansion of the CAG triplet repeat.

The way that these conditions are passed through a family can be interesting, as the amount of triplet repeat expansions can increase through successive generations and this causes increases in the severity of disease. This is known as anticipation.

In triplet repeat disorders, there are differences in how the number or stability of repeats are transmitted, depending on whether it is inherited from the mother or from the father.

Let us take the example of fragile X. This is a condition which is characterised by intellectual disability and autism spectrum disorder; it can be present in both males and females. A repeated number of the CGG triplet repeat causes the *FMR1* gene to function abnormally, resulting in changes in the way that the brain is developed and functions. A person without fragile X syndrome may have repeats of the CGG trinucleotide sequence (a normal range is between 6 and 44 repeats). In those who are carriers or have fragile X syndrome, there are more triplet repeats. This is known as a premutation, which is not clinically significant but represents a carrier. When there are 55–200 CGG repeats, this is known as the full mutation allele. Clinical features are present when there are more than 200 CGG repeats. As the *FMR1* gene is located on the X chromosome, it is not possible for a male to acquire an *FMR1* mutation from their father (they must have received the Y chromosome). The expansion size usually stays the same when passed down from father to daughter. The expansion size may become greater when passed down from mother to their offspring. Another example of a triplet expansion condition is Huntington's disease. This triplet repeat tends to expand when it is passed down from a father.

Mitochondrial DNA

Although mitochondrial DNA is not explored in depth here, it is worth mentioning that DNA is not only stored in the nucleus of cells. There is a small amount of DNA stored inside the mitochondrion of a cell. Mitochondrial DNA is only passed down from the mother. The proportion of change in the mitochondrial DNA is known as heteroplasmy. It is not possible for men with any disease resulting from mitochondrial inheritance to pass this disease on to their offspring. Conditions of mitochondrial inheritance are passed on from a genetic female to their children.

Genotype and Phenotype

The genotype describes the genetic makeup of an individual. It is objective and can be identified by testing. The phenotype is the effect that the genotype has on the individual, which can be anything physical or behavioural through to eye colour, blood type or a disease process.

The way in which the same gene is expressed in any individual can be different. This can sometimes make it challenging to counsel as to what effects could be expected in the future. It may be known that an individual has a gene for a condition and yet they do not have the phenotype for that condition. When that happens, you might say that there is low or *incomplete penetrance*. An interplay of environmental and lifestyle factors may also affect the likelihood of disease in an individual. Some conditions have *complete penetrance*, which means that in people with the gene change, all of them will have the phenotype of that condition.

Take Home Points

- DNA, genes and chromosomes describe different parts of genetic material.
- Mitosis is the process where a cell is replicated.
- Meiosis is the process where a cell divides to form a haploid sex cell.
- Errors can occur with cell replication and division.
- Disease can be inherited through families; the pattern of inheritance relates to the location of the gene change and whether it is dominant or recessive.
- The same gene change (genotype) may present differently in individuals (phenotype).

Summary

This chapter has offered a fundamental overview of how DNA, genes and chromosomes are arranged, replicate and divide in both normal and abnormal circumstances. It is not exhaustive. Chromosomal and genetic differences can often lead to complex clinical scenarios, both biologically and emotionally for the family given risk to their current and potential offspring and their wider family. The reader is encouraged to seek advice where appropriate which is likely to include the wider multidisciplinary team including midwifery, fetal medicine specialists, geneticists, genetic counsellors, genetic scientists and sonographers.

References

Peate, I. and Nair, M. (2015). *Anatomy and Physiology For Nurses at a Glance*, 2e. Oxford: Wiley-Blackwell.

Peate, I. and Nair, M. (2016). *Fundamentals of Anatomy and Physiology: For Nursing and Healthcare Students*, 2e. Oxford: Wiley-Blackwell.

Tortora, G.J. and Derrickson, B.H. (2017). *Tortora's Principles of Anatomy and Physiology*. Chichester: Wiley.

Further Reading

Kolarski, M., Ahmetovic, B., Beres, M. et al. (2017). Genetic counselling and the prenatal diagnosis of triploidy during the second trimester of pregnancy. *Medical Archives* 71: 144–147.

Finucane, B., Lincoln, S., Bailey, L., and Martin, C.L. (2017). Prognostic dilemmas and genetic counselling for prenatally detected fragile X gene expansions. *Prenatal Diagnosis* 37: 37–42.

Pritchard, D.J. and Korf, B.R. (2013). *Medical Genetics at a Glance*, 3e. Oxford: Wiley-Blackwell.

Online Resource

National Human Genome Research Institute. The Human Genome Project: https://www.genome.gov/human-genome-project.

Glossary

Acrocentric	A chromosome where the centromere is located at one end of the chromosome, which makes one arm a lot shorter than the other.
Allele	The version of a gene; we inherit one allele from our mother and one from our father. For example, a gene for eye colour could have a blue or a brown allele.
Aneuploidy	An abnormal normal number of chromosomes that is not an exact multiple of the haploid number.
Cell	The smallest unit of a living organism.
Cell membrane	The wall around a cell; it can control what leaves and enters the cell.
Centromere	Sticks the two chromosomes together.
Chromatid	One of the two halves of the chromosomes that have been replicated by cell replication.
Chromatin	Condensed tightly packed DNA.
Codon	A group of three nucleotides; codes for a protein.
Cytoplasm	The gel-like fluid that fills a cell.
Diploid	(2n) Normal amount of chromosomes (46 in humans, present in somatic cells).
Disomy	Chromosomal pair.
Euploid	Normal number of chromosomes.
Expression	The conversion of the genotype to the phenotype.
Gamete	Sex cell (contains haploid number of chromosomes); egg or sperm.
Gene	A sequence of DNA that codes for a protein or function.
Genotype	Describes the genetic material of an individual.
Haploid	(n) Half the number of chromosomes (23 in humans – eggs and sperm).
Heterozygous	When the two alleles of a gene pair are different.
Histones	Proteins around which the DNA wraps.
Homologous pair	A pair of the same chromosome (e.g. chromosome 2), one from the mother and one from the father.
Homozygous	When there are two of the same alleles in a gene pair.

Meiosis	Process of reducing a diploid cell to a haploid cell.
Messenger RNA (mRNA)	Single-stranded RNA which reads the DNA and enables synthesis of the protein within the ribosome.
Mitochondria	Where the energy for the cell is produced.
Mitosis	Process of replicating a cell so that both mother and daughter cell will have same amount of genetic material.
Monosomy	Only one copy of a chromosome.
Mosaicism	More than one genetic different sets of cells (a cell line) in an individual.
Nucleotide	A nitrogenous base, with a sugar and a phosphate group.
Nucleus	The centre of a cell which contains the genetic information.
Penetrance	The degree of the phenotype expressed in an individual with a certain phenotype.
Phenotype	Describes a feature, behaviour or appearance of an individual.
-ploidy	Referring to the whole set of chromosomes.
Ribosome	Part of a cell that makes proteins.
Sister chromatids	The identical copy of a chromosome formed when the DNA is replicated.
-somy	Referring to copies of individual chromosomes.
Telomere	Region at the end of the chromosome.
Transfer RNA (tRNA)	Matches the mRNA to the protein for which it codes.
Translation	The process that converts mRNA to protein.
Transcription	Making an RNA copy of the DNA sequence ready for translation.
Triplet/trinucleotide repeat	A group of three nitrogenous bases.
Triploid (3n)	A complete additional set of chromosomes (69 in humans).
Trisomy	Three copies of a chromosome.

Multiple Choice Questions

1. Which of the following words describes the first identified person in a family to be affected with a particular genetic condition?
   a. Dominant
   b. Mutant
   c. Proband
   d. Starter

2. What is a phenotype?
   a. An observed trait in an individual, physical or behavioural
   b. The genetic makeup of an individual
   c. The amount of people in a family with the same condition
   d. How easy it is for the trait to be passed on to the next generation

3. What is the expected phenotype of an individual whose genotype is 46XY?
   a. Female
   b. Male
   c. Neither male nor female
   d. Turner syndrome

4. What is the complementary base pair for thymine?
    a. Adenine
    b. Adenosine
    c. Guanine
    d. Cytosine

5. How many chromosomes are there in a human gamete?
    a. 11
    b. 23
    c. 46
    d. 18

6. In mRNA, the complementary base pair for adenine is what?
    a. Uracil
    b. Eumovate
    c. Thymine
    d. Cytosine

7. In triploidy, how many chromosomes are present?
    a. 3
    b. 23
    c. 46
    d. 69

8. Which sentence best describes mosaicism?
    a. The genetic material in each gamete is different as a result of 'crossing over'
    b. There is microdeletion found on chromosome 22
    c. When there are two sets of genetically different cells in one individual
    d. This has been inherited in an autosomal dominant manner

9. What is the chance of a couple having an affected child when one of the parents has an autosomal dominant condition?
    a. 1 in 2
    b. 1 in 4
    c. 1 in 3
    d. 1 in 6

10. What is the chance of a couple who are both carriers of cystic fibrosis having child affected with cystic fibrosis?
    a. 1 in 4
    b. 1 in 3
    c. 1 in 6
    d. 1 in 2

CHAPTER 6

Tissues

Iñaki Mansilla

AIM

This chapter aims to provide readers with an overview of how tissues are affected by pregnancy and to understand the anatomy and physiology of tissue during pregnancy.

LEARNING OUTCOMES

After reading this chapter, you will be able to:

- Understand the anatomy and physiology of the tissues and their main types.
- Describe the principal locations of the four types of tissues within the body.
- Understand the basics of the function of the different types of tissues.
- Understand why hormonal changes are important during pregnancy.

Test Your Prior Knowledge
1. How many tissue types are there in the body?
2. What are the main functions of the tissues in the body?
3. How can hormones directly affect the tissues in pregnancy?
4. What tissues are more affected or changed by pregnancy?

Introduction

A tissue comprises a group of cells with similar functions and structures. The cells in our body are responsible for its structure and function, and their unique specialisation enables the body to perform highly efficient processes. Although the exact number of cells in the body is unknown, it is believed that the human body has over three trillion cells (Moini 2019). Tissues can be classified into four different types (Marieb and Keller 2017; Moini 2019; Scanlon and Sanders 2018):

1. Epithelial
2. Connective

3. Muscle
4. Nervous

Pregnancy is a unique event, where all systems are involved and affected in one way or another by different hormonal changes. Tissues are also affected, playing an important part in how the body behaves. The main hormones released during pregnancy, either by the placenta or the ovaries, that affect tissues are progesterone, oestrogen, prolactin, relaxin and oxytocin (Johnson et al. 2021; Kumar and Magon 2012).

Hormones and tissues are intrinsically related throughout the pregnancy, labour and the postpartum period. It is thus important to understand the implications of tissue change in pregnancy for the mother's body and the fetus. In this chapter, we discuss how some organs and systems, such as the uterus and the breast tissue, prepare to accommodate the pregnancy, to aid your understanding of the anatomy and physiology of the tissues.

Development of Tissues

In humans, a cell starts with the division of a fertilised egg (zygote). After several rounds of cell division, embryonic cells are produced, which then compact of form a morula. This morula will develop into a blastocyst, which in turn will divide into two parts. One part will contribute to the development of the embryo, while the other part will transform into the extraembryonic tissue necessary to support the growth of the embryo in the uterus (Clift and Schuh 2013). The blastocyst then attaches to the inner tissue layer of the endometrium to invade the epithelium of the uterus and maternal circulation to form the placenta (Kim and Kim 2017). Chapter 4 gives more detail on cell differentiation.

The part of the blastocyst that contributes to the development of the fetus will form the three layers where all tissues in the body arise. These primary layers are the ectoderm, mesoderm and endoderm – the outer, middle and inner layers, respectively. Each germ layer is linked to the development of certain primitive systems during the formation of organs and tissues, which is called organogenesis (Muhr and Ackerman 2022).

The ectoderm layer will form into the tissues or organs of the epidermis, sensory system, nervous system and glands. The mesoderm layer will become the structure of the urinary system, reproductive system, circulatory system, haematopoietic system, motor system and connective tissue. Finally, the endoderm will provide growth to the development of the respiratory epithelium, intestinal epithelium and digestive gland epithelium (Gao et al. 2020).

The human body is well organised at different levels, and this starts with the cells. Cells are organised into tissues with specific characteristics and those into organs, such as the uterus, kidney or heart, and normally they perform a determined function in the body (McCance 2018).

Tissues and organs react when pregnancy occurs. Those reactions include changes in size and structure, including how they respond and function to the hormonal and metabolic responses (Napso et al. 2018). For instance, implantation in the endometrium of the blastocyst is possible because the ovaries produce oestrogen and progesterone to help prepare the uterine lining. The uterine lining becomes thicker due to oestrogen, and then progesterone matures the thickened lining, resulting in the appropriate environment for implantation (Marquardt et al. 2019). One of the main functions of the uterus is to support fertility, where the endometrium is the layer responsible for implantation to occur, supporting embryo growth and development, until the placenta provides a contact point between the fetus and the maternal circulation (Gasner and Aatsha 2022).

Hormonal Changes During Pregnancy That Affect Tissues

During pregnancy, hormonal changes occur that affect various tissues and organs. These changes are important for the growth and development of the fetus and for preparing the body for birth. Understanding these hormonal changes is crucial for managing symptoms and ensuring a healthy pregnancy outcome (Uvnäs-Moberg et al. 2019).

109

One of the primary hormones affecting tissues during pregnancy is human chorionic gonadotrophin (hCG), which is produced by the placenta. This hormone maintains the corpus luteum, which produces progesterone, a hormone necessary for maintaining a pregnancy (Betz and Fane 2022). hCG is also associated with nausea and vomiting during pregnancy in approximately 70% of pregnant women (Wang et al. 2020).

Progesterone acts on uterine tissues, promoting relaxation of the myometrium and cervical closure, peristalsis and contraction pressure (Soma-Pillay et al. 2016). Changes in the balance between uterine contraction and relaxation during pregnancy could affect pregnancy progression and result in premature or an undeveloped fetus (Buckley 2015; Patel et al. 2015; Yin et al. 2018). Additionally, progesterone helps regulate the immune system and prevent miscarriage (Coomarasamy et al. 2020).

Oestrogen, produced by the ovaries and placenta, is important for supplying adequate oxygen for fetoplacental growth and development. It also contributes to preparing breast tissue and fetal adrenal gland function (Tal and Taylor 2021). Oestrogen affects the cardiovascular system, causing increased blood volume and cardiac output by 40% at term. Insufficient uteroplacental blood flow can cause preterm birth and intrauterine growth restriction (Mandalà 2020).

Relaxin is another hormone that affects connective tissue during pregnancy. It loosens ligaments and fibrous tissue and increases mobility in joints, which may cause lower back or pelvic pain during pregnancy. Relaxin also alters the properties of cartilage and tendon and is involved in bone remodelling and healing injured ligaments and skeletal muscle. Its impact affects a significant proportion of pregnant women (between 24% and 90%; Yang et al. 2022).

Human placental lactogen is another important hormone in pregnancy, which is produced by the placenta. It has lactogenic and somatotropic effects, facilitating the growth and development of the mammary glands. It may also delay milk production until after delivery (Beesley and Johnson 2008).

While these hormonal changes can cause changes and challenges for pregnant women, they are necessary to support the growth and development of the fetus and to ensure a successful delivery.

Reflective Learning Activity

Reflect on the importance of hormonal changes during pregnancy that affect body tissues and joints. Think about what explanation would you provide to new parents about the lower back pain they may experience during pregnancy and what is the common cause.

Types of Tissues

There are four main types of tissues in the body: epithelial, connective, muscle and nervous (Wheeldon 2017). Epithelial tissues play several important roles, such as protection, absorption, filtration excretion, secretion and sensory reception.

During pregnancy, the epithelial cells of the uterus provide protection by forming a barrier that shields the fetus from potential harm (e.g. sexually transmitted infections) while allowing the exchange of nutrients and waste products through the mucus (Anahtar et al. 2018; McShane et al. 2021). Epithelial tissues also play a crucial role in absorbing, filtering and excreting nutrients and waste products through the placenta and kidneys, as well as filtering harmful substances (Biga et al. 2019b; Díaz et al. 2014; McNanley and Woods 2009). Through secretion, the mammary epithelial tissue produces and secrets human milk, including bioactive factors such as hormones, cytokines, leucocytes, immunoglobulins, lactoferrin, lysozyme, stem cells and human milk oligosaccharides (Ballard and Morrow 2013; Carr et al. 2021). Lastly, epithelial tissues detect and respond to light, taste and smell; they are located in the nose, tongue and eyes. Epithelial tissues are also found in the airway, such as the taste receptors (Dalesio et al. 2018).

Epithelial Tissue

Epithelial tissue forms the outermost layer of the body, covering the surface of the body and lining internal organs and cavities, including the skin, respiratory tract, digestive tract and reproductive system. It is also responsible for protecting internal structures (organs and systems) and forming boundaries between different environments

(Marieb and Hoehn 2019; Scanlon and Sanders 2018). Changes in epithelial tissue during pregnancy may potentially affect the function of the gastrointestinal tract, leading to common symptoms such as heartburn, nausea and vomiting (Vazquez 2015). These changes are thought to be caused by the increased production of hormones, such as progesterone, which relax the smooth muscle of the gut and slow down peristaltic movements (Alqudah et al. 2022).

Pregnancy can induce physiological changes in melanin production due to hormone stimulation. It is responsible for 50–75% of cases of melasma, a pigmentary cutaneous condition, in pregnancy (Costin and Birlea 2006),and for darkening the skin around the areola and producing the linea nigra. The linea alba is a thin band of connective tissue, whose function is to maintain the abdominal muscles close to each other (Beer et al. 2009). Hormonal influences during pregnancy can weaken its strength, and can also disrupt the dermal connective tissue of the skin, which may develop striae distensae (stretch marks), spider angiomas, palmar erythema and pruritus gravidarum (Beard and Millington 2012).

Epithelial tissue can be classified by its shape and type (Marieb and Keller 2017; Moini 2019; Scanlon and Sanders 2018; Wheeldon 2017; Table 6.1):

TABLE 6.1   Epithelial tissues.

Type of layer	Shape	Function	Organ/system
Simple (one layer)	Squamous	Diffusion/filtration	Alveoli, capillary walls, glomeruli of the kidney, heart, blood and lymph vessels (endothelium). Also covers body cavity membranes
	Cuboidal	Secretion/absorption/protection	Lining ovaries, kidneys tubules and ducts and small glands. It is also a component of the secretory portions of certain glands such as the thyroid and pancreas
	Columnar	Secretion/absorption/protection	Female reproductive tubes, uterus and most digestive tract organs
	Ciliated	Movements of fluids, mucus. The cells specialised in mucus secretion are called goblet cells	Lines the passageway of central nervous system, fallopian tubes
	Non-ciliated	Possess microvilli for absorption or secretion of mucus	Lining the digestive tract from stomach to the rectum
	Pseudostratified	Different cell height shows a false impression looking like stratified (pseudo). Absorption and secretion. Has cilia	Male reproductive system lining, lining respiratory tract
Stratified (more layers)	Squamous	Protection	Skin, mouth, uterus, vagina, anus and oesophagus
	Cuboidal	Secretion/protection	Lines mammary gland duct, sweat glands, salivary glands, pancreas, developing ovaries
	Columnar	Secretion/protection	Male urethra, ductus deferens and areas of the pharynx
	Transitional	Expansion without tearing organ	Lining urinary bladder, ureters and urethra
Glandular	Exocrine	Secretion diffuses directly into the blood vessels	Sweat and oils glands, liver and pancreas
	Endocrine	Secretion exits through ducts to the epithelial tissue surface	Thyroid, adrenals and pituitary

- Shape (Figure 6.1):
  - Squamous (flat cells)
  - Cuboidal (cube-shaped)
  - Columnar cells (tall and narrow).
- Type (Figure 6.1):
  - Simple epithelial
  - Stratified epithelial (pseudostratified and transitional epithelium)
  - Glandular.

Simple Squamous Epithelium

Simple squamous epithelium is composed of a single layer of cells. This tissue is found in structures such as the alveoli (air sacs) of the lungs, capillary walls and lining of lymph and blood vessels. Simple squamous epithelial cells are tightly packed together and form a continuous sheet (Wheeldon 2016). This type of epithelium is well-suited for processes requiring a rapid exchange of substances, such as gas exchange in the lungs and filtration and osmosis (Moini 2019; Scanlon and Sanders 2018). Although the simple squamous epithelium itself is not directly involved in the reproductive process, it is possible for the systems or organs that are lined with this tissue to be impacted. For example, as blood volume in the body increases during pregnancy, blood vessels can experience additional stress on their lining. Pre-eclampsia (Naljayan and Karumanchi 2013) may cause damage to the blood vessels, provoking changes in the simple squamous epithelium lining.

Simple Cuboidal Epithelium

Simple cuboidal epithelium is a tissue composed of a single layer of cube-shaped cells found in various parts of the body, including gland ducts, kidney tubules and ovaries (Moini 2019). The shape of the cells allows for efficient absorption and secretion of substances. During pregnancy, the cuboidal epithelium lining can change its shape to support fetal growth and development, as seen in the endometrium (Sternberg et al. 2021). Pregnancy can also cause changes in the kidney, leading to an increased workload, and changes in the size and shape of the cuboidal cells. In the liver, changes in the size and structure of bile ducts, lined with cuboidal epithelium, can occur due to increased levels of oestrogen in pregnancy, leading to impaired bile secretion and accumulation of toxic substances and resulting in pruritus (Bacq 2013; Bergman et al. 2013).

Simple Columnar Epithelium

Simple columnar epithelium is a type of tissue that is present in various parts of the body, including the lining of the uterus, the fallopian tubes and the digestive tract, and may or may not have cilia or microvilli on its surface (Hagiwara et al. 2008; Wheeldon 2016). Throughout pregnancy, this tissue experiences several alterations in response to hormonal and mechanical signals associated with the developing fetus. Columnar epithelium helps to regulate the exchange of substances between the mother and the fetus and protects the intestinal wall, helped by mucus secreted by the goblet cells from digestives enzymes (Biga et al. 2019b; Kong et al. 2018). The endometrial epithelium of the uterus, for example, experiences alterations in response to hormones such as progesterone, which help to prepare the uterus for the implantation of a fertilised egg (Sternberg et al. 2021). The uterus also experiences mechanical stretching as the fetus grows, causing alterations in its structure and function. In the digestive tract, this tissue plays an important role in absorbing nutrients from food (Kong et al. 2018). Pregnant women are recommended to consume additional amounts of calcium, iron and folic acid to meet the increased demand of the developing fetus. These essential nutrients are transported across the placenta, which can reduce the concentration levels of these nutrients in the mother's bloodstream (Brown et al. 2021; Hoenderop et al. 2005). As a result, her health and that of the developing fetus may be affected.

Pseudostratified Columnar Epithelium Tissue

Pseudostratified columnar epithelium tissue occurs at different heights above the basement membrane, which gives a false impression that is it a stratified tissue (Marieb and Keller 2017). It is found in the respiratory tract, including the trachea and bronchi, helping to regulate gas exchange. Oxygen and nutrients diffuse from maternal blood to the fetus; the gas exchange process involves the placenta, an organ key to the development of the fetus (Cenzi et al. 2019).

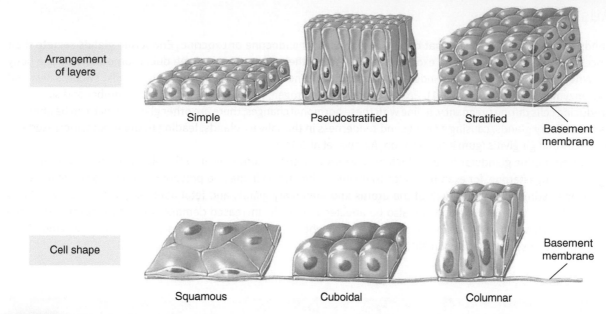

FIGURE 6.1 Epithelial tissue is classified by shape and depth. Source: Tortora and Derrickson (2017)/John Wiley & Sons.

Stratified Epithelium

Stratified epithelium is composed of multiple layers of cells, and is the most common type of epithelial tissue in the body (Marieb and Keller 2017). Its primary function is to provide extra protection against physical damage. The cells at the surface of the stratified epithelium are typically flat and scale-like, while cells deeper in the tissue are more cylindrical. These cells regenerate from the inner layer to the outer layer, pushing the older cell upwards (Wheeldon 2016). Unlike simple epithelium, stratified epithelium is typically found in structures exposed to physical stress or abrasion. It produces new cells to replace the ones worn off (e.g. in the skin and the lining of the oesophagus and vagina – non-keratinising type lining producing mucus; Scanlon and Sanders 2018).

Other types of stratified epithelium are cuboidal and columnar; however, those types are quite rare in the human body when compared with other types of tissues.

Red Flag Alert: Vaginal Itching

Any changes in vaginal pH will affect women's tissues and can mean that she is prone to vaginal infections. A woman presenting with itching in genital area, abnormal vaginal discharge or urinating frequently should be investigated rapidly.

Transitional Epithelium

Transitional epithelium is found in the urinary system, particularly in the lining of the urinary bladder, the ureters and part of the urethra. The cells in transitional epithelium can stretch and expand, allowing these organs to accommodate changes in urine volume (Marieb and Keller 2017; Moini 2019). In pregnancy, the uterus expands as the fetus grows, which can place pressure on the urinary bladder and ureters. This can cause the transitional epithelium in these organs to stretch and expand even more than usual, allowing for increased urine volume without increasing the pressure in the bladder (Marieb and Keller 2017). In addition, hormonal changes (especially increased progesterone) throughout pregnancy can also affect the urinary system, (e.g. causing relaxation of the smooth muscle in the urinary system, which can lead to increased urine retention and a higher risk of urinary tract infections; Konapala et al. 2018).

Glands

The glands are an epithelial tissue that can be categorised as endocrine or exocrine. Endocrine glands secrete their substances into the bloodstream and exocrine glands secrete their substances through ducts somewhere on the body surface (Wheeldon 2016). Exocrine glandular tissue produces and secretes substances such as milk, sweat, saliva and digestive enzymes (Freeman et al. 2021). Progesterone and oestrogen, for example, increase the number and size of the milk-producing cells during pregnancy. In line with these hormonal changes, there are other glands which can be affected, such as the salivary glands, causing swelling and tenderness in the salivary glands, leading to dry mouth, increased risk of tooth decay and gingivitis (gum inflammation; Agrawal et al. 2022).

Equally, endocrine glandular tissue, which produces and secretes hormones into the bloodstream, can be affected by pregnancy. Progesterone, for example, helps to maintain the uterine lining and prevent contractions (Yin et al. 2018), while oestrogen stimulates the growth of the uterus and mammary glands and fetal adrenal gland function (Tal and Taylor 2021). Lastly, the thyroid gland can also be affected due to the increased demand for thyroid hormones. Some women may develop hypothyroidism, causing fatigue, weight gain and other symptoms, which affects around 1% of pregnant women (Frise and Williamson 2013).

Medications Management: Uncontrolled Epithelial Cell Proliferation

Uncontrolled epithelial cell proliferation can contribute to the fertilised egg failing to implant in the endometrium. During the early stages of pregnancy, the blastocyst (fertilised egg) must implant into the uterine lining to establish a pregnancy. The endometrium changes in preparation for implantation. Uncontrolled proliferation of epithelial cells in the endometrium can lead to a thickened lining that may not be receptive to the implantation of the blastocyst, referred to as endometrial hyperplasia. A histological examination will be needed to diagnose this condition together with a biopsy of the uterine cavity. Generally, progesterone treatment works well, both continuous oral and local intrauterine progestogens (synthetic progesterone) for a minimum of six months (Royal College of Obstetricians and Gynaecologists 2016).

Certain medical conditions or hormonal imbalances causing uncontrolled epithelial cell proliferation can also contribute to infertility or failed implantation. Examples of these conditions include polycystic ovary syndrome (PCOS) and uterine fibroids. Although a cure for PCOS does not currently exist, the treatment options available are dependent on the symptoms experienced by the individual and may include the use of egg inducers and metformin in cases of diabetes. Additionally, treatment plans often involve weight management and regular exercise.

Connective Tissue

Connective tissue is the most abundant tissue in the human body. It is a diverse group of tissues providing structural protection, support, cushioning and insulation of other tissues in the body (Marieb and Keller 2017; Wheeldon 2016). This tissue has a larger extracellular matrix, which can be described as a complex structure found between cells, supporting them, combining water, protein and polysaccharides. Depending on their structural requirement in the body, such as bearing extra weight during pregnancy or withstanding stretching tissues, the properties of the extracellular matrix will change to accommodate the needs from a fluid gel-like to a firm consistency due to the abundance of collagen and elastin (Marieb and Keller 2017; McKee et al. 2019). Each connective tissue has its own specific matrix; for example, the blood has plasma (mostly water), whereas the bone matrix is made of calcium salts, which are hard and strong (Scanlon and Sanders 2018).

There are various classifications of connective tissue found in anatomical and physiology literature. However, connective tissue can be generally categorised into three types: connective tissue proper, supportive connective tissue and fluid connective tissue. Here, we describe these tissue types and their subgroups and examine how pregnancy can impact them (Biga et al. 2019b; Moini 2019; Table 6.2).

TABLE 6.2 Connective tissues summary.

Connective tissue	Type	Subtype
Proper	Dense	Dense regular
		Dense irregular
		Elastic
	Loose	Adipose tissue
		Areolar tissue
		Reticular connective tissue
	Embryonic	
Supporting	Cartilage	Hyaline
		Elastic
		Fibrous
	Bone	
Fluid	Blood	
	Lymph	

Snapshot 6.1 Oedema

Denise is a 32-year-old woman who is 22 weeks pregnant with her first child. During a routine prenatal examination, the midwife notices that she has significant swelling in her ankles and feet. She also complains of pain and stiffness in her joints, particularly her knees and wrists. On further evaluation, the midwife determined that Denise has developed oedema. Oedema is a common occurrence during pregnancy, often due to changes in connective tissue proper.

Reflective Learning Activity

Thinking about Snapshot 6.1, reflect on the following questions:

- What other antenatal examinations would you consider to exclude other issues related to oedema?
- Would you consider any other investigations to help you the evaluate signs and symptoms of Denise's condition?
- Could Denise's oedema be associated with another common issue or problem during pregnancy? It is not uncommon for there to be overlapping signs and symptoms between different conditions, yet with distinct diagnoses. What other possibilities do you think may exist?
- Until you have collated possible investigations and other examinations in this case, what non-pharmacological advice would you provide to Denise?

Connective Tissue Proper

Connective tissue proper consists of dense and loose connective tissue. Dense connective tissue forms strong structures, such as tendons and ligaments connecting skeletal muscles to bones and joints (Marieb and Keller 2017). This tissue is closely packed full of collagen fibres; it is flexible and offers great resistance to any tension. Dense connective tissue can be categorised as regular, irregular and elastic (Biga et al. 2019b). Regular connective tissue fibres are oriented in parallel, which increases their strength and makes them well suited for applications such as tendons and ligaments. Conversely, irregular connective tissue is irregular and lacks uniformity, providing greater strength overall; an example of this irregular composition is the subcutaneous layer of the skin (the dermis). Finally, elastic connective tissue allows tissues to stretch and return to their original length. This phenomenon happens during and after pregnancy, when the uterus undergoes a significant change by increasing in size, to accommodate the fetus and then returning to its normal size, due to the extra production of matrix proteins such as collagen and elastin (O'Connor et al. 2020).

Loose Connective Tissue

Loose connective tissue is softer than dense tissue. It fills spaces between organs, supports epithelial tissue and protects the specialised cells of several organs (Moini 2019). It has fewer fibres than other tissue (excluding blood) and can be classified into three subtypes, adipose, areolar and reticular connective tissue (Wheeldon 2016). Adipose tissue can comprise up to 18% of the body weight of an adult. It lies between muscles, beneath the skin and behind the eyes and is present in some membranes of the abdomen. Adipose tissue protects some organs, such as the kidneys, covering them with a capsule of fat. Adipose cell deposits are stored in the hips, abdomen and breast to be used as fuel when needed; in addition, adipose tissue cushions and helps to protect the fetus and organs (Marieb and Keller 2017; Moini 2019). The areolar type is the most abundant loose connective tissue; it contains collagen, elastic and reticular fibres. Its function is to support and bind other organs, hold body fluids, defend against infections and store nutrients as fat deposits (Marieb and Hoehn 2019). The final connective tissue subtype is reticular connective tissue; this tissue supports soft organs such as the spleen, liver and lymphatic tissue. The reticular fibres form a network on to which the cells attach, interconnecting several organs in the body (Textor et al. 2016).

Transient Connective Tissue

There is another transient type of connective tissue, the mucoidal or embryonic connective tissue found in the umbilical cord of the fetus. This tissue contains a large amount of ground substance and is rich in hyaluronic acid. Also called Wharton's jelly, its main function is to provide the blood supply to the fetus as well as biological waste removal (Stefańska et al. 2020). This tissue is no longer present after the third stage of labour has been reached. This type of tissue is only present during pregnancy (Biga et al. 2019b).

Supportive Connective Tissue

Supportive connective tissue includes cartilage and bone.

Red Flag Alert: Connective Tissue Disorders

Vaginal pressure or discharge accompanied by mild contractions could be an indicator of early labour. Pregnant women with connective tissue disorders may be at risk of preterm labour or cervical insufficiency. These women may need a cervical cerclage to prevent the cervix opening too early in pregnancy.

Cartilage

In the cartilage matrix are cells called chondrocytes or cartilage cells. There are no capillaries within the cartilage matrix; these cells are nourished by diffusion throughout the matrix, a slow process. Clinically, when the cartilage is affected or damaged, the repair will be slow or not repaired at all (Scanlon and Sanders 2018). This tissue is flexible and strong.

Cartilage serves as a shock absorber by facilitating smooth movement between bones, thereby assisting in the maintenance of their shape, or by allowing certain parts of the body to recover from impacts or pressure (Marieb and Hoehn 2019). In pregnancy, the production of cartilage in the joints increases, resulting in increased flexibility and mobility. However, the increase in weight and pressure during pregnancy for instance, in the knee joints, can be detrimental to cartilage, causing joint pain and discomfort (Chu et al. 2019; Dehghan et al. 2014). There are three types of cartilage, hyaline, fibrocartilage and elastic.

Hyaline Cartilage

Hyaline cartilage is the most common type of cartilage and is found in many joints, the soft portion of the nose and the respiratory system. It is moderately malleable, providing firm support (Wheeldon 2016). This is particularly significant because hormonal changes during pregnancy, specifically the release of relaxin, can result in increased flexibility of the pubic symphysis. This increased flexibility is necessary for the expansion of the pelvic cavity during childbirth (Biga et al. 2019b).

Fibrocartilage

Fibrocartilage is the second subtype of cartilage involved in childbirth. The pubic symphysis is a fibrocartilaginous joint covered with hyaline cartilage allowing flexibility (Fisher and Bordoni 2022) to expand the pelvic space for birth. Fibrocartilage is found in the intervertebral discs, pubic symphysis, menisci and temporomandibular joint (Benjamin and Ralphs 2004).

Elastic Cartilage

Elastic cartilage is a type of cartilage that is similar to hyaline cartilage but has elastic fibres within its matrix, allowing for greater flexibility. This type of tissue is found in the epiglottis, larynx and ear, where its resilience to pressure helps maintain the shape of these structures (Moini 2019).

117

Bone

Of all the types of connective tissues, bone is the most rigid, having the ability to support and protect the structures in the body. It comprises a matrix (also known as osteoid) consisting of 33% collagen and 67% of inorganic matter (calcium phosphate and hydroxyapatite crystal; Maas 2009). One special bone characteristic is the ability to remodel itself through resorption by the osteoclast cells and formation by osteoblasts cells. Bone is stable under physiological conditions (Chen et al. 2018). However, pregnancy and lactation are challenging periods for the mother because the fetal skeleton demands a considerable transfer of calcium, especially in the third trimester (Sanz-Salvador et al. 2015). This process is regulated by hormonal changes during pregnancy and may impact on the mother's skeleton. Recovery of calcium levels and bone structure will take some time, especially if the woman breastfeeds (Winter et al. 2020).

Snapshot 6.2   Osteoporosis

Malika is a 42-year-old woman who is 28 weeks pregnant with her second child. She has a history of osteoporosis and is concerned about the impact of pregnancy on her bone health. Malika's midwife notes that pregnancy can affect bone tissue because of the increased demand for calcium and other minerals by the developing fetus. In addition, hormonal changes during pregnancy can alter bone metabolism, leading to increased bone resorption and decreased bone formation.

Reflective Learning Activity

- As Malika had this diagnosis made before her second pregnancy, would you consider referring Malika to any other healthcare providers?
- What other investigations or examinations would you consider in this case?
- In addition to the medication (calcium) prescribed by her general practitioner, would you assess whether Malika is taking other medication to help assimilate the calcium in the body?
- As Malika is going to breastfeed her baby, will this have any impact on the length of her recovery time?

Fluid Connective Tissue

Blood and lymph are fluid connective tissues that enclose a characteristic collection of cells. Although they are connective tissues, they do not connect or provide mechanical support to any tissue (Marieb and Hoehn 2019). The matrix of the blood is the plasma, which accounts for between 52% and 62% of the total volume of the human body and is made up of dissolved salts, nutrients, gases and waste products (Scanlon and Sanders 2018). The main blood cells are:

- Red cells, which transport oxygen attached to iron in their haemoglobin.
- White cells, which defend the body against pathogens providing immunity.
- Platelets, whose function is to prevent blood loss in the body (Dean 2005).

The primary function of lymph is to protect against pathogens in the body (Wheeldon 2016). It is part of the lymphatic system together with the lymph nodes and lymph vessels (Bordoni et al. 2018). During pregnancy, changes in this system can affect women's body, causing numerous challenges such as oedema and changes in the circulation of the pregnant uterus on the inferior vena cava (Cataldo Oportus et al. 2013).

Muscle Tissue

Muscle tissues are capable of producing movements by contracting or shortening their highly specialised fibres (Marieb and Keller 2017). Muscle contraction is triggered in response to depolarisation, G protein-coupled receptor activation and other stimuli. There are three distinct types of muscle – skeletal, cardiac and smooth – each regulated by different signal pathways, depending on their cell type (Kuo and Ehrlich 2015).

Skeletal Muscle

Skeletal muscle tissue (Figure 6.2) is the only type of muscle that can have its movement controlled voluntarily. It adheres to bones; the cells are cylindrical and multinucleate, with clear striations (stripes). This type of muscle is also called

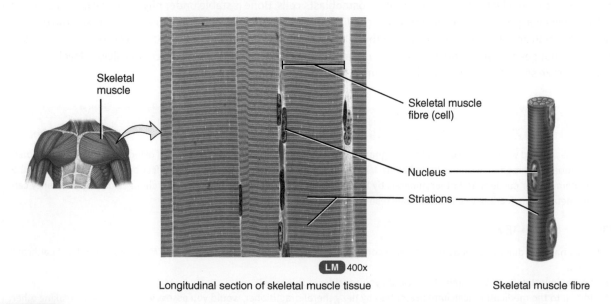

Skeletal muscle

Skeletal muscle fibre (cell)

Nucleus

Striations

LM 400x

Longitudinal section of skeletal muscle tissue

Skeletal muscle fibre

FIGURE 6.2 Skeletal muscle.

striated or voluntary muscle (Scanlon and Sanders 2018). While musculoskeletal discomfort is common among pregnant women, there is limited evidence regarding how changes in the properties of peripheral skeletal muscle may impact postural stability. However, the physical demands on the body increase with the added weight during pregnancy, which can increase the risk of injury during the later stages of pregnancy (Bey et al. 2019).

Cardiac Muscle Tissue

Cardiac muscle tissue or myocardium is a striated, involuntary muscle (Figure 6.3) that is only found in the heart. It is covered by a thick external layer called the epicardium, and an internal layer called endocardium. The cells configuring the heart are called cardiomyocytes; their primary function is to contract (Saxton et al. 2022). Changes in pregnancy affecting the cardiac muscle include the increase of cardiac output, arterial compliance and extracellular fluid volume and a decrease in blood pressure and total peripheral resistance (Hall et al. 2011). These changes are due to the hormonal relationship between the level of oestrogen and progesterone and vasodilatation (Sanghavi and Rutherford 2014).

Smooth Muscle Tissue

Smooth muscle tissue, also referred to as visceral muscle (Figure 6.4), is located in the walls of various hollow organs in the body, including the stomach, blood vessels, bladder and uterus. Unlike cardiac muscle, smooth muscle is non-striated; it also operates involuntarily. One specific characteristic of this tissue is the ability to contract and relax, which is due to the two protein molecules actin and myosin. Equally important is the calcium-containing sarcoplasmic reticulum, which helps in sustaining contractions (Hafen and Burns 2022). In pregnancy, smooth muscle tissue regulates uterus contractility, which is of vital importance for maintaining the pregnancy and helping during labour (Pehlivanoğlu et al. 2013).

119

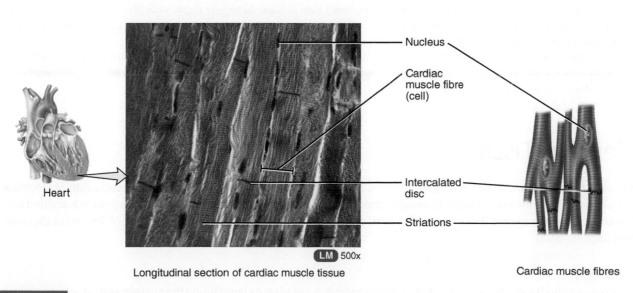

Heart

Nucleus

Cardiac muscle fibre (cell)

Intercalated disc

Striations

LM 500x

Longitudinal section of cardiac muscle tissue

Cardiac muscle fibres

FIGURE 6.3 Cardiac muscle.

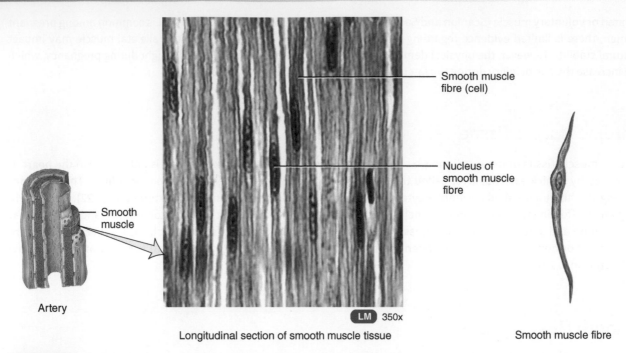

Smooth muscle
fibre (cell)

Nucleus of
smooth muscle
fibre

Smooth
muscle

Artery

LM 350x

Longitudinal section of smooth muscle tissue

Smooth muscle fibre

FIGURE 6.4 Smooth muscle.

120

Medication Management: Palpitations During Pregnancy

Palpitations, or the feeling of a rapid or irregular heartbeat, can be common during pregnancy because of hormonal changes and increased blood volume. However, it is important to have any new or persistent palpitations evaluated by a cardiologist to rule out any underlying cardiac issues.

Treatment for palpitations during pregnancy will depend on the underlying cause and severity of the symptoms. In some cases, lifestyle changes such as reducing caffeine intake or managing stress can be helpful in reducing palpitations. However, if the palpitations are caused by an underlying cardiac issue, medication may be necessary to manage the symptoms.

For example, if the palpitations are due to an arrhythmia such as supraventricular tachycardia (SVT), medications such as beta-blockers or calcium channel blockers may be prescribed to control the heart rate and prevent episodes of SVT. In some cases, cardioversion may be necessary, which is safe during pregnancy (Adamson and Nelson-Piercy 2008).

It is important to note that not all medications or procedures are safe during pregnancy. The risks and benefits of any medication must be carefully considered before it is prescribed. The healthcare provider should work very closely with pregnant women to develop a treatment plan that is safe and effective.

Nervous Tissue

Nervous tissue consists of two cell types, neurons and glial cells, which are specialised for the conduction of electrical impulses from one area of the body to another and the nervous system (Moini 2019). The nervous system is divided into the central nervous system (brain and spinal cord) and the peripheral nervous system, consisting of the nerves (Scanlon and Sanders 2018).

Neurons

Neurons vary in shape. They can be differentiated into bodies called soma (containing the nucleus and cytoplasm), axons (transmitting information among other neurons) and dendrites (message receivers from other neurons); where the neurons and the target cell meet is called a synapse (Biga et al. 2019a).

Glial Cells

Cells or neuroglia are cells insulating, supporting and protecting the neurons in the structures of the nervous system – brain, spinal cord and nerves (Marieb and Keller 2017). During pregnancy, hormonal changes exert a profound impact on the maternal brain. Specifically, steroid hormones, as well as peptide hormones such as prolactin and human platelet lysate, are transported into the brain and can interact with receptors expressed in various brain regions. Notably, the hypothalamus represents a specific target of these hormones, allowing the brain to modulate a wide range of autonomic nervous system targets and, consequently, affect multiple body systems (Grattan and Ladyman 2020).

Reflective Learning Activity

Pregnancy can have a significant impact on the nervous system and can result in various symptoms for women. Due to the hormonal changes that occur during pregnancy, nervous tissue is particularly susceptible to alterations. Common symptoms that women may experience include:

- Decreased attention span
- Mood changes
- Increased irritability or tearfulness
- Muscle tension
- Headaches
- Fatigue

How would you explain these changes to pregnant parents?

Tissue Repair

Tissue repair refers to the natural process of healing and restoring damaged tissues in the body. Although all tissue types discussed can regenerate and replace the cells damaged by trauma, disease or other events, there is a greater degree of success in some tissues over others (Wheeldon 2016). A well-vascularised tissue will heal more quickly than cartilage tissue. The first sign of tissue damage is inflammation, which manifests as pain, heat, redness and swelling. In its acute response, inflammation does not normally require treatment other than painkillers while the damage is naturally repaired (Perretti and Montero-Melendez 2017).

In response to tissue injury, the body originates a chemical signalling cascade that encourages responses aimed at healing affected tissues. These signals activate leucocyte chemotaxis from the general circulation to sites of damage. These activated leucocytes produce cytokines that induce inflammatory responses (Chen et al. 2018). During the process of birth, for example, a woman can naturally tear, damaging connective or muscle tissue. When repairing the damaged tissue surgically, it is important to know the anatomy of the female external genitalia (Nguyen and Duong 2022).

Take Home Points

- All cells and tissues in the body originate from three germ layers: the ectoderm, mesoderm and endoderm – outer, middle and inner layers, respectively. Each germ layer will be linked to the development of certain primitive systems during the formation of organs and tissues.
- The different types of epithelial tissues are characterised by their cellular shapes and arrangements: squamous, cuboidal or columnar epithelia. Single-cell layers form simple epithelia whereas stacked cells form stratified epithelia. The main functions of epithelia are protection from the environment, coverage, secretion, excretion, absorption and filtration.

- The major types of connective tissue are connective tissue proper, supportive tissue and fluid tissue. Cartilage and bone are supportive tissue and are classified as hyaline, fibrocartilage and elastic cartilage.
- Fluid tissue such as blood and lymph is characterised by a liquid matrix and no supporting fibres. Exocrine glands release their products through ducts. Endocrine glands secrete hormones directly into the interstitial fluid and bloodstream.
- The three types of muscle cells are skeletal, cardiac and smooth. Their morphologies are equal to their specific functions in the body. Cardiac muscle cells contract autonomously and involuntarily. Smooth muscle is involuntary. Skeletal muscle is voluntary and responds to conscious stimuli.
- The cells from nervous tissue are neurons and glia cells. Characterised by its ability to receive stimuli and respond by generating an electrical signal.

Summary

Tissues play a crucial role in pregnancy, both in the development of the fetus and in the changes occurring in a woman's body. During pregnancy, the placenta, a specialised tissue, forms to provide the growing fetus with nutrients and oxygen while also removing waste products.

Other tissues, such as the uterine lining and the cervix, undergo significant changes to support the developing fetus and prepare for childbirth. Hormonal changes also affect various tissues in the mother's body, leading to changes in blood volume, breast tissue development, and increased joint mobility.

Understanding the changes occurring in the woman's tissues during pregnancy is crucial in providing appropriate antenatal care and managing any complications that may arise. Additionally, being aware of the interactions between fetal and maternal tissues is essential in improving our understanding of pregnancy and fetal development, leading to better outcomes for mother and child.

References

Adamson, D.L. and Nelson-Piercy, C. (2008). Managing palpitations and arrhythmias during pregnancy. *Postgraduate Medical Journal* 84 (988): 66–72.

Agrawal, A.T., Hande, A., Reche, A., and Paul, P. (2022). Appraisal of saliva and its sensory perception in reproductive transitions of women: a review. *Cureus* 14 (11): e31614. https://doi.org/10.7759/cureus.31614.

Alqudah, M., Al-Shboul, O., Al-Dwairi, A. et al. (2022). Progesterone inhibitory role on gastrointestinal motility. *Physiological Research* 71 (2): 193–198. https://doi.org/10.33549/physiolres.934824.

Anahtar, M.N., Gootenberg, D.B., Mitchell, C.M., and Kwon, D.S. (2018). Cervicovaginal microbiota and reproductive health: the virtue of simplicity. *Cell Host and Microbe* 23 (2): 159–168. https://doi.org/10.1016/j.chom.2018.01.013.

Bacq, Y. (2013). The liver in normal pregnancy. In: *Madame Curie: Bioscience Database*. Austin, TX: Landes Bioscience https://www.ncbi.nlm.nih.gov/books/NBK6005.

Ballard, O. and Morrow, A.L. (2013). Human milk composition. Nutrients and bioactive factors. *Pediatric Clinics of North America* 60 (1): 49–74.

Beard, M.P. and Millington, G.W.M. (2012). Recent developments in the specific dermatoses of pregnancy. *Clinical and Experimental Dermatology* 37 (1): 1–5.

Beer, G.M., Schuster, A., Seifert, B. et al. (2009). The normal width of the linea alba in nulliparous women. *Clinical Anatomy* 22 (6): 706–711. https://doi.org/10.1002/ca.20836.

Beesley, R.D. and Johnson, J.V. (2008). The breast during pregnancy and lactation. *Global Library of Women's Medicine* https://doi.org/10.3843/glowm.10305.

Benjamin, M. and Ralphs, J.R. (2004). Biology of fibrocartilage cells. *International Review of Cytology* 233: 1–45. https://doi.org/10.1016/S0074-7696(04)33001-9.

Bergman, H., Melamed, N., and Koren, G. (2013). Pruritus in pregnancy: treatment of dermatoses unique to pregnancy. *Canadian Family Physician* 59 (12): 1290–1294. College of Family Physicians of Canada. /pmc/articles/PMC3860924/.

Betz, D. and Fane, K. (2022). *Human Chorionic Gonadotropin*. Treasure Island, FL: StatPearls https://www.ncbi.nlm.nih.gov/books/NBK532950. https://doi.org/10.1016/C2010-0-65647-1.

Bey, M.E., Marzilger, R., Hinkson, L. et al. (2019). Vastus lateralis architecture changes during pregnancy – a longitudinal study. *Frontiers in Physiology* 10: 1163. https://doi.org/10.3389/fphys.2019.01163.

Biga, L.M., Dawson, S., Harwell, A. et al. (2019a). Connective tissue supports and protects. In: *Anatomy & Physiology*. Corvallis, OR: OpenStax/Oregon State University https://open.oregonstate.education/aandp/chapter/4-3-connective-tissue-supports-and-protects.

Biga, L.M., Dawson, S., Harwell, A. et al. (2019b). Epithelial tissue. In: *Anatomy & Physiology*. Corvallis, OR: OpenStax/Oregon State University https://open.oregonstate.education/aandp/chapter/4-2-epithelial-tissue.

Bordoni, B., Marelli, F., Morabito, B., and Castagna, R. (2018). A new concept of biotensegrity incorporating liquid tissues: blood and lymph. *Journal of Evidence-Based Integrative Medicine* 23: 1–10. https://doi.org/10.1177/2515690X18792838.

Brown, L.V.L., Cohen, B.E., Edwards, E. et al. (2021). Physiological need for calcium, iron, and folic acid for women of various subpopulations during pregnancy and beyond. *Journal of Women's Health* 30 (2): 207–211. https://doi.org/10.1089/jwh.2020.8873.

Buckley, S.J. (2015). Executive summary of hormonal physiology of childbearing: evidence and implications for women, babies, and maternity care. *The Journal of Perinatal Education* 24 (3): 145–153. https://doi.org/10.1891/1058-1243.24.3.145.

Carr, L.E., Virmani, M.D., Rosa, F. et al. (2021). Role of human milk bioactives on infants' gut and immune health. *Frontiers in Immunology* 12: 290. https://doi.org/10.3389/fimmu.2021.604080.

Cataldo Oportus, S., de Paiva Rodrigues, L., de Pereira Godoy, J.M., and de Guerreiro Godoy, M.F. (2013). Lymph drainage in pregnant women. *Nursing Research and Practice* 2013: 1–3. https://doi.org/10.1155/2013/364582.

Cenzi, J.R., Albuquerque, C., and Mady, C.E.K. (2019). Phenomenological and thermodynamic model of gas exchanges in the placenta during pregnancy: a case study of intoxication of carbon monoxide. *International Journal of Environmental Research and Public Health* 16 (21): https://doi.org/10.3390/ijerph16214138.

Chen, L., Deng, H., Cui, H. et al. (2018). Inflammatory responses and inflammation-associated diseases in organs. *Oncotarget* 9 (6): 7204–7218. https://doi.org/10.18632/oncotarget.23208.

Chu, S.R., Boyer, E.H., Beynnon, B., and Segal, N.A. (2019). Pregnancy results in lasting changes in knee joint laxity. *PM and R* 11 (2): 117–124. https://doi.org/10.1016/j.pmrj.2018.06.012.

Clift, D. and Schuh, M. (2013). Restarting life: fertilization and the transition from meiosis to mitosis. *Nature Reviews Molecular Cell Biology* 14 (9): 549–562. https://doi.org/10.1038/nrm3643.

Coomarasamy, A., Harb, H.M., Devall, A.J. et al. (2020). Progesterone to prevent miscarriage in women with early pregnancy bleeding: the PRISM RCT. *Health Technology Assessment* 24 (33): 1–70. https://doi.org/10.3310/hta24330.

Costin, G.E. and Birlea, S.A. (2006). Is there an answer? What is the mechanism for melasma that so commonly accompanies human pregnancy? *IUBMB Life* 58 (1): 55–57. https://doi.org/10.1080/15216540500417020.

Dalesio, N.M., Barreto Ortiz, S.F., Pluznick, J.L., and Berkowitz, D.E. (2018). Olfactory, taste, and photo sensory receptors in non-sensory organs: it just makes sense. *Frontiers in Physiology* 9: 1–19. https://doi.org/10.3389/fphys.2018.01673.

Dean, L. (2005). Blood and the cells it contains. In: *Blood Groups and Red Cell Antigens*, 1–6. National Center for Biotechnology Information (US) https://www.ncbi.nlm.nih.gov/books/NBK2263.

Dehghan, F., Haerian, B.S., Muniandy, S. et al. (2014). The effect of relaxin on the musculoskeletal system. *Scandinavian Journal of Medicine and Science in Sports* 24 (4): e220. https://doi.org/10.1111/sms.12149.

Díaz, P., Powell, T.L., and Jansson, T. (2014). The role of placental nutrient sensing in maternal-fetal resource allocation. *Biology of Reproduction* 91 (4): 82–83. https://doi.org/10.1095/biolreprod.114.121798.

Fisher, M. and Bordoni, B. (2022). *Anatomy, Bony Pelvis and Lower Limb, Pelvic Joints*. Treasure Island, FL: StatPearls Publishing https://www.ncbi.nlm.nih.gov/books/NBK538523.

Freeman, S.C., Malik, A., and Basit, H. (2021). *Physiology, Exocrine Gland*. Treasure Island, FL: StatPearls Publishing https://www.ncbi.nlm.nih.gov/books/NBK542322.

Frise, C.J. and Williamson, C. (2013). Endocrine disease in pregnancy. *Clinical Medicine Journal* 13 (2): 176–181. https://doi.org/10.7861/clinmedicine.13-2-176.

Gao, X., Cui, X., Zhang, X. et al. (2020). Differential genetic mutations of ectoderm, mesoderm, and endoderm-derived tumors in TCGA database. *Cancer Cell International* 20 (1): 1–14. https://doi.org/10.1186/S12935-020-01678-x.

Gasner, A. and Aatsha, P.A. (2022). *Physiology, Uterus*. Treasure Island, FL: StatPearls Publishing https://www.ncbi.nlm.nih.gov/books/NBK557575.

Grattan, D.R. and Ladyman, S.R. (2020). Neurophysiological and cognitive changes in pregnancy. *Handbook of Clinical Neurology* 171: 25–55. https://doi.org/10.1016/B978-0-444-64239-4.00002-3.

Hafen, B.B. and Burns, B. (2022). *Physiology, Smooth Muscle*. Treasure Island, FL: StatPearls Publishing https://www.ncbi.nlm.nih.gov/books/NBK526125.

Hagiwara, H., Ohwada, N., Aoki, T. et al. (2008). The primary cilia of secretory cells in the human oviduct mucosa. *Medical Molecular Morphology* 41 (4): 193–198. https://doi.org/10.1007/s00795-008-0421-z.

123

Hall, M.E., George, E.M., and Granger, J.P. (2011). El corazón durante el embarazo. *Revista Espanola de Cardiologia* 64 (11): 1045–1050. https://doi.org/10.1016/j.recesp.2011.07.009.

Hoenderop, J.G.J., Nilius, B., and Bindels, R.J.M. (2005). Calcium absorption across epithelia. *Physiological Reviews* 85 (1): 373–422. https://doi.org/10.1152/physrev.00003.2004.

Johnson, M.S., Jackson, D.L., and Schust, D.J. (2021). Endocrinology of pregnancy. In: *Encyclopedia of Reproduction, Volume 2*, 2e (ed. M.K. Skinner), 469–476. Cambridge, MA: Academic Press https://doi.org/10.1016/B978-0-12-801238-3.64672-X.

Kim, S.-M. and Kim, J.-S. (2017). A review of mechanisms of implantation. *Development & Reproduction* 21 (4): 351–359. https://doi.org/10.12717/dr.2017.21.4.351.

Konapala, L.A., Vesalapu, V., Kiran Kolakota, R. et al. (2018). Pregnancy and hormonal effects on urinary tract infections in women: a scoping review. *International Journal of Research and Review* 5 (10): 407.

Kong, S., Zhang, Y.H., and Zhang, W. (2018). Regulation of intestinal epithelial cells properties and functions by amino acids. *BioMed Research International* 2018: 2819154. https://doi.org/10.1155/2018/2819154.

Kumar, P. and Magon, N. (2012). Hormones in pregnancy. *Nigerian Medical Journal* 53 (4): 179. https://doi.org/10.4103/0300-1652.107549.

Kuo, I.Y. and Ehrlich, B.E. (2015). Signaling in muscle contraction. *Cold Spring Harbor Perspectives in Biology* 7 (2): https://doi.org/10.1101/cshperspect.a006023.

Maas, M.C. (2009). Bones and teeth, histology of. In: *Encyclopedia of Marine Mammals*, 2e (ed. W.F. Perrin, B. Würsig, and J.G.M. Thewissen), 124–129. Cambridge, MA: Academic Press https://doi.org/10.1016/B978-0-12-373553-9.00034-1.

Mandalà, M. (2020). Influence of estrogens on uterine vascular adaptation in normal and preeclamptic pregnancies. *International Journal of Molecular Sciences* 21 (7): 2592. https://doi.org/10.3390/ijms21072592.

Marieb, E.N. and Hoehn, K.N. (2019). Tissue: the living fabric, Chapter 4. In: *Human Anatomy & Psysiology*, 11e. Harlow: Pearson Education.

Marieb, E.N. and Keller, S.M. (2017). Cells and tissues, Chapter 3. In: *Essentials of Human Anatomy and Physiology*, 12e, 657. Harlow: Pearson Education.

Marquardt, R.M., Kim, T.H., Shin, J.H., and Jeong, J.W. (2019). Progesterone and estrogen signaling in the endometrium: what goes wrong in endometriosis? *International Journal of Molecular Sciences* 20 (15): https://doi.org/10.3390/ijms20153822.

McCance, K.L. (2018). The Cell. In: *Pathophysiology: The Biologic Basis for Disease in Adults and Children*, 8e, 1–45. St. Louis, MO: Mosby.

McKee, T.J., Perlman, G., Morris, M., and Komarova, S.V. (2019). Extracellular matrix composition of connective tissues: a systematic review and meta-analysis. *Scientific Reports* 9 (1): 1–15. https://doi.org/10.1038/s41598-019-46896-0.

McNanley, T. and Woods, J. (2009). Placental physiology. *Global Library of Women's Medicine* https://doi.org/10.3843/glowm.10195.

McShane, A., Bath, J., Jaramillo, A.M. et al. (2021). Mucus. *Current Biology* 31 (15): R938–R945. https://doi.org/10.1016/j.cub.2021.06.093.

Moini, J. (2019). Tissues, Chapter 5. In: *Anatomy and Physiology for Health Professionals*, 3e. Sudbury, MA: Jones & Bartlett Learning.

Muhr, J. and Ackerman, K.M. (2022). *Embryology, Gastrulation*. StatPearls; StatPearls Publishing https://www.ncbi.nlm.nih.gov/books/NBK554394.

Naljayan, M.V. and Karumanchi, S.A. (2013). New developments in the pathogenesis of preeclampsia. *Advances in Chronic Kidney Disease* 20 (3): 265–270. https://doi.org/10.1053/j.ackd.2013.02.003.

Napso, T., Yong, H.E.J., Lopez-Tello, J., and Sferruzzi-Perri, A.N. (2018). The role of placental hormones in mediating maternal adaptations to support pregnancy and lactation. *Frontiers in Physiology* 9 (AUG): 1091. https://doi.org/10.3389/fphys.2018.01091.

Nguyen, J.D. and Duong, H. (2022). *Anatomy, Abdomen and Pelvis, Female External Genitalia*. Treasure Island, FL: StatPearls Publishing https://www.ncbi.nlm.nih.gov/books/NBK547703.

O'Connor, B.B., Pope, B.D., Peters, M.M. et al. (2020). The role of extracellular matrix in normal and pathological pregnancy: future applications of microphysiological systems in reproductive medicine. *Experimental Biology and Medicine* 245 (13): 1163–1174. https://doi.org/10.1177/1535370220938741.

Patel, B., Elguero, S., Thakore, S. et al. (2015). Role of nuclear progesterone receptor isoforms in uterine pathophysiology. *Human Reproduction Update* 21 (2): 155–173. https://doi.org/10.1093/humupd/dmu056.

Pehlivanoğlu, B., Bayrak, S., and Doğan, M. (2013). Myometriyumun kasilma ve gevşeme mekanizmalarinda kalsiyumun rolü. *Journal of the Turkish German Gynecology Association* 14 (4): 230–234. https://doi.org/10.5152/jtgga.2013.67763.

Perretti, M. and Montero-Melendez, T. (2017). Resolution in an "over-inflamed" era. *Biochemist* 39 (4): 4–7. https://doi.org/10.1042/bio03904004.

Royal College of Obstetricians and Gynaecologists (2016). *Management of Endometrial Hyperplasia*. Green-top Guideline No. 67. London: Royal College of Obstetricians and Gynaecologists.

Sanghavi, M. and Rutherford, J.D. (2014). Cardiovascular physiology of pregnancy. *Circulation* 130 (12): 1003–1008. https://doi.org/10.1161/CIRCULATIONAHA.114.009029.

Sanz-Salvador, L., García-Pérez, M.A., Tarín, J.J., and Cano, A. (2015). Bone metabolic changes during pregnancy: a period of vulnerability to osteoporosis and fracture. *European Journal of Endocrinology* 172 (2): R53–R65. https://doi.org/10.1530/EJE-14-0424.

Saxton, A., Tariq, M.A., and Bordoni, B. (2022). *Anatomy, Thorax, Cardiac Muscle*. Treasure Island, FL: StatPearls Publishing https://www.ncbi.nlm.nih.gov/books/NBK535355.

Scanlon, V. and Sanders, T. (2018). Tissues and membranes. In: *Essentials of Anatomy and Physiology*, 8e, 17. Philadelphia, PA: F. A. Davis Company.

Soma-Pillay, P., Nelson-Piercy, C., Tolppanen, H., and Mebazaa, A. (2016). Physiological changes in pregnancy. *Cardiovascular Journal of Africa* 27 (2): 89–94. https://doi.org/10.5830/CVJA-2016-021.

Stefańska, K., Ożegowska, K., Hutchings, G. et al. (2020). Human Wharton's Jelly – cellular specificity, stemness potency, animal models, and current application in human clinical trials. *Journal of Clinical Medicine* 9 (4): 1102. https://doi.org/10.3390/jcm9041102.

Sternberg, A.K., Buck, V.U., Classen-Linke, I., and Leube, R.E. (2021). How mechanical forces change the human endometrium during the menstrual cycle in preparation for embryo implantation. *Cells* 10 (8): 2008. https://doi.org/10.3390/cells10082008.

Tal, R. and Taylor, H.S. (2021). Endocrinology of pregnancy. In: *Endotext,* 469–476. South Dartmouth, MA: MDText.com, Inc. https://www.ncbi.nlm.nih.gov/books/NBK278962.

Textor, J., Mandl, J.N., and de Boer, R.J. (2016). The reticular cell network: a robust backbone for immune responses. *PLoS Biology* 14 (10): https://doi.org/10.1371/journal.pbio.2000827.

Tortora, G.J. and Derrickson, B.H. (2017). *Tortora's Principles of Anatomy and Physiology*. Chichester: Wiley.

Uvnäs-Moberg, K., Ekström-Bergström, A., Berg, M. et al. (2019). Maternal plasma levels of oxytocin during physiological childbirth – a systematic review with implications for uterine contractions and central actions of oxytocin. *BMC Pregnancy and Childbirth* 19 (1): 1–17. https://doi.org/10.1186/s12884-019-2365-9.

Vazquez, J.C. (2015). Heartburn in pregnancy. *BMJ Clinical Evidence* 1411: https://doi.org/10.1136/dtb.28.3.11.

Wang, Y., Li, H., Peng, W. et al. (2020). Non-pharmacological interventions for postpartum depression: a protocol for systematic review and network meta-analysis. *Medicine* 99 (31): e21496. https://doi.org/10.1097/MD.0000000000021496.

Wheeldon, A. (2016). Tissue. In: *Fundamentals of Anatomy and Physiology for Nursing and Healthcare Students*, 2e (ed. I. Peate and M. Nair), 139–164. Chichester: Wiley.

Wheeldon, A. (2017). Cell and body tissue physiology. In: *Fundamentals of Applied Pathophysiology : An Essential Guide for Nursing and Healthcare Students*, 2e (ed. I. Peate), 33–47. Chichester: Wiley.

Winter, E.M., Ireland, A., Butterfield, N.C. et al. (2020). Pregnancy and lactation, a challenge for the skeleton. *Endocrine Connections* 9 (6): R143. https://doi.org/10.1530/EC-20-0055.

Yang, J., Wang, Y., Xu, J. et al. (2022). Acupuncture for low back and/or pelvic pain during pregnancy: a systematic review and meta-analysis of randomised controlled trials. *BMJ Open* 12 (12): e056878. https://doi.org/10.1136/bmjopen-2021-056878.

Yin, Z., Li, Y., He, W. et al. (2018). Progesterone inhibits contraction and increases TREK-1 potassium channel expression in late pregnant rat uterus. *Oncotarget* 9 (1): 651–661. https://doi.org/10.18632/oncotarget.23084.

Glossary

Bronchi	Large tubes that connect the trachea and direct the air to the lungs.
Cilia	Hair-like projections moving microbes and debris out of the body.
Chemotaxis	Movement of an organism in response to a chemical stimulus.
Depolarisation	Opening of sodium ion channels within the plasma membrane.
Gingivitis	Gum inflammation.
Gland	A structure that manufactures a product.
Goblet cells	Intestinal mucosal epithelial cells that synthetise and secrete mucus.
Hormones	Chemicals coordinating different functions in the body (molecules).
Hypothalamus	Control coordinating centre in the brain.
Lactogenic	Stimulating lactation.
Microvilli	Finger-like membrane protrusions found on some cell types.
Miscarriage	Loss of a pregnancy during the first 23 weeks.
Palmar erythema	Skin condition making the palms turning red.
Pathogens	Organism causing disease to its host.
Peristalsis	Wave-like muscle movement.

Pruritus	Itchy skin with irritating sensation.
Somatotrophic cell	Cell that produces growth hormone.
Osmosis	Spontaneous passage or diffusion of water or other solvents through a semipermeable membrane.
Synapse	Neuronal junction; site of transmission of electric nerve impulse.
Oedema	Fluid outside the cell or fluid retention.
Secretion	Product or substance discharged by a cell.
Spider angioma	Vascular lesion, small red to purple mark in the skin.
Supraventricular	Above the ventricles.

Multiple Choice Questions

1. Which part of a neuron contains the nucleus?
   a. Dendrite
   b. Synapse
   c. Soma
   d. Axon

2. Cells are arranged in a single layer and look tall and narrow in what type of epithelial tissue?
   a. Squamous
   b. Stratified
   c. Columnar
   d. Transitional

3. Which connective tissue specialises in the storage of fat?
   a. Adipose tissue
   b. Reticular tissue
   c. Dense connective tissue
   d. Tendon

4. The layer covering structures such as the circulatory system, urinary system or motor system including is what type of connective tissue?
   a. Mesoderm
   b. Ectoderm
   c. Endoderm
   d. Estraderm

5. In bone, what are the main cells?
   a. Lymphocytes
   b. Osteocytes
   c. Chondrocytes
   d. Fibroblasts

6. The nervous system consists of what type of cells?
   a. Glia cells
   b. Epithelial cells
   c. Neurons
   d. Glial cells and neurons

7. Which cells responsible for the transmission of the nerve impulse?
   a. Neurons
   b. Oligodendrocytes
   c. Microglia
   d. Astrocytes

8. Which of the following processes is **not** a cardinal sign of inflammation?
   a. Heat
   b. Redness
   c. Swelling
   d. Fever

9. Which organ produces oestrogen and progesterone to make possible the implantation of the blastocyst?
   a. Fallopian tube
   b. Ovaries
   c. Uterus
   d. Endometrium

10. What stratified tissue protects the skin, mouth, vagina, uterus, anus and oesophagus?
    a. Transitional
    b. Squamous
    c. Cuboidal
    d. Columnar

CHAPTER 7

The Placenta

Antonio Sierra

AIM

The aim of this chapter is to provide a comprehensive understanding of the anatomy and physiology of the placenta and its role in enabling pregnancy, while sustaining and preserving fetal life during the childbearing period.

LEARNING OUTCOMES

On completion of this chapter, you will be able to:

- Have an awareness of the social and medical history behind placental studies.
- Enhance your knowledge around placental anatomy and physiology, to help better understand pregnancy-related processes and changes.
- Increase your knowledge of abnormal placental functioning.
- Have insight into the role of the midwife as an autonomous practitioner in the detection of deviations from placenta-related, physiological processes.
- Reflect and apply learning in the clinical environment.

Test Your Prior Knowledge

1. An acknowledgement of embryology is crucial in supporting understanding the role of the placenta and placental malfunctioning. Draw a chronology highlighting key events of placental formation and development, from implantation to birth.
2. Can you name and describe the most common placenta-related disorders and their potential implications to the mother and fetus?
3. How would you explain uterine involution to a postnatal mother who is at home after giving birth three days ago?
4. After learning about the different types of placental anomalies, can you name and briefly describe the most common placentation, vascular and umbilical cord anomalies?

Fundamentals of Maternal Anatomy and Physiology, First Edition. Edited by Ian Peate and Claire Leader.
© 2024 John Wiley & Sons Ltd. Published 2024 by John Wiley & Sons Ltd.

Introduction

Pregnancy is often at the core of human conversations and interactions that involve discussions about life and social events. A mother and baby can be referred to as forming a unique symbiosis that ultimately leads to parenthood. While reciprocal, physiological interactions between both parties are necessary in the process; there is an added entity without which fetal life would simply not be accomplished (the existence of viviparous beings is only possible because of it) – the placenta. This is an organ responsible for the development of mammals in utero through the provision of oxygen and nutrients; it is key to pregnancy and life itself.

This chapter discusses the placenta. We briefly outline some history before discussing the anatomy and physiology of this essential pregnancy-enabling organ. Pathophysiology of the most common placental abnormalities which lead to women experiencing life-threatening pregnancy-related conditions are explored. We navigate all stages of pregnancy with a focus on the placenta, highlighting the role of the midwife and multidisciplinary team during the childbearing period.

Background

The Latin word placenta derives from the Greek term *plakuos*, which means 'flat cake', in reference to its morphological shape. Mossman (1937) originally defined the normal placenta in mammals as 'an opposition or fusion of the fetal membranes to the uterine mucosa for physiological exchange' (Mossman 1937, cited by Burton and Foden 2015). The placenta has historically been a focal point of attention for individuals with an interest in medical science, but it has also been subject of artistic representations dating back to Egyptian times (Romero 2015). The birth of a baby surrounded by amniotic fluid and intact placental membranes has been considered as lucky in some cultures for centuries. The placenta has also had a crucial role in traditional Chinese medicine, where the benefits of placental tissues in treating a range of illnesses continues to be supported by medical journal publications since the sixteenth century (Silini et al. 2015). Its unique role in growing and preserving fetal life has led to numerous investigations in neonatal intervention, attempting to mimic physiological oxygenation processes in infants born severely premature (Schoberer et al. 2012).

Understanding of the placenta and its functions in contemporary medicine began to develop in the second part of the eighteenth century. This began with the revelation of the existence of separate fetal and maternal placental circulations, a discovery by John Hunter and Colin Mackenzie in 1754. It would be in the twentieth century that the placenta would gain acknowledgement for its holistic role, acting as a multifunctional organ for the growing fetus. Specifically, but not limited to, it has a role in sustaining circulation, oxygenation, metabolism and other key physiological functions, as well as facilitating removal of fetal waste products (Roberts et al. 2016). Equally important, the placenta would be found to contribute to fetal protection. This is done by selectively filtering and partly acting as a barrier to a number of external agents, while regulating key functions to support healthy development of the fetus. Anomalies in the anatomy or functioning of the placenta can therefore negatively impact the development of a healthy pregnancy, thus potentially affecting the wellbeing of the mother and the unborn infant (Jauniaux et al. 2022). Despite the advances in knowledge, human understanding of placental development, physiology and pathophysiology continues to have limitations. The following sections aim to help the reader to expand their understanding of the physiological development and functioning of the placenta.

Placental Anatomy and Physiology

Formation and Development

Placental formation is originally triggered by the blastocyst, which is the fertilised egg containing embryonic and trophoblast stem cells. Following fertilisation, which occurs in the distal part of the fallopian tube, the production and release of human chorionic gonadotrophin (hCG) starts preparing the endometrium for implantation. Structural changes lead to the development of enhanced venous and arterial connections. As a result, the decidua becomes more vascular, which will later support intraplacental flow. During this time, development of the fertilised egg has been supported by the secretion of glycogen and other nutrients from the uterine glands.

The blastocyst undergoes a process of cell division (mitosis) while it travels through the fallopian tube, forming two main layers of cells called the embryoblast (which will subsequently form the embryo) and the trophoblast (outer layer of cells). Approximately seven days after conception takes place, the blastocyst makes contact with the decidua. This is known as the prelacunar stage and marks the start of implantation. As the blastocyst embeds itself into the endometrium, the trophoblast differentiates itself into two layers: the cytotrophoblast (inner, cellular layer) and the syncytiotrophoblast (outer, acellular layer). During the lacunar stage, a number of chemical and hormonal reactions will lead to further development of syncytiotrophoblasts surrounding the blastocyst. As a result, small lacunae form within the cells, creating intervillous spaces. At this point, the decidua provides nutrients to the fertilised egg due to its secretory function and supported by the hormonal release of progesterone (Bailey 2014).

Vascular adaptations, alongside immunological ones, are crucial at supporting placental development until intraplacental blood flow is complete at around 10–12 weeks. At the end of the second week, the cytotrophoblast start to expand into the syncytiotrophoblast, which leads to the formation of primary chorionic villi. These structures are finger-like projections and consist of membranes surrounding the embryo; they contain blood vessels and will later form the chorionic villous tree. Although the initial vessels develop from progenitor cells, their additional development will lead to the creation of a vascular system interconnecting all vessels via the umbilical vein and arteries. This is gradually achieved early in the third week due to the formation of secondary chorionic villi, entailing the growth of extra embryonic mesoderm into the villi, forming a main loose connective tissue early in the third week (Jauniaux et al. 2022). Figure 7.1 illustrates chorionic villi and Figure 7.2 shows the blood flow around the chorionic villi.

By the end of the third week, embryonic vessels begin to form, leading to the development of tertiary chorionic villi. From there, cytotrophoblast cells continue to grow towards the decidua basalis, spreading across and establishing the anchoring and branch villi (Figure 7.3). This will ultimately serve as the main site for gas exchange between the fetus and the mother. While fetal blood flow is initiated by week 4, fetoplacental circulation will not be fully established until week 8.

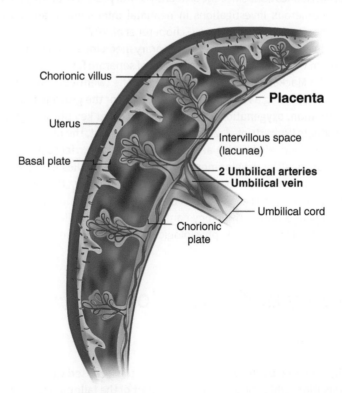

FIGURE 7.1   Chorionic villi. Source: Sakurra/Adobe Stock Photos.

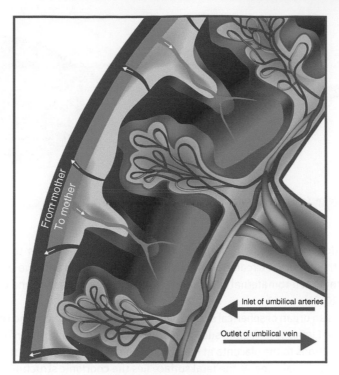

FIGURE 7.2 Blood flow around the chorionic villi. Source: Sakurra/Adobe Stock Photos.

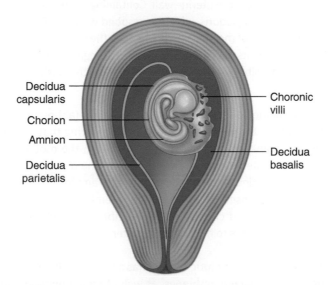

FIGURE 7.3 Site of implantation at week 3.

During the first trimester of pregnancy, placental metabolism is rarely reliant on oxygen to protect the fetus from electrons and oxygen free radicals. At this point, fetomaternal circulation allows deoxygenated blood to be transported from the fetus to the placenta. This is done via umbilical arteries, which extend in the form of branches into the chorionic villi prior to dispersing into capillary networks at the terminal ends. From there, carbon dioxide and waste products from the fetus are removed via the placental membranes and transferred to maternal blood and the intervillous space. Concomitantly, oxygenated blood and nutrients are transported across the placental membranes from maternal blood to

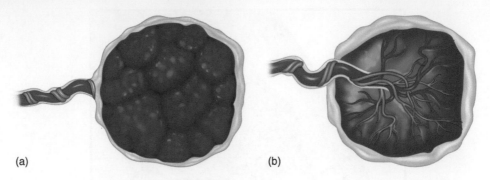

(a)   (b)

FIGURE 7.4   The placenta at term. (a) Maternal surface. (b) Fetal surface.

the fetal capillaries. This is done via veins, which join to form a single umbilical vein that is connected to the fetus. Thereafter, blood returns to the maternal circulation through endometrial veins and due to the pressure of the arterial blood arriving. It is at this point that fetomaternal circulation is functionally established and circulatory reciprocity finally achieved (Turco and Moffett 2019).

The placenta at full term is an organ of spherical shape, with a diameter of 20–22 cm and thickness of 2.5 cm in its core, and an average weight of 470 g (Figure 7.4). Factors such as mode of birth and timing of cord clamping at birth may cause weight and morphological variations to the placenta at macroscopic inspection. The placenta has significant morphological differences in its fetal and maternal sites. At the fetal surface lies the chorionic structure covered by the amnion. The umbilical cord is usually sited centrally and comprises a network of vessels forms by chorionic veins (providing blood to the single umbilical vein) and arteries (supplying the villous trees). The maternal surface of the placenta is formed by the basal plate and results from its separation from the uterine wall. Containing a number of cells, this structure is dark red in colour and is formed of 10–40 lobes called cotyledons, which correspond with 60–70 villous trees in a full-term placenta. Findings related to microscopic examination of the placenta are beyond the scope of this chapter, but further corroborate the anatomical complexity of this organ and its development from early pregnancy to term (Huppertz 2008).

Pregnancy and birth would not be possible without the crucial role that the cord, placental membranes and amniotic fluid play:

- The umbilical cord is 1–2 cm in diameter and around 50 cm in length, (although this varies). It is responsible for transporting oxygen and nutrients to the developing fetus, while ensuring that waste products are removed from circulation. It contains one vein (transporting oxygenated blood from the mother to the fetus) and two arteries (transporting carbon dioxide and waste products from the baby to the mother). These vessels are surrounded by Wharton's jelly, which serves as protection, and an extended layer of amnion.
- The chorioamnion membrane is composed of amnion (inner membrane containing amniotic fluid and prostaglandin E2, which helps start labour) and chorion (outer membrane, which produces enzymes to help reduce levels of progesterone as well as hormones to help stimulate uterine activity such as prostaglandins and oxytocin; Figure 7.5).
- The amniotic fluid is contained within the amniotic sac and has a clear or yellowish colour. It originates mainly from maternal circulation through the placental membranes, as well as fetal lung fluid and urine. The amniotic fluid is mostly formed of water (99%), as well as some particulates from waste products. Its volume increases from 20 ml at 10 weeks to an average 500 ml at term (Bailey 2014).

Placental Functions

The placenta has four main functions to fulfil to make pregnancy and fetal life possible: gas exchange, metabolism, endocrine or hormonal secretion and provision of immunity.

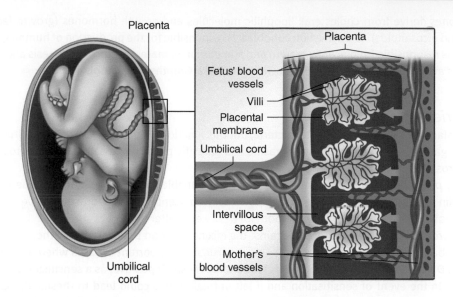

Placenta

Placenta

Fetus' blood
vessels

Villi

Placental
membrane

Umbilical cord

Intervillous
space

Mother's
blood vessels

Umbilical
cord

FIGURE 7.5   The chorioamnion membrane. Bailey (2014)/Elsevier.

Gas Exchange

Fetomaternal exchange of gases takes place through the placenta, which becomes primarily responsible for the transfer of oxygen and removal of carbon dioxide in the developing fetus. Transfer of oxygen and carbon dioxide is mainly passive and depends on the pressure gradient between maternal (in the intervillous space) and fetal blood (in the umbilical arteries), respectively. Thus, oxygen crosses the placenta via diffusion and assisted by fetal haemoglobin, which has higher concentration and affinity for oxygen to sustain oxygenation. The process is complemented by the role of deoxygenated blood in being able to transport high amounts of carbon dioxide (Macnab 2022)

Metabolic Function

The placenta has the ability to synthesise glycogen, protein, cholesterol and fatty acids, among other substances.

- *Glucose*: since the fetus has limited capacity to generate glucose from non-carbohydrate sources, the placenta maximises the supply of maternal glucose to the fetus via the placenta by using glucose transporters.
- *Amino acids*: a number of proteins transport amino acids from the mother to the fetus, which will later facilitate the synthesis of protein. This process is often assisted by sodium molecules to help transfer amino acids into the cells.
- *Fatty acids* have an essential role in cell signalling and the production of phospholipids, membranes and myelin. To activate this process, lipoprotein (present on the maternal surface of the placenta) breaks down lipoproteins into free fatty acids, which, alongside glycerol, are later transported to the fetus.
- *Electrolytes, vitamins and water*: sodium, chloride, calcium, iron, vitamins and water are transferred across the placenta to further support metabolism and fetal growth (Griffiths and Campbell 2015).

Endocrine Function

The placenta is responsible for the production of peptide and steroid hormones, to mitigate the lack of nerve supply:

- *Peptide hormones* are mostly produced by the trophoblast cells within the chorionic villi: hCG (produced in early pregnancy by the syncytiotrophoblast to stimulate progesterone release to help make pregnancy viable), human placenta lactogen (hPL, produced by the syncytiotrophoblast to reduce maternal insulin sensitivity, hence increasing glucose levels in maternal blood, as well as stimulating the production of surfactant fluid and breast development to assist with milk production), insulin-like growth factor and corticotrophin-releasing hormone.

133

- *Steroid hormones* derive from cholesterol: lipophilic molecules and growth hormones (growth factor, cytokines, chemokines and eicosanoids). The syncytiotrophoblast is responsible for the production of human growth hormone variant, which is responsible for placental growth and stimulation of maternal gluconeogenesis and lipolysis to help make nutrients available to the developing fetus (Macnab 2022; Griffiths and Campbell 2015).

Protective Barrier/Immune Function

- *Infection*: the placenta can act as barrier to bacteria, but this function is limited. Indeed, many viruses (such as HIV, human cytomegalovirus, rubella) and some parasitic and parasitic protozoan diseases (such as toxoplasmosis and malaria) can cross the placenta.
- *Immunological protection*: the vast majority of proteins are unable to cross the placenta due to their size, but immunoglobulin (IgG) antibodies from the mother do cross the placenta. This is a form of passive immunity from the mother to the baby, which will protect the newborn for 6–12 weeks after birth.
- *Resus disease protection*: natural protection against the mixing of blood between the mother and fetus is possible because of the barrier function of the placenta. This is particularly important in cases where the mother is known to be of rhesus D negative blood and the fetus is found to be rhesus D positive, as a sensitising event could lead to rhesus conflict. In the event of sensitisation and if left untreated, this could lead to rhesus disease – a condition where fetal blood enters the maternal circulation, activating maternal antibodies to fight against fetal antigens and cells, which can ultimately lead to fetal malformations and death.
- *Pharmacological and recreational drugs*: the placenta is only able to filter high molecular weight substances. Some pharmacological components and substances contained within recreational drugs (alcohol, smoking, chemical drugs) will cross the placenta, which may impair fetal growth and health (Griffiths and Campbell 2015; Bailey 2014).

Reflective Learning Activity

Thinking of the key functions of the placenta. How would you would explain these functions to an expectant mother/couple who tell you that they do not understand how nutrients, oxygen and protection are provided to a baby in the womb?

Placental Anomalies and Pathophysiology

Knowledge of placental anomalies and early diagnosis has been made possible due to advances in ultrasound. Availability of resources and accessibility will vary in different healthcare systems and settings. The existence of placental abnormalities in pregnancy has the potential to negatively influence pregnancy viability and affect maternal and fetal/neonatal morbidity and mortality. Early diagnosis and appropriate management can mitigate some of the risk.

Placental Anomalies

Placental anomalies may be differentiated into those caused by placentation itself, those of a vascular origin and those that relate to the umbilical cord.

Placentation Anomalies

The location of a placenta can often be seen in a pregnancy dating ultrasound scan. However, it becomes particularly significant and is often reported during the routine anomaly scan, recommended between 18+0 and 20+6 weeks of gestation according to the NHS England FAST programme (NHSE 2023, NHSE 2022). Although placentation will be uneventful for most pregnancies, implantation anomalies may lead to conditions that can significantly complicate pregnancies.

TABLE 7.1   Types of placenta praevia.

Grade	Classification	Extent
1	Minor praevia	Lower edge inside the lower segment
2	Marginal praevia	Lower edge reaching the internal os
3	Partial praevia	Covering the cervix partially
4	Complete praevia	Covering the cervix fully

Source: Adapted from RCOG (2018).

Placenta Praevia

Placenta praevia refers to a placenta that implants and develops in the lower uterine segment, either fully or partially, and is within 20 mm of the internal os. Depending on the proximity between the placental edge and the os of the cervix, placenta praevia can be classified as grades 1–4, with increasing severity and risks (Table 7.1). In instances where the placental edge is more than 20 mm but less than 35 mm from the internal os, placentas are defined as 'low lying'.

The incidence of placenta praevia is 4–5 per 1000 pregnancies in the UK and worldwide (Jauniaux et al. 2018; Cresswell et al. 2013). Risk factors such as previous caesarean section, assisted reproduction and smoking increase the chances of placenta praevia. Although rare, the condition can trigger maternal complications (including antepartum/ postpartum haemorrhage and septicaemia), as well as fetal and neonatal complications (including preterm birth and fetal death). Where a placenta is found to be low lying, a placental location scan is usually recommended in the third trimester to redefine location (Jansen et al. 2020; Jauniaux et al. 2018).

135

Placenta Accreta

Placenta accreta is a spectrum referring to a placenta that partially or completely adheres to the underlying uterine wall. Depending on the extent of the invasion of the villi into the myometrium, it is further classified as adherent or creta (superficial adherence), increta (deep invasion into the myometrium and serosa) and percreta (perforation of the uterine wall and adherence to other organs).

Histopathological examinations by means of modern ultrasonography is essential in the identification and diagnosis of placentation abnormalities, which supports management options. The lack of universal access to imaging resources contributes to the uncertainty in the reported incidence of placenta accreta, with variations ranging from 1 in 300–2000 pregnancies. This has in some cases led to professionals using 'misleading' terminology that is outcome based, such as the term 'morbidly adherent placenta' when referring to retained placentas that result in clinical complications. For clarify and consistency, the Royal College of Obstetricians and Gynaecologists (RCOG) advocates the use of the term *placenta accreta spectrum* (Jansen et al. 2020; Jauniaux et al. 2018).

Vascular Abnormalities

Defective placentation may cause impairment in uteroplacental circulation, which can lead to the development of placental vascular abnormalities. These are often divided into maternal and fetal vascular abnormalities. The conditions listed here are common vascular abnormalities.

Haematomas

Haematomas can occur because of accidental leakage of either maternal or fetal blood. This process is also known as extravasation and, depending on the focus of bleeding, the haemorrhage may be subamniotic, subchorionic or retroplacental. Maternal bleeding can be identified on ultrasound in 1% of all early pregnancies. Bleeding beyond seven weeks increases the risk of miscarriage, preterm birth, abruption and low birth weight.

Thrombosis and Infarcts

Thrombosis and infarcts are more often seen in the third trimester. A thrombosis is a blood clot that often originates in the intervillous space and travels through placental circulation to a more central point, causing an obstruction. A placental infarction is the interruption of blood supply to a given area of the placenta, causing local necrosis. Thrombosis and infarcts may be caused by pregnancy complications such as essential hypertension or pre-eclampsia and can lead to fetal growth restriction and fetal death (Kovo et al. 2013; Jauniaux et al. 2022).

Anomalies of the Umbilical Cord

The two most common umbilical cord-related anomalies are the presence of single umbilical artery and vasa praevia.

Single Umbilical Artery

The incidence of single umbilical artery is 1% of all pregnancies. It can be identified at the anomaly scan, prompting further follow-up and investigations. Although rare, the presence of a single umbilical artery can be associated with fetal malformation and velamentous insertion. Following birth, the neonatologist may request follow-up investigations to exclude the presence of other undiagnosed anomalies related to the heart, kidneys or other organs.

Vasa Praevia

Vasa praevia is defined as the presence of fetal vessels running through the membranes unprotected by the placental tissue or umbilical cord. This means that they are not supported by Wharton's jelly, a mucoid connective tissue (see Chapter 6). Because of this, they are subject to potential compression changes, especially in instances where cervical dilation has taken place and the presenting fetal part has descended (e.g. where spontaneous rupture of membranes takes place combined with cervical dilation or where an artificial rupture of membranes may be required). Vasa praevia usually occurs as a result of velamentous insertion and is more commonly seen in women with placentation abnormalities (e.g. placenta praevia; Jauniaux et al. 2022)

Placenta-related Disorders

Many pregnancy-related diseases have traditionally been defined around the placenta as a vascular network. This is the case because placental anomalies will often affect its vascular function, causing a reduction in blood supply and therefore affecting the transport of oxygen and nutrients. Placental disorders are often divided into ischaemic and non-ischaemic (Maltepe and Fisher 2015). We cover only some of the more common disorders affecting pregnancy here.

Pulmonary Embolism

Pulmonary embolism is defined as the obstruction of the pulmonary arterial system by one of more emboli, which leads to severe respiratory dysfunction. A pulmonary embolism can be provoked, where it occurs following a recent (within three months) and transient risk factor, or unprovoked (when the condition happens in the absence of transient risk factors) (NICE 2023c). Pulmonary embolism is a leading direct cause of maternal death in the UK and many other countries, with 70–89% having identifiable risks factors.

Pregnancy may increase the risk of pulmonary embolism due to inadequate vascular remodelling of maternal uterine spiral arterioles. This can lead to two main complications. First, the presence of defective endovascular formation causes damage to the chorionic villi (due to increased pressure), leading to the release of clotting factor into maternal circulation. Second, impaired vascularisation increased resistance in the uterine arteries, reducing blood flow to the placenta and fetus.

The exacerbation of these complications can lead to systemic vasculitis and hypertension, characteristics of pulmonary embolism (Maltepe and Fisher 2015). Women who are identified to be at risk of pulmonary embolism should be under obstetric care. Preventive treatment is often recommended in the form of thromboprophylaxis with low molecular weight heparin (RCOG 2015).

Medications Management: Deep Vein Thrombosis and Pulmonary Embolism

In the event of suspected venous thromboembolism, anticoagulant LMWH treatment is recommended, unless contraindicated (RCOG 2015). The dose of LMWH should be titrated according to the woman's weight.

In the event of pulmonary embolism and collapse, NHS trust guidelines should be followed. Management options often include the use of intravenous unfractionated heparin (preferred treatment), thrombolytic therapy and thoracotomy and surgical embolectomy.

A multidisciplinary approach to managing pulmonary embolism is crucial and would normally include obstetricians, radiologists, physicians, anaesthetists and midwives.

Non-pharmacological interventions support diagnosis and treatment, including diagnostic testing, such an echocardiogram or computed tomography pulmonary angiogram. Treatment options may include elastic compression stockings to reduce oedema, mobilisation (when possible) and hydration (where not contraindicated).

Vitamin K antagonists (like warfarin) are contraindicated to treat venous thromboembolism antenatally due to their potential adverse effects on the fetus.

Intrauterine Growth Restriction

Intrauterine growth restriction (IUGR) refers to an abnormal impairment of the growth potential of a fetus (for maternal, placental, fetal or extrinsic reasons). IUGR should not be mistaken with small-for-gestational age, which refers to babies who are born with a birth weight less than the 10th centile (RCOG 2014) but may just be constitutionally small (based on maternal or fetal characteristics). Severe vascular insufficiency is commonly seen in pregnancies with IUGR. Clinical examination and ultrasound fetal measurements are used in the identification and subsequent management of IUGR. Fetal growth restriction can ultimately result in complications in pregnancy. Once diagnosis is made, more specific testing to monitor IUGR may include cardiotocography, uterine fetal Doppler and ultrasound to assess biophysical activity. These investigations help to plan the best timing for delivery (RCOG 2014).

Preterm Labour

Preterm labour refers to pregnancies where labour commences before 37 weeks of gestation and can lead to preterm birth, where a baby is born before term. The rate of preterm birth is around 8% (World Health Organization 2022). The aetiology of preterm labour can be multifactorial. From a placental perspective, trophoblast invasion, vascular remodelling and the presence of placental and intrauterine infections can lead to preterm labour and birth. The management and care of a woman with threatened or confirmed preterm labour may include the use of corticosteroids to enhance fetal lung maturity, magnesium sulphate for fetal neuroprotection, amnioinfusion and labour care interventions, including continuous fetal monitoring and neonatal involvement (Thomson 2019).

Hypertensive Disorders

Some hypertensive disorders can appear before, during of after pregnancy. Pre-eclampsia (previously known as pre-eclamptic toxaemia) is a condition that appears during second trimester of pregnancy and is characterised by hypertension and proteinuria and/or evidence of maternal acute kidney injury, liver dysfunction, neurological features, haemolysis, thrombocytopenia and/or fetal growth restriction. The condition affect up to 5% of UK pregnant women. Although its aetiology is not fully understood, some theories pinpoint inadequate development of the placenta as the leading reason for defective fetomaternal blood supply – this is known as uteroplacental ischaemia. Symptoms include severe headache, problems with vision (blurred vision/flashing lights), severe epigastric pain, vomiting and sudden oedema of the face, hands and/or feet. Pre-eclampsia must be treated to ensure maternal and fetal wellbeing. Severe pre-eclampsia can result in maternal eclamptic seizure and fetal death (Brown et al. 2018; NICE 2019a).

Medications Management: Severe Pre-eclampsia and Eclampsia

Antihypertensive pharmacological treatment is offered to women with blood pressure readings above 140/90 mm/Hg (NICE 2023a). In the event of unstable or uncontrolled blood pressure, admission may be required so that further diagnostic tests can be used. Urinalysis is offered to rule out proteinuria. Blood tests allow monitoring of renal function and full blood count. Fetal assessment is also undertaken in the form of a cardiotocography (CTG) where appropriate.

In terms of pharmacological treatment, labetalol is often used to treat hypertension in pregnancy in women with confirmed pre-eclampsia. Women for whom labetalol may not be suitable can be offered nifedipine or methyldopa.

Depending on the severity of the condition and gestational age, conversations regarding time of birth will contribute to safety for both mother and their unborn child.

Eclampsia is treated with anticonvulsants and antihypertensives. These include:

- Anticonvulsants: magnesium sulphate (loading dose, infusion and recurrent doses where necessary); diazepam, phenytoin or other anticonvulsants are not recommended.
- Antihypertensives: commonly labetalol (oral/intravenous), nifedipine (oral) or hydralazine (intravenous).
- Crystalloid fluids may also be considered, alongside corticosteroid to help mature the fetal lungs. A strict fluid input/output balance is crucial to assist with blood pressure management, without causing any further kidney damage.

Emergency procedures and referral to critical care and the multidisciplinary and interdisciplinary team will be required in the event of eclampsia.

The Midwife and the Placenta: Care and Considerations

Role of the Midwife

Midwives are autonomous practitioners who provide care and support women and birthing people through the pregnancy journey. They do this by leading pregnancy care in the absence of complications and working alongside the wider multidisciplinary team, where obstetric/medical support is required. Working alongside the pregnancy continuum places midwives in a crucial position to support physiological processes and detect deviations from the norm, working within their scope of practice and referring to other healthcare professionals where necessary (Nursing and Midwifery Council 2018, 2021).

The standards of proficiency for midwives (2019a) and those of preregistration of midwifery programmes (2019b) highlight the role of the midwife in assessing, screening and care planning. Specifically, the standards highlight a midwife's responsibility in supporting the birth of the placenta and membranes, as well as its clinical inspection following the birth, to assess completeness. In addition, the standards identify the role that midwives play in initiating first-line management of any potential emergencies and supporting the multidisciplinary team when manual removal of the placenta is required (Nursing and Midwifery Council 2019a,b).

Within the role of a midwife in providing effective, holistic and evidence-based care during the childbearing period, there are a number of considerations in relation to the placenta as an organ that need to be taken into account.

Pregnancy

As coordinators of care, midwives are responsible for completing health and risk assessments during the pregnancy journey. In matters that affect placental health, midwives regularly enquire about vaginal bleeding, fetal movements and arrange ultrasound scans. These scans will include a dating and anomaly scan, when these are offered and accepted by the woman.

Where risk factors are present that will prompt closer monitoring and/or investigations, women are referred to obstetricians and other members of the multidisciplinary/interdisciplinary team (e.g. anaesthetists, endocrinologists, cardiologists, neonatologists, sonographers) to support care provision (NICE 2019). In instances where placental anomalies are identified, women may need to be referred to a tertiary centre with specialist services that provide specialist testing, advice and counselling. Women may be advised to give birth in specialised units, depending on the level of severity of the concern, type and level of maternity and neonatal units where the woman is receiving care, chosen/expected timing and mode of birth and extent of the diagnosis.

Offering antenatal education to women about Braxton Hicks (latent phase) contractions and active labour contractions, as well as their expected frequency, is crucial in supporting women make informed choices and know when to ask for midwifery support or self-refer to an obstetric unit. The NHS website has information available to women regarding complications that can affect the normal functioning the placenta (NICE 2023b; NHS England 2022).

Labour and Birth

Assessment of uterine activity during labour is crucial to support normal placental functioning (and therefore maternal and fetal health) while prompting identification of placental functional anomalies. As part of the initial labour assessment, midwives enquire about the length, strength and frequency of uterine contractions, as well as the level of pain experienced by women. This assessment will also include monitoring of any vaginal loss and other haemodynamic parameters (maternal pulse, blood pressure and temperature), all of which support the holistic assessment of the pregnant woman. Monitoring of the fetal heart by means of intermittent auscultation or continuous fetal monitoring, depending on risk assessment and the individual needs and wishes of the woman, indirectly contribute to assessment of normal placental functioning. Uterine activity will be monitored and documented at least half-hourly during the first and second stages of labour to help confirm normality or detect deviations from it (i.e. presence of irregular contractions that may prompt recommendation for medical intervention). This documentation is often complete in the woman's intrapartum records (printed notes and/or digital). In the event of bleeding, continuous pain or excessive uterine tone (tachysystole, hypersystole, hyperstimulation), midwives are expected to follow local policy and activate emergency referral pathways, escalating concerns to the obstetric and anaesthetic teams (NICE 2023b).

Snapshot 7.1   Placental Abruption

As a student midwife, you are allocated to work alongside a midwife during a shift on labour ward. You are caring for an expectant mother who is a primigravida and is undergoing continuous electronic fetal monitoring as she had some antenatal bleeding on admission. She is currently 5 cm dilated and the midwife asks you to exclude placental abruption.

Reflective Learning Activity

Taking into account what you have learned about the role of the midwife during pregnancy and birth, and within the scope of the subject of this chapter:

- What antenatal information and admission details might you review to exclude abnormal placentation?
- What parameters within a CTG could provide you with information about uterine activity?
- How else could you observe and search for evidence of bleeding?
- What other considerations might you need to take into account when completing the assessment (i.e. maternal consent and intact membranes)?
- How would you document your findings?

Imminent Postnatal Period

Following the birth of a baby, the third stage of labour commences and involves the delivery of the placenta and membranes. This process is driven by the release of oxytocin, causing the uterine muscles to continue to contract. During the second stage of labour, the uterus starts decreasing as the fetus descends through the birth canal. The reduction in size of the site where the placenta is attached, alongside a reduction in its vascularity, causes the placenta to begin to separate from the uterine wall. The type of placental separation will vary depending on the position of the placenta. Further uterine contractions will help the placenta to move to the lower uterine segment and into the vagina. Membranes follow and the umbilical cord may be seen to lengthen. As the placenta sits in the lower segment of the uterus, it stimulates physiological maternal pushing which, alongside gravity, will aid the birth of the placenta and membranes. The bleeding that follows the birth of the placenta is the result of blood vessels in the decidua rupturing due to increased pressure and some blood loss (normal up to 500 ml) in the third stage of labour. The third stage is complete when the bleeding is controlled (Kirwan 2022)

In terms of management of the third stage of labour, there are generally two ways in which the process can take place, with benefits and risks associated with both (NICE 2023b):

1. *Physiologically*, where the placenta and membranes are delivered by maternal effort without using uterotonic medication and without the clamping and cutting of the cord until it stops pulsating. This process may take up to one hour from the birth. Physiological management of the third stage is less likely to produce nausea (90/1000), but it does increase the risk of haemorrhage of more than 500 ml (188/1000) and the need for further uteronics (247/1000) and blood transfusion (35/1000; NICE 2023b).

2. *Actively*, where uterotonic medication is provided alongside mechanical actions such as controlled cord traction and deferred cord clamping and cutting, to facilitate the delivery of the placenta and membranes. The process should be complete within 30 minutes following on from the birth. Active management of the third stage increases the risk of nausea and vomiting (186/1000) but reduces the risk of haemorrhage of more than 500 ml (13/1000) and the need for uteronics (47/1000) and blood transfusion (68/1000) (NICE 2023b).

In the UK, the majority of women will experience an active management of the third stage of labour. Physiological management of the third stage is often seen as a choice that is mostly offered to women who have had an uneventful pregnancy and a birth without or with minimal interventions. Most research studies on management of the third stage of labour undertaken to date have been based in obstetric settings. Thus, there is little understanding on best management approach for women who choose to birth at home or in midwifery units, who are at low risk of suffering from a postpartum haemorrhage (Baker et al. 2021).

Midwives may facilitate delivery of the placenta by encouraging the woman to mobilise (where possible) and empty her bladder. In instances where delivery of the placenta does not take place after 30 minutes following active management or after 60 minutes in physiological management, a diagnosis of prolonged or delayed third stage of labour is made. At this point, a multidisciplinary discussion takes place to assist in planning and offering interventions to help deliver the placenta and membranes and avoid further complications. This would normally involve insertion of an intravenous cannula and administration of fluids, vaginal examination to determine the location of the placenta, insertion of a urinary catheter to help reduce bladder size, and administration of further uterotonic medication. Where delivery of the placenta and membranes is attempted but unsuccessful, a diagnosis of retained placenta is made. At this point, transfer to the operating theatre and manual removal of products of conception under a regional anaesthesia may be required. Failed timely separation and delivery of the placenta increases the risk of postpartum haemorrhage; the multidisciplinary team should be prepared to manage this potential complication, which would include the use of further uterotonic medication, fluid replacement, bimanual compression and potentially the need for blood transfusion.

Midwives are responsible for completing an examination of the placenta and membranes after birth, confirming completeness of the placenta and membranes and detecting any anomalies related to excessive blood loss (Nursing and Midwifery Council 2019a). As part of this process, midwives will ensure an assessment of the structure of the placenta, its condition, the presence of cord vessels and that it is complete at delivery (that is, the amnion and chorion are present, with no cotyledons missing and no ragged or missing membranes). Any placental blood sampling that may be indicated can be completed at this point (e.g. paired cord gases from a doubly clamped cord or cord blood for any other purposes, such as rhesus isoimmunisation, thyroid or any other indication) with maternal consent. Where no anomalies are detected, the placenta and membranes will be disposed of following local policies.

Should the examination of the placenta and membranes identify any anomalies, the woman would be referred to obstetric care. In some instances, products of conception may need to undergo histopathological analysis to exclude further anomalies. Local guidelines and standard operating procedures should be followed (NICE 2023b).

Red Flag Alerts: Delayed Third Stage

Where delivery of the placenta does not take place after 30 minutes following active management or after 60 minutes in physiological management, a diagnosis of prolonged or delayed third stage of labour is made. Failed timely separation and delivery of the placenta increases the risk of postpartum haemorrhage.

Snapshot 7.2   Delivery of the Placenta

You are looking after an expectant couple having their first child and undergoing induction of labour. They have arrived to delivery suite and you commence care by introducing yourself and reviewing their care plan. You notice that the parents have documented they prefer a 'physiological delivery of the placenta, using oxytocin'.

Reflective Learning Activity

- How would you approach the subject and test understanding in a non-judgemental way?
- How can you ensure that the couple have the necessary information they need to make an informed choice?
- What information will you provide them with?
- How would you proceed to document the outcome of your discussion?

Postnatal Period

Following the birth of the placenta and membranes, physiological uterine involution commences, causing the uterine cavity to progressively decrease in size. As part of maternal health checks in the immediate postnatal period, midwives have traditionally undertaken an abdominal palpation to confirm that the uterus is central and well contracted. This check is part of the assessment of placental completeness and to assess the risk of postpartum haemorrhage, although evidence in this area is not conclusive. Monitoring of uterine involution by using a tape measure is not evidence based.

Involution is also assessed in terms of vaginal loss during the postnatal period, with bleeding minimising over time until it becomes light (Fraser and Cullen 2009). NICE (2021) guidelines no longer include routine abdominal palpation to confirm uterine involution in the wellbeing assessment of the postnatal mother. Although involution will be different form woman to woman, it is generally accepted that, by 10th postnatal day, the uterus will no longer be palpable. Midwives must continue to apply their judgement and monitor for signs of retained placenta, sepsis and haemorrhage.

Reflective Learning Activity

Reflect on the role of the midwife in relation to the placenta during pregnancy, birth and the postnatal period. Identify examples from clinical placement where you feel that your practice, advice or actions would be different as a result of the learning acquired through this chapter.

- What was your previous approach and why is there a need for you to practice differently?
- How will you ensure that your acquired knowledge and newly adopted practice will be sustained moving forward?
- How could you share your learning with your colleagues?

Take Home Points

- Placental formation is triggered by the blastocyst and the release of hCG, causing the decidua to become more vascular and preparing for intraplacental flow. Structural adjustments following contact between the decidua and the blastocyst will trigger vascular changes that will later lead to uterofetal vascularisation.
- At full term, the placenta has a diameter of 20–22 cm, a thickness of 2.5 cm and weighs an average of 470 g. It has a fetal site, containing the chorion, amnion and cord, as well as a maternal site, including placental lobes.
- The placenta has a number of vital functions, including:
  - Gas exchange
  - Metabolic
  - Endocrine
  - Protective barrier.
- Anomalies of the placenta lead to an increase in fetal and maternal morbidity and mortality. Early diagnosis, follow-up with investigations and multidisciplinary interventions are crucial in pregnancy and birth management.
- Placenta-related disorders can also negatively affect maternal and fetal health. These may include pulmonary embolism, IUGR, preterm labour and hypertensive disorders.
- Midwives have a vital role in supporting women from the early stages of pregnancy, through labour and birth. By offering women investigations to confirm the healthy functioning of a placenta and detect anomalies, midwives activate referrals to other members of the multidisciplinary team. In their role as birth experts and collaborating with other through teamwork, midwives enhance surveillance and thereafter safety for mothers and their babies during pregnancy, birth and the postnatal period. This is achieved through risk assessments, monitoring and safeguarding during the birth and facilitation of delivery of the placenta and membranes.

142

Summary

The placenta is a transient but crucial organ that supports human life from its origin until birth. Anatomically speaking, its structural complexity is the end result of hormonal and physiological changes driven by fertilisation to serve the purpose of growing fetal life. Physiologically, it is the interceptor between the mother and the embryo, supporting vital body functions without which fetal live may not be fulfilled. In instances, anomalies in implantation or vascularisation can lead to placenta-related complications that may compromise a healthy pregnancy and put both the mother and the unborn child at risk. Midwives play a crucial role in monitoring fetomaternal wellbeing, supporting physiological processes, initiating investigations and referrals where necessary, so that the multidisciplinary team can work together to support physiological processes and manage deviations from normality.

References

Bailey, J. (2014). The placenta. In: *Myles' Textbook for Midwives* (ed. J.E. Marshal and D.M. Raynor), 91–100. Amsterdam: Elsevier Health Sciences.

Baker, K., Stephenson, J., Leeming, D., and Soltani, H. (2021). A review of the third stage of labour care guidance. *British Journal of Midwifery* 29 (10): 557–563.

Brown, M.A., Magee, L.A., Kenny, L.C. et al. (2018). The hypertensive disorders of pregnancy: ISSHP classification, diagnosis & management recommendations for international practice. *Pregnancy Hypertension* 13: 291–310. https://doi.org/10.1016/j.preghy.2018.05.004.

Burton, G.J. and Fowden, A.L. (2015). The placenta: a multifaceted, transient organ. *Philosophical Transactions of the Royal Society B* 370 (1663): 1–8. https://doi.org/10.1098/rstb.2014.0066.

Cresswell, J.A., Ronsmans, C., Calvert, C., and Filippi, V. (2013). Prevalence of placenta praevia by world region: a systematic review and meta-analysis. *Trompical Medicine and International Health* 18 (6): 712–724.

Fraser, D. and Cullen, L. (2009). Postnatal management and breastfeeding. *Obstetrics, Gynaecology and Reproductive Medicine* 19 (1): 7–12.

Griffiths, S.K. and Campbell, J.P. (2015). Placental structure, function and drug transfer. *Continuing Education in Anaesthesia Critical Care & Pain* 15 (2): 84–89. https://doi.org/10.1093/bjaceaccp/mku013.

Huppertz, B. (2008). The anatomy of the normal placenta. *Journal of Clinical Pathology* 61 (12): 1296–1302.

Jansen, C.H.J.R., Kastelein, A.W., Kleinrouweler, C.E. et al. (2020). Development of placental abnormalities in location. *Acta Obstetricia et Gynecologica Scandinavica* 99 (8): 983–993. https://doi.org/10.1111/aogs.13834.

Jauniaux, E.R.M., Alfirevic, A., Bhide, A.G. et al. (2018). Placenta praevia and placenta acreta: diagnosis and management. Green-top Guideline No. 27a. *BJOG* 126 (1): e1–e48.

Jauniaux, E., Bide, A., and Burton, G.J. (2022). The placenta. Chapter 9. In: *Oxford Textbook of Obstetrics and Gynaecology* (ed. S. Arulkumaran, W. Ledger, L. Denny, and S. Doumouchtsis), 120–132. Oxford: Oxford Academic https://doi.org/10.1093/med/9780198766360.003.0009.

Kirwan, C. (2022). The third stage of labour: part 1. The physiology. *Student Midwife* 5 (1): https://www.all4maternity.com/the-third-stage-of-labour-part-1-the-physiology.

Kovo, M., Schreiber, L., and Bar, J. (2013). Placental vascular pathology as a mechanism of disease in pregnancy complications. *Thrombosis Research* 131 (Suppl 1): s. 18–s. 21.

Macnab, W.R. (2022). Physiology: functions of the placenta. *Anaesthesia and Intensive Care Medicine* 23 (6): 344–346. https://doi.org/10.1016/j.mpaic.2022.03.003.

Maltepe, E. and Fisher, S.J. (2015). Placenta: the forgotten organ. *Annual Review of Cell and Developmental Biology* 31: 523–552. https://doi.org/10.1146/annurev-cellbio-100814-125620.

Mossman, H.W. (1937). Comparative morphogenesis of the fetal membranes and accessory uterine structures. *Contributions to Embryology* 26: 129–146.

NHS England (2023). 20-week screening scan. https://www.gov.uk/government/publications/fetal-anomaly-screening-programme-handbook/20-week-screening-scan (accessed 14 January 2024).

NHS England (2022b). What complications can affect the placenta? https://www.nhs.uk/pregnancy/labour-and-birth/what-happens/placenta-complications (accessed 27 October 2023).

NICE (2019). *Intrapartum Care for Women with Existing Medical Conditions or Obstetric Complications and their Babies*. NICE Guideline NG121. London: National Institute for Health and Care Excellence.

NICE (2021). *Postnatal Care*. NICE Guideline NG194. London: National Institute for Health and Care Excellence.

NICE (2023a). *Hypertension in Pregnancy: Diagnosis and Management*. NICE Guideline NG133. London: National Institute for Health and Care Excellence.

NICE (2023b). *Intrapartum Care*. Clinical Guideline NG235. London: National Institute for Health and Care Excellence.

NICE (2023c). Pulmonary embolism. Clinical Knowledge Summaries. London: National Institute for Health and Care Excellence. https://cks.nice.org.uk/topics/pulmonary-embolism (accessed 27 October 2023).

Nursing and Midwifery Council (2018). *The Code: Professional Standards of Practice and Behaviour for Nurses, Midwives and Nursing Associates*. London: Nursing and Midwifery Council.

Nursing and Midwifery Council (2019a). *Standards of Proficiency for Midwives*. London: Nursing and Midwifery Council.

Nursing and Midwifery Council (2019b). *Standards for Pre-registration Midwifery Programmes*. London: Nursing and Midwifery Council.

Nursing and Midwifery Council (2021). *Practising as a Midwife in the UK*. London: Nursing and Midwifery Council.

RCOG (2014). *The Investigation and Management of the Small-for-Gestational-Age Fetus*. Green-top Guideline No.31, 2e. London: Royal College of Obstetricians and Gynaecologists.

RCOG (2015). *Reducing the Risk of Venous Thromboembolism during Pregnancy and the Puerperium*. Green-top Guideline No.37a. London: Royal College of Obstetricians and Gynaecologists.

RCOG (2018). *Placenta Praevia and Placenta Accreta: Diagnosis and Management*. Green-top Guideline No. 27a. London: Royal College of Obstetricians and Gynaecologists.

Roberts, R.M., Green, J.A., and Schulz, L. (2016). The evolution of the placenta. *Reproduction* 152 (5): 179–189.

Romero, R. (2015). Images of the human placenta. *American Journal of Obstetrics and Gynecology* 213 (4): S1–S2. https://doi.org/10.1016/j.ajog.2015.08.039.

Schoberer, M., Arens, J., Lohr, A. et al. (2012). Fifty years of work on the artificial placenta: milestones in the history of extracorporeal support of the premature newborn. *Artificial Organs* 36 (3): 512–516. https://doi-org.ezproxy.herts.ac.uk/10.1111/j.1525-1594.2011.01404.x.

Silini, A.R., Cargnoni, A., Magatti, M. et al. (2015). The long path of human placenta and its derivatives, in regenerative medicine. *Frontiers in Bioengineering and Biotechnology* 3 (162): 1–16.

Thomson, A.J. (2019). Care of women presenting with suspected preterm prelabour rupture of membranes from 24+0 weeks of gestation: Green-top Guideline No. 73. *BJOG* 126: e152–e166.

Turco, M.Y. and Moffett, A. (2019). Development of the human placenta. *Development* 146 (22): dev163428. https://doi.org/10.1242/dev.163428.

WHO World Health Organization (2022). Preterm birth. Fact sheet. https://www.who.int/news-room/fact-sheets/detail/preterm-birth (accessed 27 October 2023).

Glossary

Blastocyst	Cluster of cells that originates following multiple cell divisions following fertilisation.
Cytotrophoblast	Inner layer of the trophoblast, also the interior of the syncytiotrophoblast and the outer layer of the fetal component of the human placenta.
Decidua	The endometrium in pregnancy.
Human chorionic gonadotrophin (hCG)	A hormone produced by trophoblast cells that will ultimately lead to the formation of the placenta.
Hyperstimulation	Presence of more than 5 contractions per 10 minutes, associated with fetal heart rate features indicative of fetal distress.
Hypersystole/hypertonicity	A contraction lasting for more than two minutes.
Interdisciplinary team	A group of health and care staff from different specialties who build on the expertise of each discipline to elaborate decisions/recommendations regarding care pathways.
Mitosis	Process of miosis in a fertilised egg; division of a cell into two genetically identical cells.
Multidisciplinary team	A group of health and care staff that work together within their professional boundaries, by drawing on their expert knowledge to elaborate decisions/recommendations regarding care pathways of individuals.
Organ	Collection of tissues that are part of an organism and has a number of specific vital functions.
Premature infant	A baby born before 37 weeks of pregnancy.
Tachysystole	Presence of more than 5 contractions per 10 minutes.
Term infant	A baby born from 37 to 42 weeks of pregnancy.
Uterotonic	Pharmacological medication (or group of medications) used to increase the tonicity of the uterus.
Viviparous	Able to develop an embryo inside the body of the mother, leading to the growth and birth of living young.

144

Multiple Choice Questions

1. Which of these statements is correct?
   a. The embryoblast contains a cytotrophoblast and syncytiotrophoblast.
   b. The trophoblast is composed of a blastocyst and embryoblast.
   c. An embryoblast and trophoblast form a blastocyst and a cytotrophoblast and syncytiotrophoblast form a trophoblast.
   d. A trophoblast and syncytiotrophoblast form a blastocyst; a cytotrophoblast and embryoblast form a trophoblast.

2. Which of the following statements is **not** correct about the placenta, membranes and the cord?
   a. The time of cord clamping and mode of birth may affect the weight and morphology of the placenta.
   b. The fetal surface of the placenta has the chorionic structure and the cord, which is usually sited centrally.
   c. The umbilical cord has a 1–2 cm diameter and contains two arteries and one vein.
   d. The total volume of amniotic fluid increases from 20 ml at 10 weeks of gestation to around 500 ml at the end of pregnancy.

3. Which of these is not a function of the placenta?
   a. Gast exchange.
   b. Metabolism.
   c. Motor.
   d. Endocrine.

4. A low-lying placenta is how many millimetres (mm) from the os?
   a. Less than 20 mm.
   b. More than 10 mm.
   c. Between 10 and 35 mm.
   d. More than 20 mm and less than 35 mm.

5. Which of these is not a type of placenta accreta?
   a. Placenta percreta.
   b. Placenta creta.
   c. Placenta increta.
   d. Placenta praevia.

6. Which of these statements about vasa praevia is incorrect?
   a. Vasa praevia occurs due to velamentous insertion.
   b. In vasa praevia, the fetal vessels are unprotected.
   c. The incidence of vasa praevia is higher in women with placentation abnormalities.
   d. In vasa praevia, fetal vessels are protected by Wharton's jelly.

7. Which of these is a common placenta-related disorder?
   a. Pulmonary oedema.
   b. Pulmonary embolism.
   c. Pulmonary fibrosis.
   d. Pulmonary arterial hypertension.

8. What volume of blood loss is considered normal in the third stage of delivery?
   a. Up to 1 litre.
   b. Up to 750 ml.
   c. Up to 500 ml.
   d. Up to 250 ml.

9. Physiological management of the third stage should be completed how long after the birth of the baby?
   a. 2 hours.
   b. 1 hour.
   c. 1.5 hours.
   d. 30 minutes.

10. Which of these statements about completion of an examination of the placenta and membranes after birth is true?
   a. Midwives are not responsible for examining the placenta and membranes.
   b. The presence of any anomalies within the examination is irrelevant, as baby would now be delivered and the mother would have entered the postnatal period.
   c. The examination of the placenta should ensure assessment of its structure, condition, presence of cord vessels (and numbers) and completeness.
   d. In some instances, the placenta and membranes may be sent to histopathology for further analysis to exclude anomalies.

CHAPTER **8**

The Musculoskeletal System

Suzanne Britt

AIM

This chapter provides an overview of the structure and function of the musculoskeletal system, outlining areas for health promotion and exploring selected considerations for midwifery practice.

LEARNING OUTCOMES

At the end of this chapter, you will be able to:

- Describe the structure and function of the human skeleton and its components.
- Explain the different types of muscle tissue and how a muscle contracts.
- Understand how diet and exercise supports a healthy musculoskeletal system.
- Consider the effects of pregnancy and childbearing on selected elements of the musculoskeletal system.

Introduction

Human movement relies on interaction between the structures of the musculoskeletal system, these being the bones, muscles, joints, ligaments, tendons and connective tissue. This complex body system is also integral to controlling cardiac function, respiration, digestion and temperature regulation. It also has an important role to play in supporting pregnancy and the processes involved in giving birth.

The Human Skeleton

The human skeleton is made up of 206 bones, although this figure can vary depending on individual variations in ribs, vertebrae and digits. It is important to make the distinction between the *bones* of the skeletal system and the material *bone* as a biomaterial, which is dynamic and metabolically active (Hart et al. 2020). The latter is discussed in detail later in this chapter.

Fundamentals of Maternal Anatomy and Physiology, First Edition. Edited by Ian Peate and Claire Leader.
© 2024 John Wiley & Sons Ltd. Published 2024 by John Wiley & Sons Ltd.

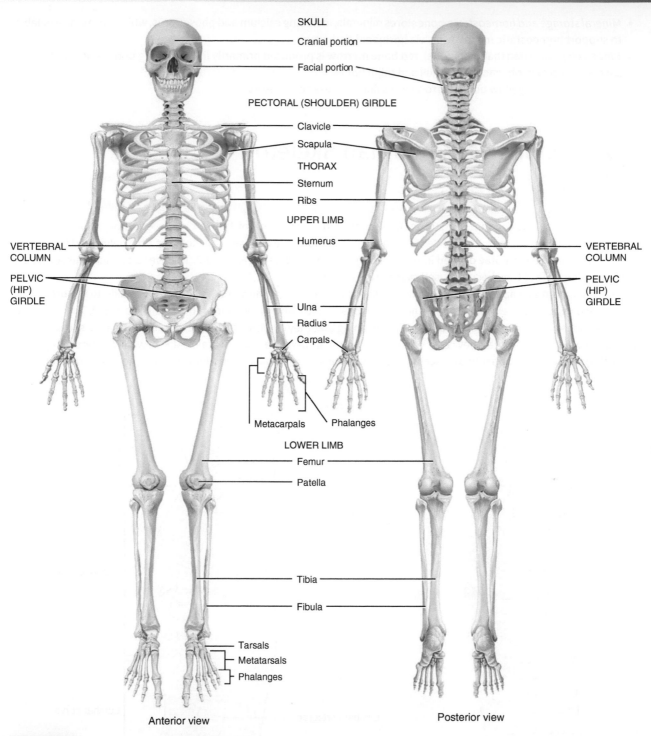

SKULL
— Cranial portion
— Facial portion

PECTORAL (SHOULDER) GIRDLE
— Clavicle
— Scapula

THORAX
— Sternum
— Ribs

UPPER LIMB
— Humerus

VERTEBRAL
COLUMN

PELVIC
(HIP)
GIRDLE

VERTEBRAL
COLUMN

PELVIC
(HIP)
GIRDLE

— Ulna
— Radius
— Carpals

Metacarpals   Phalanges

LOWER LIMB
— Femur
— Patella

— Tibia
— Fibula

— Tarsals
— Metatarsals
— Phalanges

Anterior view   Posterior view

FIGURE 8.1 The axial (blue) and the appendicular skeleton (brown).

The skeleton is divided into the *axial skeleton* and the *appendicular skeleton* (Figure 8.1). The skeletal system has several vital functions:

- *Support*: the skeleton provides a framework for the body and supports soft tissues and skeletal muscle.
- *Protection*: the skeleton protects internal organs such as the brain, the heart and the lungs.
- *Movement*: muscles and bones work together to produce movement, across articulations known as joints.

- *Mineral storage and homeostasis*: bone stores minerals, including calcium and phosphorus, which are made available to support homeostatic mechanisms via hormonal pathways.
- *Blood cell production* (haemopoiesis): red bone marrow is produced primarily in developing bones and adult bones such as the pelvis, rib, backbone, skull and thigh bones.
- *Storage of energy*: yellow bone marrow stores lipids as an energy reserve.

Key Divisions of the Human Skeleton

The Vertebral (Spinal) Column

The vertebral or spinal column is a strong, flexible structure consisting of bones called vertebrae, which allow for movement in different planes. It protects the spinal cord, supports the head and anchors the ribs, pelvis and back muscles. The spine has 33 vertebrae divided into five sections, shown in detail in Figure 8.2. The five sacral and four coccygeal vertebrae differ, in that they become fused over the life course.

The spine normally appears straight when viewed from the back. If the spine curves from one side to the other, this indicates scoliosis. However, the spine has normal gradual curves when viewed from the side (Figure 8.2). The neck and lumbar sections of the spine have a lordotic curve, meaning that they curve inwards. The thoracic and sacral sections have a kyphotic curve, meaning that they curve outwards. The spinal curves help to maintain balance while the body is upright, supporting the head and upper body. Excessive curvature can cause imbalance, resulting in pain and reduced mobility.

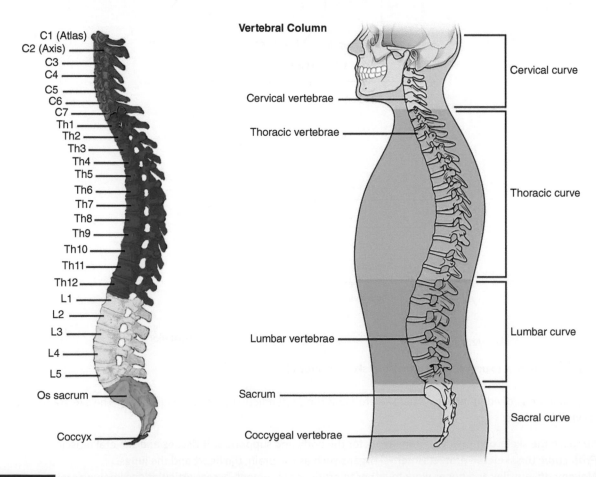

FIGURE 8.2   The spinal column and its normal curvature.

Pregnancy Considerations

As pregnancy progresses, the increase in gestational weight accompanied by the softening of ligaments and connective tissue is associated with postural changes, although the extent and nature of these changes is debated (Conder et al. 2019). As the mass of the growing abdomen and breasts increases, the body's centre of gravity is shifted anteriorly, which can increase the forward tilt of the pelvis and the lordosis (inward curvature) of the spine. Any resulting strain on the musculature of the back might increase lower back pain (Schroder et al. 2016), a common complaint in about 50% of pregnancies. These changes are accompanied by several compensatory changes in posture and gait, which affect both the neck and chest area as well as the lower leg, resulting in the common 'leaning back' 'waddling' and 'sway' associated with late pregnancy (Fiat et al. 2022). These changes are summarised in Figure 8.3, together with corrective advice.

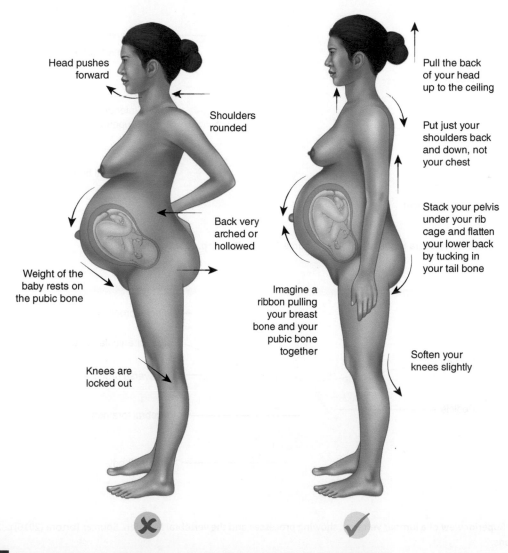

FIGURE 8.3 Postural changes in pregnancy. Source: Health Service Executive, Ireland (2021).

The Spinal Vertebrae

Figures 8.4 and 8.5 show the anatomical structure of a typical vertebra. While there are differences in anatomical structure within each area of the spinal column, there are many common elements, these being the body, the arch and several processes.

The vertebral body is the weight-bearing element of the spinal column. On its upper and lower surfaces there is a rough area, which allows for the attachment of intervertebral discs. Together with the vertebral arch, the vertebral body surrounds the spinal cord, forming the vertebral foramen. The processes which arise from the vertebral arch serve several functions, either as the point of attachment for muscles or as part of joint formation with other vertebrae.

Intervertebral discs are found between vertebrae from the second cervical vertebrae down to the sacrum; they account for around one-quarter of the height of the spinal column. Each disc comprises an outer fibrous cartilage ring and an inner soft pulpy substance called the nucleus. Compression occurs in the vertebral discs during waking activities, but rehydration and decompression occurs during sleep and certain stretching activities such as yoga (Tortora 2016).

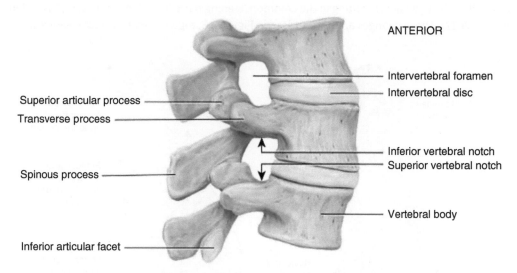

FIGURE 8.4   The lumbar vertebra (right lateral view). Source: Tortora (2016) : p. 223/John Wiley & Sons.

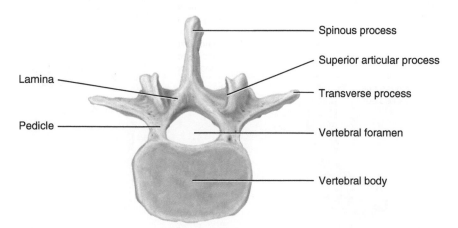

FIGURE 8.5   Superior view of a lumbar vertebra, showing processes and the vertebral foramen. Source: Tortora (2016) p. 223/ John Wiley & Sons.

The Pelvis

The pelvic (hip) girdle is part of the appendicular skeleton. It comprises two hip bones, which are connected to the axial skeleton posteriorly at the sacrum. Anteriorly, the two hipbones meet at the pubic symphysis joint. Taken together, these structures form the basin of the pelvis. The pelvis is divided into the greater (false) pelvis, which lies above the pelvic brim, and the lesser (true) pelvis below the brim.

In a newborn, the two hip bones are subdivided into the ilium, the ischium and the pubis. These bones fuse in adulthood, the site of fusion and ossification being a deep socket called the acetabulum, which receives the head of the femur to form a ball-and-socket joint. The bones of the hip are shown in Figures 8.6 and 8.7.

Reflective Learning Activity

Think for a moment about the differences between the male and female pelvis. What significant structural differences would you expect to find and why? Note down your answers before you read the next section.

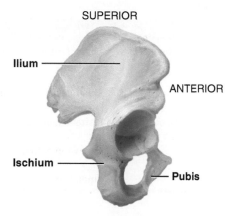

FIGURE 8.6 Lateral view of the hip bone of the pelvis. Source: Tortora (2016), p. 244/John Wiley & Sons.

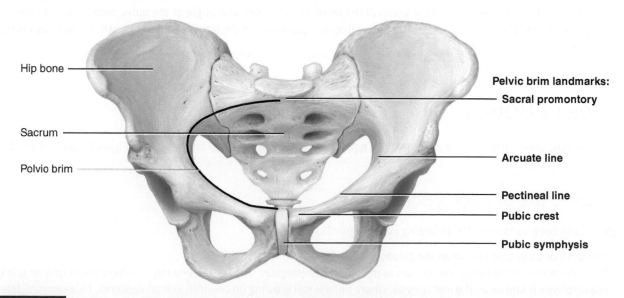

FIGURE 8.7 Anterior view of the female pelvis. Source: Tortora (2016), p. 246/John Wiley & Sons.

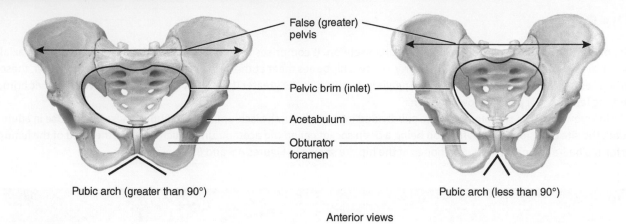

False (greater)
pelvis

Pelvic brim (inlet)

Acetabulum

Obturator
foramen

Pubic arch (greater than 90°)

Pubic arch (less than 90°)

Anterior views

FIGURE 8.8   Structural difference between male (right) and female (left) pelvis. Source: Tortora (2016), p. 248/John Wiley & Sons.

TABLE 8.1   **Types of bones in the skeleton.**

Bone shape	Examples	Structure
Long	Femur, humerus, tibia, radius, fibula	Characterised by a central section between two end points or epiphyses
Short	Ankle and wrist bones	Spherical or conical shape
Flat	Sternum, cranium, ilium, ischium, pubis	Flattened, broad surfaces
Irregular	Vertebrae	Take various shapes
Sesamoid	Patella	Small and round

The distinction between the false and true pelvis is an important consideration for the function of pregnancy and childbearing. There are some key structural differences between the female and male pelvis, seen most clearly in the depth of the greater (false) pelvis and the width of the lesser (true) pelvis. The angle of the pubic arch is also greater in the female pelvis and the sacral curve shorter and wider, to accommodate the fetal head during birth. These differences are shown in Figure 8.8.

Types of Bones

The bones of the skeleton may be classified into five types: long, short, flat, irregular and sesamoid (Figure 8.9 and Table 8.1).

The Structure of a Long Bone

A typical long bone consists of the following parts (Figure 8.10):

- The shaft or body also known as the diaphysis.
- The extremities of the bone, also known as the epiphyses (singular: epiphysis). The region where the diaphysis joins the epiphysis is known as the metaphysis. Where bone is still growing (in children and adolescents, for example), this region will be a layer of cartilage known as the epiphyseal (growth) plate.

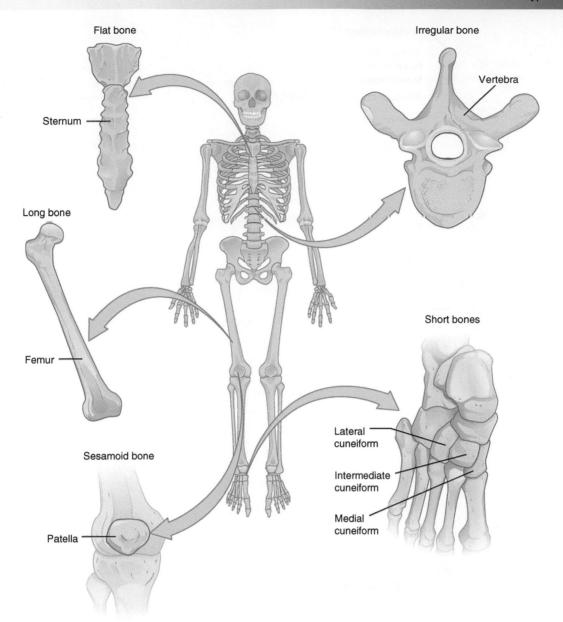

FIGURE 8.9 Types of bones. Source: Tortora (2016), p. 197/John Wiley & Sons.

- Articular cartilage is a thin layer covering the epiphysis where bones meet to form a joint. It reduces friction and absorbs shock. Where there is no articular cartilage, the surface of the long bone is covered by the periosteum, a tough membrane. The periosteum comprises tissue blood vessels and nerves and bone cells, serving an important function in protecting and nourishing the long bone. It also forms the attachment point for ligaments and tendons.
- The medullary or marrow cavity, the site of yellow marrow production.

Bone is often perceived as a solid substance but it is structurally complex. It must yield to substantial forces acting upon it and must facilitate continuous delivery of nutrients for cell repair and replacement. Different parts of the skeleton determine the type of osseous tissue found in each type of bone. Spongy or cancellous bone is also known as trabecular bone (Figure 8.10). It makes up most of the bone tissue of short flat and irregular bones and most of the epiphyses of long bones. Trabecular bone resembles a spongy meshwork of interconnecting spaces containing red bone marrow in some locations. The spongy nature of trabecular bone enables it to withstand substantial force without breaking.

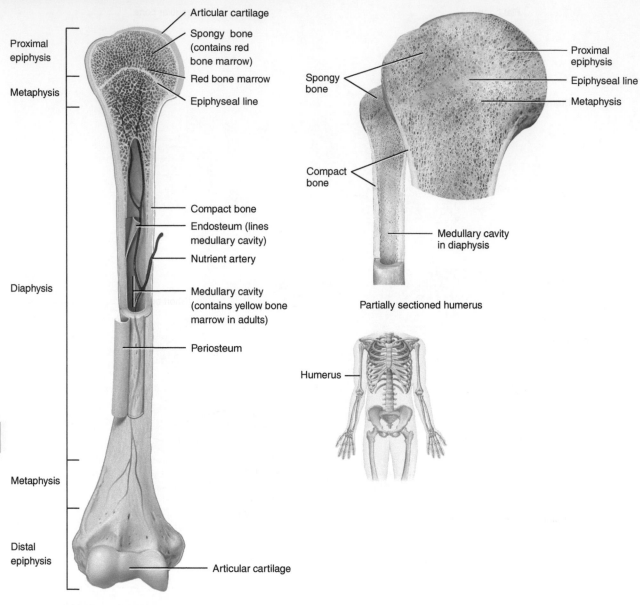

Proximal epiphysis

Metaphysis

Diaphysis

Metaphysis

Distal epiphysis

Articular cartilage

Spongy bone (contains red bone marrow)

Red bone marrow

Epiphyseal line

Compact bone

Endosteum (lines medullary cavity)

Nutrient artery

Medullary cavity (contains yellow bone marrow in adults)

Periosteum

Articular cartilage

Partially sectioned humerus (arm bone)

Spongy bone

Compact bone

Proximal epiphysis

Epiphyseal line

Metaphysis

Medullary cavity in diaphysis

Partially sectioned humerus

Humerus

FIGURE 8.10   The anatomy of a long bone. Source: Tortora (2016), p. 173/John Wiley & Sons.

Compact bone, also known as cortical bone, forms the superficial layer of all bones. It is highly mineralised, densely packed, rigid and smooth, with high resistance to sudden impact forces, approximately 25% stronger than spongy or trabecular bone (Augat and Schorlemmer 2006). Compact bone consists of tiny cells called osteons (Figure 8.11), which are bundled tightly together in an arrangement that provides their great strength. Each osteon comprises a central canal (Haversian canal) housing blood vessels and nerves, which is surrounded by concentric layers of tissue (lamellae). Gaps in the tissue (lacunae) contain osteocyte cells, which keep the bone matrix healthy and replenished.

Throughout a person's life course, bone development and mineralisation occur at varying rates. Childhood and adolescence are critical times for bone growth, although the process is not linear, with the appendicular skeleton growing more rapidly before puberty and spinal growth occurring mostly later. After reaching peak bone mass in adulthood, bone remodelling achieves more balance, with bone mass being stable for decades until age-related bone loss begins later in life (Langdahl et al. 2016). Bone formation, maintenance and remodelling involve three types of cells: osteoblasts, osteoclasts and osteocytes.

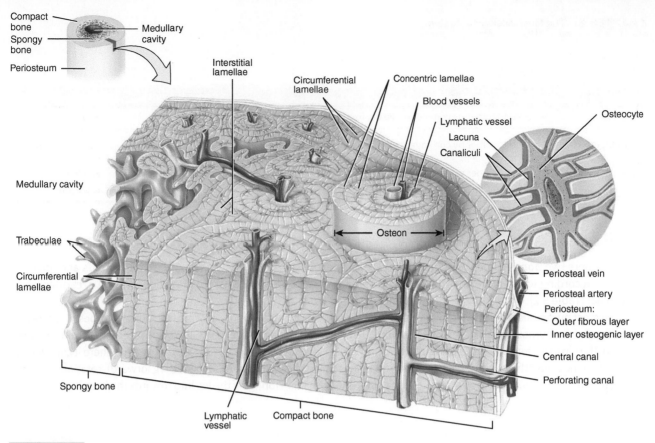

FIGURE 8.11 Compact and spongy bone. Source: Tortora (2016), p. 176/John Wiley & Sons.

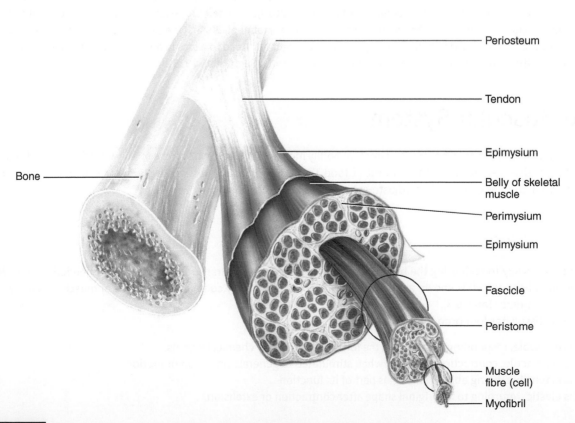

FIGURE 8.12 Cellular structure of muscle cells and attachment point of muscle to bone at tendon.

TABLE 8.2 **Types of joints.**

Joint	Structure	Synovial cavity	Examples
Fibrous	Held together by connective tissue, fixed in nature	No	Skull bones
Cartilaginous	Held together by cartilage, semi moveable in nature	No	Pubic symphysis
Synovial	Held together via a joint capsule and ligaments, allowing for movement	Yes, contains synovial fluid	Hip joint Knee joint

Where Bones Meet: Joints and Articulations

The site where two bones come together is called a joint or articulation. The body has more than 300 joints and they are classified according to structure and the type of movement that they allow. Joints are classified as fibrous, cartilaginous or synovial (Table 8.2).

The most numerous and versatile joints are synovial joints, which come in various forms. Their diverse types facilitate the capabilities of the human body in terms of different movements. Joints hinge, slide, pivot, glide and rotate depending on their function; the hip joint, for example, is a complex ball-and-socket joint, allowing for a wide range of motion where it connects to the femur in the upper thigh. It supports extension (pushing the leg back), flexion (bringing the leg forward), rotation (twisting the leg round), abduction (moving the leg out to the side) and adduction (bringing the leg into towards the body).

Pregnancy Considerations

Relaxin, a polypeptide hormone, is considered significant in stimulating uterine growth in pregnancy (Rankin 2017). It is also thought to act on the connective tissue in muscles, tendons and ligaments, increasing joint laxity, especially noticeable during the second trimester of pregnancy (Cherni et al. 2019). Elevated progesterone levels also contribute to this, potentially precipitating musculoskeletal pain and discomfort (Fiat et al. 2022). One unexpected effect may be a change in foot structure, as increased joint laxity and gestational weight gain lead to a loss in foot arch height and changes in foot length and width. Some of these changes may persist postnatally (Segal et al. 2013).

The Muscular System

The muscular system creates external and internal bodily movement. It generates force to allow motion across bones and joints, but is also responsible for the transit of food through the gastrointestinal system, for controlling cardiac and respiratory function as well as micro adjustments such as pupil dilation in the eye.

Muscle Tissue

Muscle tissue is key to stabilising the body, storing vital substances and transporting them when needed, alongside the generation of heat, which is known as thermogenesis. The human body contains three types of muscle tissue, skeletal, smooth and cardiac (Table 8.3).

Muscle tissue has four properties:

- It is excitable, responding to stimuli in the form of electrical or chemical signals.
- It is contractile, contracting forcefully when stimulated to generate an action or motion.
- It is extensible, being able to stretch as part of its function.
- It is elastic, returning to its original shape after contraction or extension.

TABLE 8.3 Types of muscle tissue.

Muscle tissue	Description
Skeletal	The majority of muscle tissue is skeletal or striated muscle. Characterised by striations or bands of highly organised muscle fibres. Main type of muscle tissue associated with skeletal movement. Most skeletal muscles are under voluntary control, but some act without us being aware (diaphragm)
Smooth	Located in internal structures, such as the walls of the intestine, blood vessels and skin. Has no striations and is therefore described as smooth. Under involuntary control
Cardiac	Also striated, but its action is not under conscious control

Skeletal muscle forms the majority of the body's muscle tissue. It is important, therefore, to explore its structure and function. The basic functional unit of skeletal muscle is the myofiber or muscle cell. These cells are elongated and grouped into bundles called fascicles. Each fascicle is surrounded by connective tissue called the perimysium and each group of fascicles is enclosed in turn within connective tissue known as the endomysium. The epimysium encloses the whole muscle (Figure 8.12).

The elongated muscle fibre is enclosed within a membrane called the sarcolemma, which encloses the sarcoplasm, a cytoplasm containing mitochondria, proteins and other elements required for muscular contraction. Each muscle fibre contains cylindrical structures called myofibrils, which are in turn made up of thick (myosin) and thin (actin) filaments. These filaments do not stretch along the length of the myofibril, but are instead arranged in basic units called sarcomeres, which give the muscle its striated or striped appearance under a microscope (Figure 8.13).

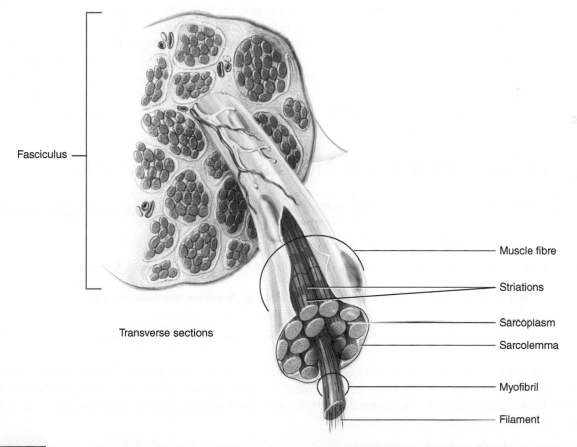

FIGURE 8.13 Microscopic structure of a muscle fibre. Source: Tortora (2016), p. 296/John Wiley & Sons.

The Organisation of the Muscular System

Human movement relies on muscles interacting with skeletal structures at joints and articulations. There are between 600-700 muscles in the body and most will produce movement, but some will act to stabilise the body to facilitate or even prevent harmful motion. Muscles are attached to bones by tendons seen in Figure 8.12, made up of strong inelastic connective tissue, which assist in generating pulling forces. They are distinguished from ligaments, which are flexible and elastic fibrous bands connecting bone to bone. Muscles are grouped according to their primary functions in different body regions, shown in detail in Figures 8.14 and 8.15.

Key Muscle Group: Abdominal Muscles

The abdominal muscles support the trunk, allow movement and hold organs in place by regulating abdominal pressure. There are three main anterior abdominal muscles comprising three flat muscular sheets, which extend laterally. These muscles are the external oblique, the internal oblique and the deep transverse abdominis. The sheath-like tendons of these three muscles, also known as aponeuroses, fuse medially to form the rectus sheath, which in turn encloses the long vertical rectus abdominis muscle (Flynn and Vickerton 2022). The rectus sheath meets at the linea alba, a fibrous white band that runs down the centre of the abdominal wall. The posterior wall of the abdominal musculature is formed by the paraspinal muscles, supporting the stability of the lower back and helping to maintain good postural alignment. Figure 8.16 shows the detailed structure of the anterior abdominal musculature, the pectoralis muscles of the chest and the latissimus dorsi muscles of the upper back.

Considerations for Pregnancy and the Postnatal Period

Pregnancy affects the abdominal muscles significantly. In most people, the linea alba will darken under the influence of melanin, enough to be visible in the midline of the abdomen by the second trimester. The abdominal muscles will essentially house the growing uterus as it emerges from the pelvis to become an abdominal organ. These muscles also play an important role in providing spinal stability as body shape changes and the centre of gravity shifts (Swanson 2001), so it may be important to stress the role of strong core abdominal muscles, even during the preconception period. While it might be assumed that strong abdominal muscles could help with the expulsive phase of labour, studies suggest that training the abdominal muscles has no effect on birth outcome (Rise et al. 2019), although research is scant.

Physical Activity and the Musculoskeletal System

Reflective Learning Activity

Consider the following questions before you read this section.

- How do you build physical activity into your life? Are you active enough? What are the barriers you face and do these affect the people you care for?
- How confident do you feel about advising families about physical activity? Do you feel that this is the role of the midwife?

Read de Vivo and Mills (2019) if you are interested in this topic.

Physical activity offers numerous health benefits, including the prevention and management of chronic diseases, enhancing overall wellbeing and improving cognitive function (World Health Organization 2022). While many are familiar with the effects of physical activity on the cardiovascular system, it also significantly improves musculoskeletal function, contributing to a better quality of life. Benefits include:

- Improved joint lubrication and nourishment
- Improved flexibility

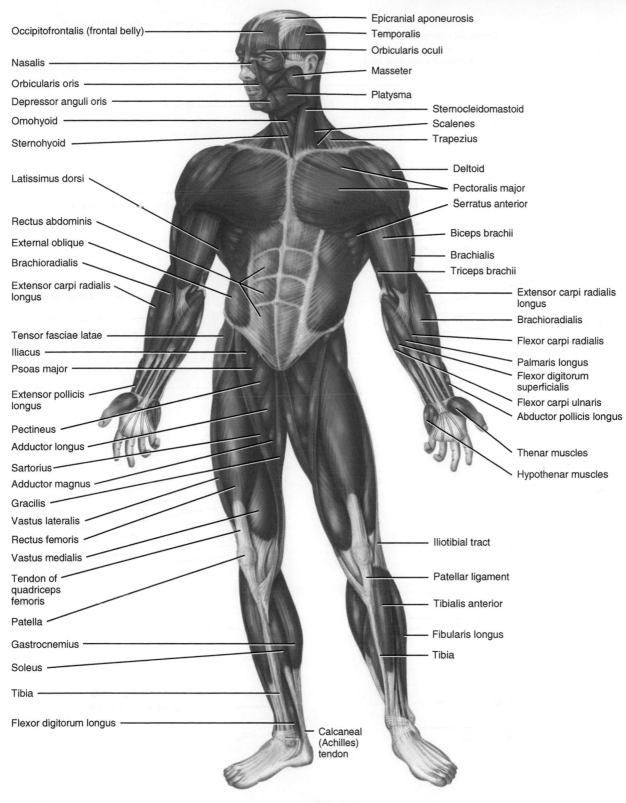

Occipitofrontalis (frontal belly)

Nasalis

Orbicularis oris

Depressor anguli oris

Omohyoid

Sternohyoid

Latissimus dorsi

Rectus abdominis

External oblique

Brachioradialis

Extensor carpi radialis longus

Tensor fasciae latae

Iliacus

Psoas major

Extensor pollicis longus

Pectineus

Adductor longus

Sartorius

Adductor magnus

Gracilis

Vastus lateralis

Rectus femoris

Vastus medialis

Tendon of quadriceps femoris

Patella

Gastrocnemius

Soleus

Tibia

Flexor digitorum longus

Epicranial aponeurosis

Temporalis

Orbicularis oculi

Masseter

Platysma

Sternocleidomastoid

Scalenes

Trapezius

Deltoid

Pectoralis major

Serratus anterior

Biceps brachii

Brachialis

Triceps brachii

Extensor carpi radialis longus

Brachioradialis

Flexor carpi radialis

Palmaris longus

Flexor digitorum superficialis

Flexor carpi ulnaris

Abductor pollicis longus

Thenar muscles

Hypothenar muscles

Iliotibial tract

Patellar ligament

Tibialis anterior

Fibularis longus

Tibia

Calcaneal (Achilles) tendon

Anterior view

FIGURE 8.14 Anterior view of muscles.

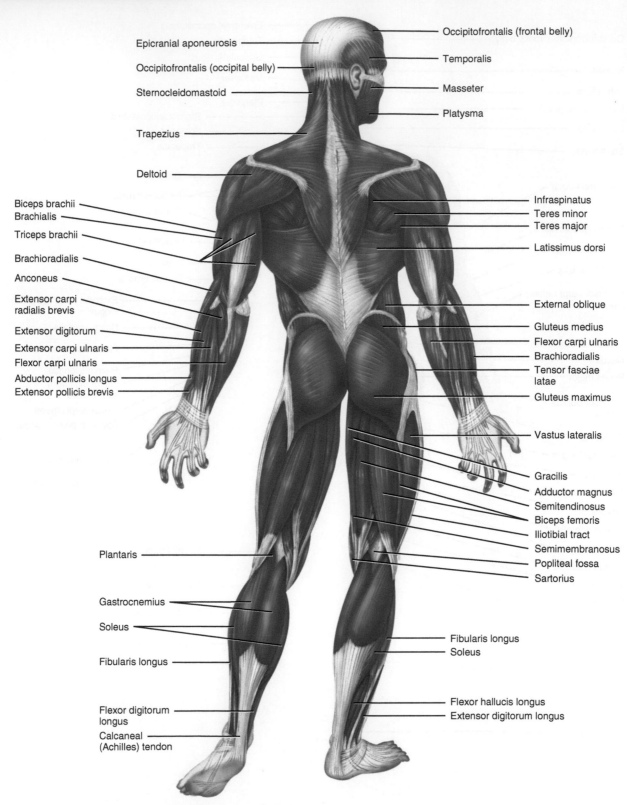

Posterior view

FIGURE 8.15   Posterior view of muscles.

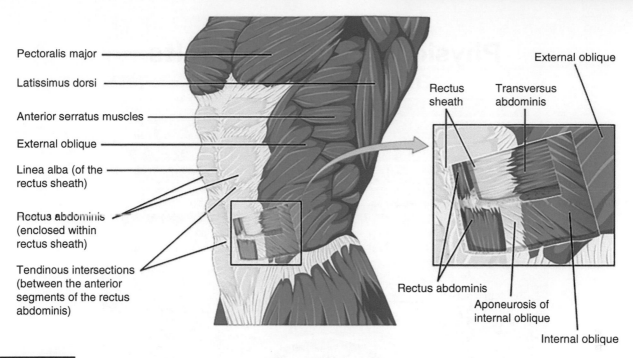

Pectoralis major

Latissimus dorsi

Anterior serratus muscles

External oblique

Linea alba (of the
rectus sheath)

Rectus abdominis
(enclosed within
rectus sheath)

Tendinous intersections
(between the anterior
segments of the rectus
abdominis)

External oblique

Rectus
sheath

Transversus
abdominis

Rectus abdominis

Aponeurosis of
internal oblique

Internal oblique

FIGURE 8.16   Muscles of the abdomen (anterior view). Source: OpenStax College/Wikimedia/CCBY 3.0/public domain.

- Greater levels of muscular strength
- Improved balance and posture
- Enhanced bone density
- Preservation of muscle mass into older age.

Activities that are linked to enhanced musculoskeletal function encompass resistance training and flexibility-focused exercises like yoga and pilates. Engaging in cardiovascular exercises such as swimming, cycling and walking have a beneficial impact on the metabolic processes in skeletal muscles, notably in terms of glucose uptake. However, weight-bearing activities such as running, dancing, racket games and high-impact training have the most effect on bone mass density and tendon strength (Manaye et al. 2023).

Many governments issue public health guidance that can be used to guide health professionals in advising the population. In the UK, this guidance is issued by the Chief Medical Officers (2023; Figure 8.17).

During pregnancy and the postpartum period, healthcare professionals play a significant part in addressing the benefits of physical activity as part of their public health role. Guidance from the National Institute for Health and Care Excellence (NICE 2021) recommends that physical activity should form part of health and wellbeing discussions at the pregnancy booking visit and during postnatal contacts. Hopkinson et al.'s (2018) study, however, suggested that mid-wives' confidence in their knowledge of physical activity guidance for pregnancy might be misplaced, with only 2% of midwives identifying them correctly. While most women do not meet the current recommendations for physical activity before pregnancy, many tend to become even less physically active when they become pregnant (Hinman et al. 2015). Fear of potential risks to the fetus, notably hyperthermia, fetal distress, miscarriage and trauma to the maternal abdomen may contribute to decreased activity levels (Hammer et al. 2000). Nevertheless, the decision by the American College of Obstetricians and Gynecologists in 1994 to issue guidelines around this issue has meant that advice is available to families and healthcare professionals around physical activity during pregnancy and lactation (Artal and O'Toole 2003).

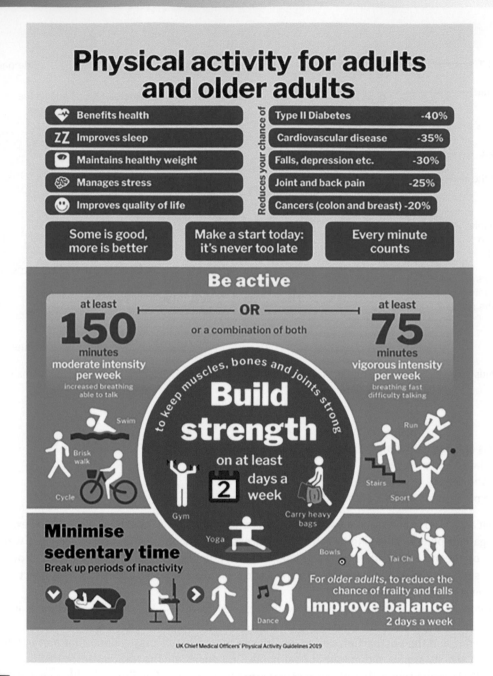

FIGURE 8.17 Physical activity guidelines for adults and older adults Source: UK Chief Medical Officers (2019)/Crown copyright/ CCBY 3.0/public domain.

In an umbrella review, DiPietro et al. (2019) reviewed 76 systematic reviews and meta-analyses on physical activity during pregnancy and the postpartum period. Their findings suggested strong evidence that moderately intense physical activity reduced the risk of excessive gestational weight gain, gestational diabetes and postpartum depression symptoms. There was limited evidence of reduction in risks of pre-eclampsia, gestational hypertension and antenatal anxiety symptoms. There was insufficient evidence to determine the impact of physical activity on postnatal weight loss or postnatal anxiety, with more research needed in these areas. Current UK guidance for both pregnancy and the period after birth is shown in Figures 8.18 and 8.19.

Red Flag Alerts: Pregnancy and Exercise

Contraindications to moderate to vigorous physical activity in pregnancy are traditionally classified as 'absolute' or 'relative'. In an evidence review, Meah et al. (2020) evaluated existing evidence of harm. The study proposed that the following conditions be viewed as having a strong potential for adverse effects for the mother and/or fetus:

- Severe respiratory diseases (e.g. chronic obstructive pulmonary disease, restrictive lung disease and cystic fibrosis)
- Severe acquired or congenital heart disease with exercise intolerance
- Uncontrolled or severe arrhythmia
- Placental abruption
- Vasa previa
- Uncontrolled type 1 diabetes
- Intrauterine growth restriction (IUGR)
- Active preterm labour
- Severe pre-eclampsia
- Cervical insufficiency.

Meah et al. (2020) propose that some conditions merit a discussion between an obstetric healthcare professional and the woman about risks and benefits of continuing physical activity. This might involve discussing reducing the intensity, duration or volume of exercise or could mean complete avoidance. These conditions include:

- Mild respiratory disorders
- Mild congenital or acquired cardiovascular disease
- Well-controlled type 1 diabetes
- Mild pre-eclampsia
- Preterm premature rupture of membranes
- Placenta previa after 28 weeks
- Untreated thyroid disease
- Symptomatic, severe eating disorder
- Multiple nutrient deficiencies and/or chronic undernutrition
- Moderate to heavy smoking (> 20 cigarettes/day) in the presence of comorbidities.

According to the same review, conditions such as anaemia, multiple pregnancy, obesity and history of spontaneous preterm labour should not preclude participation in physical activity, the traditionally prescribed bedrest for many conditions being possibly detrimental. However, the authors do acknowledge limited evidence in many cases and call for high-quality research to inform future advice. In the meantime, some general guidelines are supported by the most recent UK CMOs' physical activity (UK Chief Medical Officers 2019; Figure 8.17) and American College of Obstetricians and Gynecologists (2020) guidelines, summarised here:

- Physical activity can safely be recommended during and after pregnancy and has no negative impact on breastfeeding.
- Physical activity choices should reflect activity levels pre-pregnancy and should include strength training.
- Vigorous activity is not recommended for previously inactive women. After the six-to-eight-week postnatal check and depending on the woman's feelings, more intense activities can gradually be introduced, with a slow build-up over a minimum period of at least three months.
- Women should avoid doing exercises that involve lying on their back after the first trimester of pregnancy because this position restricts blood flow to the uterus and fetus. They should avoid contact or collision sports and activities with high risk of falling or abdominal trauma. Scuba diving should be avoided. Updated guidance from the NHS can be found at https://www.nhs.uk/pregnancy/keeping-well/exercise.

164

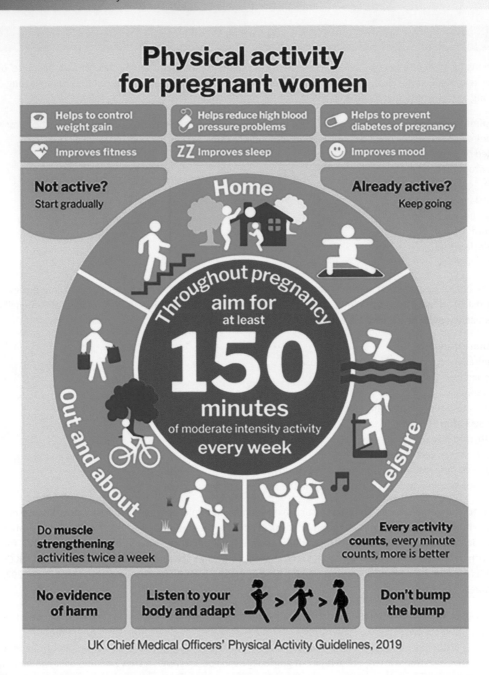

FIGURE 8.18 Physical activity for pregnant women. Source: UK Chief Medical Officers (2019)/Crown copyright/CCBY 3.0/public domain).

Eating for Healthier Bones

Reflective Learning Activity

Consider these questions before reading this section:

- What dietary advice have you seen given to pregnant women in practice?
- How confident do you feel about giving nutritional advice to those in your care?
- Has the advice you give made you change your habits at all? How?

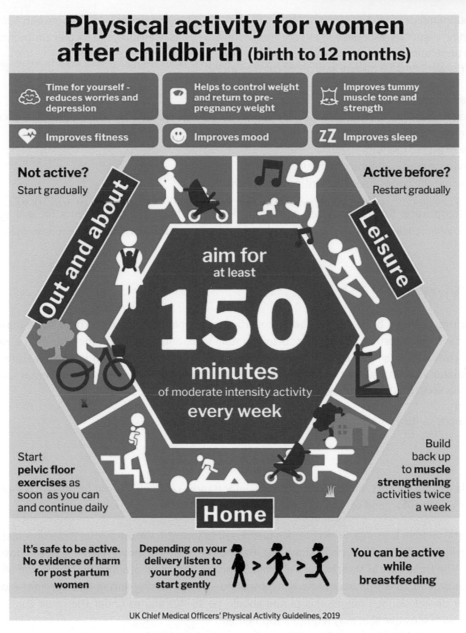

Physical activity for women after childbirth (birth to 12 months)

Time for yourself - reduces worries and depression

Helps to control weight and return to pre-pregnancy weight

Improves tummy muscle tone and strength

Improves fitness

Improves mood

ZZ Improves sleep

Not active?
Start gradually

Out and about

Active before?
Restart gradually

Leisure

aim for
at least

150
minutes
of moderate intensity activity
every week

Start
pelvic floor
exercises as
soon as you can
and continue daily

Build
back up
to muscle
strengthening
activities twice
a week

Home

It's safe to be active. No evidence of harm for post partum women

Depending on your delivery listen to your body and start gently

You can be active while breastfeeding

UK Chief Medical Officers' Physical Activity Guidelines, 2019

FIGURE 8.19 Guidance for PA during the year after birth. Source: UK Chief Medical Officers (2019)/Crown copyright/CCBY 3.0/ public domain.

The osseous tissues of the skeletal system form a complex living organ, continually breaking down and rebuilding, storing vital mineral deposits needed for broader metabolic functioning within the body. As we age, bone tissue weakens, but many modifiable factors influence optimum bone health throughout life. Avoiding smoking and alcohol are crucial considerations, but nutrition plays a significant role in maintaining bone strength. Nutrition provides bone-forming minerals, ensuring growth and the supply of vitamins involved in controlling calcium and phosphate levels (Ward 2013).

Calcium and vitamin D are essential for bone growth and mineralisation. Calcium is critical to bone structure. When blood calcium levels are low, threatening many cellular processes, the parathyroid gland resorbs calcium from bone tissue and replenishes the bloodstream's supplies. Bone stores of calcium require replenishing through the diet or in certain cases by supplementation. According to Anderson et al. (2019), an intake of calcium between 500 and 1250 mg/day is needed to meet demands. Excessive supplementation, however, has been linked to cardiac problems, although the evidence remains uncertain (Morelli et al. 2020).

According to the NHS (2020a) dietary sources of calcium include:

- Milk, cheese and other dairy foods
- Green leafy vegetables – such as curly kale, okra but not spinach (spinach does contain high levels of calcium but the body cannot digest it all)
- Soya drinks with added calcium
- Bread and anything made with fortified flour
- Fish where you eat the bones – such as sardines and pilchards.

The Royal Osteoporosis Society provides a calcium-rich food-chooser with amounts for average potions at: https://theros.org.uk/information-and-support/bone-health/nutrition-for-bones/calcium/calcium-rich-food-chooser.

The Role of Vitamin D (Calciferol)

When the equilibrium between bone calcium being resorbed and replenished is disturbed, bone mineral density is affected and skeletal fragility results. Vitamin D acts to maintain equilibrium, allowing the intestinal absorption of calcium favouring its storage through bone calcium deposition. When the parathyroid gland acts to restore blood calcium levels, it also stimulates vitamin D activation to indirectly support absorption of calcium from external sources.

According to the NHS (2020b) the following are sources of vitamin D:

- Oily fish – salmon, sardines, herring and mackerel
- Red meat
- Liver
- Egg yolks
- Fortified foods – some spreads and breakfast cereals. Importantly, cow's milk is not fortified in the UK, unlike some other countries, so is not a good source. Some plant milks are fortified.

Sunlight is a vital vitamin D source. When the skin is exposed to sunlight, the ultraviolet B rays interact with a protein in the skin, converting it to the active form of vitamin D. Balance is important, however, since overexposure to sunlight can be dangerous. The University of Manchester's vitamin D and sunlight team propose that 'little and often' is the best approach and recommend 10–15 minutes of daily exposure to sunlight during spring and summer months for light-skinned people; for darker-skinned people this period should be 25–40 minutes under the same conditions (Burchell et al. 2019). People with sensitive skin may require a supplement.

Vitamin D is also crucial for the formation of strong bones, teeth and optimum heart and nerve function. Pregnant women should take 10 µg (400 iu) daily and this should be continued if breastfeeding (Carter 2022). Vitamin D deficiency disproportionately affects those from black, Asian and minority ethnic groups, as well as those with chronic illnesses. While there are evidence gaps around dosage and other potential benefits, a Cochrane review (Palacios et al. 2019) proposed the potential additional advantages of vitamin D supplementation in pregnancy:

- Probably reduces the risk of pre-eclampsia and gestational diabetes.
- May reduce the risk of having a low-birthweight baby.
- May reduce the risk of severe bleeding after birth.
- May make little or no difference to the risk of preterm birth before 37 weeks.

Snapshot 8.1   Restless Legs Syndrome

Ria is 34 weeks pregnant. She has been increasingly unable to sleep because of cramps in her legs. Sometimes she also feels as though she cannot keep her legs still in bed at night. She feels exhausted and tearful.

- What questions would you ask Ria?
- What would your initial concerns be? How would you decide what action to take next?

After you have spoken to Ria, she describes the pains as being in both legs and much worse at night than during the day. She is still working and gets very little time to rest. Her pregnancy has been normal to date, and she has not required any extra medications or supplements. She is a regular exerciser and a non-smoker.

- Have your concerns changed at all?
- What do you think is the problem here?
- How will you advise Ria?

Psychological Wellbeing and Sleep – Orange Flag

Lack of sleep can lead to the inability to complete tasks and maintain focus, as well as weakening the immune system. Poor sleep affects emotional regulation, meaning that individuals may be less able to manage stress and may be more likely to experience anxiety and depression (Vandekerckhove and Wang 2018). Perinatal anxiety and depression are leading causes of morbidity in childbearing women, with long-ranging effects on the whole family (Howard and Kalifeh 2020).

Further Considerations

Ria may be experiencing restless legs syndrome or Willis–Ekbom disease, which affects up to one-third of pregnant women. Symptoms may peak in the third trimester and usually disappear after birth. The condition can lead to poor sleep quality and compromised daytime functioning. Low serum ferritin (50–75 µg/l) has been suggested as an underlying cause and supplementation may be appropriate in consultation with obstetric care providers (NICE 2022).

Leg cramps are a painful muscular contraction affecting the foot, the calf or both. They are classified as a sleep-related movement disorder and are likely to be idiopathic in pregnancy. According to Hensley (2009), practitioners face a challenge in discovering whether the symptoms indicate a more serious disorder, particularly a deep vein thrombosis (DVT). Benign leg cramps occur unilaterally during sleep (Walters 2007). Evidence to support any interventions is very weak (Luo et al. 2020) and midwives should focus on offering reassurance and listening to concerns, once other serious disorders have been ruled out (Hensley 2009).

167

Red Flag Alert: Deep Vein Thrombosis

Unilateral leg pain is also a symptom of DVT. Examination of the lower extremities for a calf-circumference size discrepancy (and/or oedema) is the physical examination sign that is most reliable in establishing the diagnosis of DVT. There may also be lower abdominal pain, redness and heat with extreme local tenderness (RCOG 2015). Venous thromboembolism, which includes DVT and pulmonary embolism, is a leading cause of maternal mortality and any suspicion requires prompt investigation.

Medications Management: the Musculoskeletal System

A number of prescription medications are used medicines are used to treat musculoskeletal pain and disorders, and midwives need an overview of them for their practice, as they may care for women taking these medications for musculoskeletal pain. The following resources will help you to find up-to-date information:

- Bumps: Best Use of Medicines in Pregnancy: https://www.medicinesinpregnancy.org
- Breastfeeding Network. Drugs in breastmilk factsheets: www.breastfeedingnetwork.org.uk/drugs-factsheets
- UKTIS. UK Teratology Information Service: https://uktis.org

Research the most common medication types and make notes on their other names, <u>their applications, and any pregnancy and lactation issues:</u>

- Paracetamol
- Non-steroidal anti-inflammatory drugs
- Tramadol
- Morphine
- Codeine
- Duloxetine
- Amitriptyline
- Gabapentin.

Take Home Points

- The musculoskeletal system is integral to facilitating movement, controlling cardiac function, respiration, digestion and regulating temperature.
- Some of the changes to the musculoskeletal system in the childbearing period have the potential to disrupt quality of life, and a compassionate, listening approach is required from caregivers.
- Knowledge of the musculoskeletal system allows midwives to fulfil their role as public health practitioners, as well as helping them to identify possible deviations from the norm.
- Physical activity and adequate nutrition have an important function in maintaining a healthy musculoskeletal system and guidelines exist to support healthcare professionals in giving advice.

References

American College of Obstetricians and Gynecologists (2020). *Physical Activity and Exercise During Pregnancy and the Postpartum Period.* Committee Opinion No. 804. Washington DC: American College of Obstetricians and Gynecologists https://www.acog.org/clinical/clinical-guidance/committee-opinion/articles/2020/04/physical-activity-and-exercise-during-pregnancy-and-the-postpartum-period.

Anderson, P., Jeray, K., Lane, J., and Binkley, N. (2019). Bone health optimization: beyond own the bone: AOA critical issues. *Journal of Bone and Joint Surgery* 101: 1413–1419. https://doi.org/10.2106/JBJS.18.01229.

Artal, R. and O'Toole, M. (2003). Guidelines of the American College of Obstetricians and Gynecologists for exercise during pregnancy and the postpartum period. *British Journal of Sports Medicine* 37: 6. https://doi.org/10.1136/bjsm.37.1.6.

Augat, P. and Schorlemmer, S. (2006). The role of cortical bone and its microstructure in bone strength. *Age and Ageing* 35 (suppl 2): ii27–ii31.

Burchell, K., Webb, A., and Rhodes, L. (2019). Sunlight exposure and vitamin D: Getting the balance right: sunlight exposure advice that ensures adequate vitamin D while minimising the risk of sunburn and cancer. policy@http://manchester.ac.uk

Carter, E. (2022). Vitamin D supplements in pregnancy: what's the latest evidence? Evidently Cochrane 6 January [blog post]. https://www.evidentlycochrane.net/vitamin-d-supplements-in-pregnancy-whats-the-latest-evidence(accessed 27 October 2023).

Cherni, Y., Desseauve, D., Decatoire, A. et al. (2019). Evaluation of ligament laxity during pregnancy. *Journal of Gynaecology Obstetrics and Human Reproduction* 48: 351–353. https://doi.org/10.1016/j.jogoh.2019.02.009.

Conder, R., Zamani, R., and Akrami, M. (2019). The biomechanics of pregnancy: a systematic review. *Journal of Functional Morphology and Kinesiology* 4 (4): 72. https://doi.org/10.3390/jfmk4040072.

Dipietro, L., Evenson, K.R., Bloodgood, B. et al. (2019). Benefits of physical activity during pregnancy and postpartum: an umbrella review. *Medicine and Science in Sports and Exercise* 51 (6): 1292–1302.

Fiat, F., Merghes, P.E., Scurtu, A.D. et al. (2022). The main changes in pregnancy: therapeutic approach to musculoskeletal pain. *Medicina* 58 (8): 1115. https://doi-org.nottingham.idm.oclc.org/10.3390/medicina58081115.

Flynn, W. and Vickerton, P. (2022). *Anatomy, Abdomen and Pelvis, Abdominal Wall.* Treasure Island (FL): StatPearls Publishing.

Hammer, R.L., Perkins, J., and Parr, R. (2000). Exercise during the childbearing year. *The Journal of Perinatal Education* 9 (1): 1–14.

Hart, N.H., Newton, R.U., Tan, J. et al. (2020). Biological basis of bone strength: anatomy, physiology and measurement. *Journal of Musculoskeletal & Neuronal Interactions* 20 (3): 347–371.

Health Service Executive, Ireland (2021). Back pain in pregnancy. https://www2.hse.ie/conditions/back-pain/back-pain-in-pregnancy/#:~:text=Back%20pain%20is%20caused%20by,pelvis%20and%20back%20feel%20weaker (accessed 28 October 2023).

Hensley, J.G. (2009). Leg cramps and restless legs syndrome during pregnancy. *Journal of Midwifery & Women's Health* 54 (3): 211–218.

Hinman, S.K., Smith, K.B., Quillen, D.M., and Smith, M.S. (2015). Exercise in pregnancy: a clinical review. *Sports Health* 7 (6): 527–531.

Hopkinson, Y., Hill, D.M., Fellows, L., and Fryer, S. (2018). Midwives understanding of physical activity guidelines during pregnancy. *Midwifery* 59: 23–26.

Howard, L.M. and Khalifeh, H. (2020). Perinatal mental health: a review of progress and challenges. *World Psychiatry* 19 (3): 313–327.

Langdahl, B., Ferrari, S., and Dempster, D.W. (2016). Bone modelling and remodelling: potential as therapeutic targets for the treatment of osteoporosis. *Therapeutic Advances in Musculoskeletal Disease* 8 (6): 225–235. https://doi.org/10.1177/1759720X16670154.

Luo, L., Zhou, K., Zhang, J. et al. (2020). Interventions for leg cramps in pregnancy. *Cochrane Database of Systematic Reviews* (12): CD010655.

Manaye, S., Cheran, K., Murthy, C. et al. (2023). The role of high-intensity and high-impact exercises in improving bone health in postmenopausal women: a systematic review. *Cureus* 15 (2): e34644.

Meah, V.L., Davies, G.A., and Davenport, M.H. (2020). Why can't I exercise during pregnancy? Time to revisit medical 'absolute' and 'relative' contraindications: systematic review of evidence of harm and a call to action. *British Journal of Sports Medicine* 54: 1395–1404.

Morelli, M.B., Santulli, G., and Gambardella, J. (2020). Calcium supplements: good for the bone, bad for the heart? A systematic updated appraisal. *Atherosclerosis* 296: 68–73.

NHS. (2020a). Calcium. https://www.nhs.uk/conditions/vitamins-and-minerals/calcium (accessed 27 October 2023).

NHS. (2020b). Vitamin D. https://www.nhs.uk/conditions/vitamins-and-minerals/vitamin-d (accessed 27 October 2023).

NICE (2021). *Antenatal Care. NICE Guideline NG201.* London: National Institute for Health and Care Excellence https://www.nice.org.uk/guidance/ng201/chapter/recommendations#information-about-antenatal-care (accessed 27 October 2023).

NICE (2022). *Restless Legs Syndrome. Clinical Knowledge Summaries.* London: National Institute for Health and Care Excellence https://cks.nice.org.uk/topics/restless-legs-syndrome.

Palacios, C., Kostiuk, L.K., and Peña-Rosas, J.P. (2019). Vitamin D supplementation for women during pregnancy. *Cochrane Database of Systematic Reviews* (7): e34644.

Rankin, J. (2017). *Physiology in Childbearing,* 4e. Philadelphia, PA: Elsevier.

RCOG (2015). *Reducing the Risk of Thrombosis and Embolism during Pregnancy and the Puerperium.* Green-top Guideline No. 37a. London: Royal College of Obstetricians and Gynaecologists.

Rise, E., Bø, K., and Nystad, W. (2019). Is there any association between abdominal strength training before and during pregnancy and delivery outcome? The Norwegian mother and child cohort study. *Brazilian Journal of Physical Therapy* 23 (2): 108–115. https://doi-org.nottingham.idm.oclc.org/10.1016/j.bjpt.2018.06.006.

Schröder, G., Kundt, G., Otte, M. et al. (2016). Impact of pregnancy on back pain and body posture in women. *Journal of Physical Therapy Science* 28 (4): 1199–1207. https://doi.org/10.1589/jpts.28.1199.

Segal, N.A., Boyer, E.R., Teran-Yengle, P. et al. (2013). Pregnancy leads to lasting changes in foot structure. *American Journal of Physical Medicine & Rehabilitation* 92 (3): 232–240. https://doi-org.nottingham.idm.oclc.org/10.1097/PHM.0b013e31827443a9.

Swanson, S. (2001). Abdominal muscles in pregnancy and the postpartum period. *International Journal of Childbirth Education* 16 (4): 12.

Tortora, G.J. (2016). *Principles of Anatomy and Physiology,* 6e. Oxford: Wiley-Blackwell.

UK Chief Medical Officers. (2019) *UK Chief Medical Officers' Physical Activity Guidelines.* London: Department of Health and Social Care. https://www.gov.uk/government/publications/physical-activity-guidelines-uk-chief-medical-officers-report (accessed 27 October 2023).

UK Chief Medical Officers (2023). *UK CMOs' Physical Activity Guidelines Communications Framework: Main Guidance.* London: Department of Health and Social Care https://www.gov.uk/government/publications/uk-chief-medical-officers-physical-activity-guidelines-communications-framework/uk-cmos-physical-activity-guidelines-communications-framework-main-guidance.

Vandekerckhove, M. and Wang, Y. (2018). Emotion, emotion regulation and sleep: An intimate relationship. *Neuroscience* 5 (1): 1–17. doi: 10.3934/Neuroscience.2018.1.1.

de Vivo, M. and Mills, H. (2019). They turn to you first for everything: insights into midwives' perspectives of providing physical activity advice and guidance to pregnant women. *BMC Pregnancy and Childbirth* 19: 462. https://doi.org/10.1186/s12884-019-2607-x.

Walters, A.S. (2007). Clinical identification of the simple sleep-related movement disorders. *Chest* 131 (4): 1260–1266.

Ward, K.A. (2013). A life course approach to healthy musculoskeletal ageing. In: *A Life Course Approach to Healthy Ageing, Life Course Approach to Adult Health* (ed. D. Kuh). Oxford: Oxford Academic.

World Health Organization. (2022). Physical activity. https://www.who.int/news-room/fact-sheets/detail/physical-activity (27 October 2023).

Further Reading

Clarke, B. (2008). Normal bone anatomy and physiology. *Clinical Journal of the American Society of Nephrology* 3 (Suppl 3): S131–S139. https://doi.org/10.2215/CJN.04151206.

Ding, X.X., Wu, Y.L., Xu, S.J. et al. (2014). A systematic review and quantitative assessment of sleep-disordered breathing during pregnancy and perinatal outcomes. *Sleep & Breathing* 18: 703–713. https://doi-org.nottingham.idm.oclc.org/10.1007/s11325-014-0946-4.

Distefano, G. and Goodpaster, B.H. (2018). Effects of exercise and aging on skeletal muscle. *Cold Spring Harbor Perspectives in Medicine* 8 (3): a029785. https://doi-org.nottingham.idm.oclc.org/10.1101/cshperspect.a029785.

Dunietz, G.L., Lisabeth, L.D., Shedden, K. et al. (2017). Restless legs syndrome and sleep-wake disturbances in pregnancy. *Journal of Clinical Sleep Medicine* 13 (7): 863–870.

Frontera, W.R. and Ochala, J. (2015). Skeletal muscle: a brief review of structure and function. *Calcified Tissue International* 96: 183–195. https://doi-org.nottingham.idm.oclc.org/10.1007/s00223-014-9915-y.

Gilleard, W.L. and Brown, J.M. (1996). Structure and function of the abdominal muscles in primigravid subjects during pregnancy and the immediate postbirth period. *Physical Therapy* 76 (7): 750–762.

Heazell, A., Li, M., Budd, J. et al. (2018). Association between maternal sleep practices and late stillbirth – findings from a stillbirth case-control study. *BJOG* 125 (2): 254–262.

Huxley, A.F. and Niedergerke, R. (1954). Structural changes in muscle during contraction: interference microscopy of living muscle fibres. *Nature* 173 (4412): 971–973.

Kuliukas, A., Kuliukas, L., Franklin, D., and Flavel, A. (2015). Female pelvic shape: distinct types or nebulous cloud? *British Journal of Midwifery* 23: 490–496. https://doi.org/10.12968/bjom.2015.23.7.490.

Maggioli, C. and Stagi, S. (2017). Bone modeling, remodelling, and skeletal health in children and adolescents: mineral accrual, assessment and treatment. *Annals of Pediatric Endocrinology and Metabolism* 22 (1): 1–5. https://doi.org/10.6065/apem.2017.22.1.1.

McArdle, W.D. et al. (2010). *Exercise Physiology : Nutrition, Energy and Human Performance*, 7e, International ed. Philadelphia, PA: Wolters Kluwer/Lippincott Williams & Wilkins.

Michalska, A., Rokita, W., Wolder, D. et al. (2018). Diastasis recti abdominis – a review of treatment methods. *Ginekologia Polska* 89 (2): 97–101.

Mindell, J.A., Cook, R.A., and Nikolovski, J. (2015). Sleep patterns and sleep disturbances across pregnancy. *Sleep Medicine* 16 (4): 483–488.

Mota, P., Pascoal, A.G., Carita, A.I., and Bø, K. (2015). The immediate effects on inter-rectus distance of abdominal crunch and drawing-in exercises during pregnancy and the postpartum period. *Journal of Orthopaedic and Sports Physical Therapy* 45 (10): 781–788.

Olsson, A., Kiwanuka, O., Wilhelmsson, S. et al. (2021). Surgical repair of diastasis recti abdominis provides long-term improvement of abdominal core function and quality of life: a 3-year follow-up. *BJS Open* 5 (5): zrab085. https://doi-org.nottingham.idm.oclc.org/10.1093/bjsopen/zrab085.

Radhakrishnan, M. and Ramamurthy, K. (2022). Efficacy and challenges in the treatment of diastasis recti abdominis-a scoping review on the current trends and future perspectives. *Diagnostics* 12 (9): 2044.

Vandekerckhove, M. and Wang, Y.L. (2018). Emotion, emotion regulation and sleep: an intimate relationship. *AIMS Neuroscience* 5 (1): 1–17.

VanSickle, C., Liese, K.L., and Rutherford, J.N. (2022). Textbook typologies: challenging the myth of the perfect obstetric pelvis. *Anatomical Record* 305 (4): 952–967. https://doi-org.nottingham.idm.oclc.org/10.1002/ar.24880.

Glossary

Abduction	Movement away from the midline of the body.
Actin	Protein found in muscle cells, playing a crucial role in muscle contraction and movement.
Adduction	Movement towards the midline of the body.
Appendicular skeleton	The bones of the limbs, the shoulder and pelvic girdles.
Axial skeleton	The central part of the skeleton, consisting of the skull, vertebral column and ribcage.
Bone	Osseous tissue; a biomaterial, which is dynamic and metabolically active.
Bone marrow	Soft, spongy tissue found in the cavities of bones. It produces blood cells and stores fat.
Bones	Calcified structures forming the skeletal framework of the body, providing support and protection to internal organs.
Cartilage	Flexible connective tissue found in joints and other structures, acting as a cushion, reducing friction and absorbing shock.
Extension	Straightening movement that increases the angle between bones at a joint.
Flexion	Bending movement that decreases the angle between bones at a joint.
Joint	Junction where bones meet, allowing movement and flexibility.
Kyphosis	An exaggerated outward curvature of the spine, leading to a rounded back posture.
Ligament	Strong connective tissue that connects bones to other bones, providing stability and preventing excessive movement.
Lordosis	An exaggerated inward curvature of the spine, commonly seen in the lower back.
Mineralisation	The process of depositing minerals, particularly calcium and phosphorus, into the bone matrix.
Muscle atrophy	A decrease in muscle size and strength due to disuse or injury.
Muscle hypertrophy	The enlargement and increase in size of muscle fibres, typically resulting from strength training exercises.
Muscles	Contractile tissues responsible for generating force and movement.
Muscular strength	The maximum force a muscle or group of muscles can generate during a single contraction or effort.
Myosin	Protein found in muscle cells, responsible for the interaction with actin during muscle contraction.
Osteoblasts	Specialised cells responsible for bone formation.
Osteoclasts	Cells responsible for bone resorption, breaking down old or damaged bone tissue.
Osteocytes	Mature bone cells embedded within the bone matrix. They maintain bone tissue.
Range of motion	The extent to which a joint can move through its full capacity.
Resorption	Process of breaking down bone tissue by osteoclasts, releasing minerals into the bloodstream.
Rotation	Movement around a central axis.
Scoliosis	A lateral curvature of the spine.
Tendons	Dense connective tissues attaching muscles to bones.
Vitamin D	A fat-soluble vitamin, essential for bone health and mineralisation.

Multiple Choice Questions

1. Approximately how many bones are in the human body?
   a. 193
   b. 106
   c. 206
   d. 285

2. Bones are attached to bones by what structure?
   a. Ligaments
   b. Vertebrae
   c. Tendons
   d. Cords

3. The joints of the hip and the shoulder are what type of joint?
   a. Hinge
   b. Ball and socket
   c. Fused
   d. Sliding

4. Spongy bone is also known as what?
   a. Cortical bone
   b. Osteon bone
   c. Trabecular bone
   d. Cuboidal bone

5. Which bones form part of the axial skeleton?
   a. Femur
   b. Scapula
   c. Phalanges
   d. Rib cage

6. Which of the following statements is TRUE?
   a. The angle of the pubic arch is smaller in the female pelvis
   b. The female pelvis has a wider true pelvis
   c. There are only minor differences between the male and female pelvis
   d. The male pelvis has a wider true pelvis

7. Which of the following bone cells make up most of the bone matrix?
   a. Osteoblasts
   b. Osteoclasts
   c. Osteoprogenitor cells
   d. Osteocytes

8. Which of the following is a function of the muscular system?
   a. It transports food through the gastrointestinal system
   b. It produces motion across bones and joints
   c. It generates heat in a process known as thermogenesis
   d. It does all of the above

9. During pregnancy, what is the site of the separation of the abdominal muscles?
   a. The linea alba
   b. The external oblique muscles
   c. The latissimus dorsi
   d. The pelvic floor

10. How many days a week does the Department of Health and Social Care recommend that adults engage in strength-building activities?
    a. 5
    b. 3
    c. 2
    d. 4

CHAPTER 9

The Circulatory System

Kate Nash

AIM

This chapter describes the components and functions of the circulatory system and explains changes that take place in response to pregnancy, and during the perinatal period.

LEARNING OUTCOMES

On completion of this chapter, you will be able to:

- Define the structure and function of the systemic, pulmonary, portal and fetal circulatory systems.
- Discuss the physiological adaptations that occur to meet the specific requirements of the mother and fetus during pregnancy and childbirth.
- Explain the associated midwifery care to ensure optimal functioning of the circulatory system during pregnancy.
- Identify some of the pathological considerations associated with the circulatory system and associated midwifery actions.

Test Your Prior Knowledge
1. List the main functions of the circulatory system.
2. Describe the key changes to red blood cells and plasma that occur during pregnancy.
3. List four signs and symptoms of venous thromboembolism.
4. Describe why it is important to screen for iron deficiency anaemia during pregnancy.

Introduction

The circulatory system is a complex distribution system permitting blood and lymph to transport nutrients, gases (oxygen, carbon dioxide, nitrogen), hormones and blood cells to and from cells within the body (Peate and Evans 2020). The heart, blood vessels and blood are integral components of this system. The heart is a pump that is essential for distributing blood via the blood vessels around the body.

Fundamentals of Maternal Anatomy and Physiology, First Edition. Edited by Ian Peate and Claire Leader.
© 2024 John Wiley & Sons Ltd. Published 2024 by John Wiley & Sons Ltd.

The Circulatory System

The circulatory system has a vital and complex role in preserving life and maintaining homeostasis to ensure a stable equilibrium exists between the physiological processes within the body. Physiological and anatomical adaptations of the circulatory and cardiovascular systems occur during pregnancy, designed to support fetal growth and development and enhance maternal wellbeing. Although most changes occur during pregnancy, significant changes also occur during labour and immediately following delivery of the baby.

Specific functions of the circulatory system are outlined here and discussed throughout this chapter as the adaptations that occur during pregnancy are explained:

- Circulation of oxygenated blood to cells and removal of waste products of metabolism (e.g. carbon dioxide and nitrogen via elimination sites including kidneys and lungs).
- Transportation of hormones from endocrine organs to corresponding target hormones through the circulatory system.
- Stabilisation of the body temperature through absorption and distribution of body heat produced by cellular chemical activity.
- Maintenance of blood pH by the excretion or reabsorption of hydrogen ions and bicarbonate ions.
- Prevention of infection and fighting disease within the body via actions of white blood cells, antibodies and complement proteins.
- Preservation of circulating blood volume.
- Protection against blood loss and body fluids through the mechanism of clotting, in which platelets and plasma proteins play a vital role in the coagulation pathway.

The circulatory system encompasses the systemic, pulmonary and portal circulations in addition to the fetal and placental circulation established during pregnancy. Central to the circulatory system is the heart, a muscular pump that moves approximately 4000–7000 l of blood through the body each day (Shier et al. 2016). Blood is transported on a continual basis through the heart, arteries, arterioles, veins, venules and a capillary network.

175

The Systemic and Pulmonary Circulations

Through the systemic circulation, oxygen-rich (oxygenated) blood is pumped away from the heart via arteries to provide oxygen for all living cells, and veins carry deoxygenated blood back to the heart, where it is pumped to the lungs for reoxygenation via the pulmonary circulatory system. The pulmonary circulation refers to the part of the circulatory system that circulates deoxygenated blood returning from the body from the right side of the heart to the lungs for oxygenation and then to the left side of the heart where it begins its journey back via the systemic circulation. As well as enabling oxygenation of the blood, the pulmonary circuit also permits carbon dioxide to be released and exhaled from the body via the lungs.

Figure 9.1 shows a diagram of the circulatory system, depicting the heart and major blood vessels. The arteries (red) carry oxygenated blood from the heart, and the veins (blue) carry deoxygenated blood back to the heart. Blood is transported through the circulatory system largely because of the pressure generated by the contractions of the heart (Wylie 2005). Stroke volume, heart rate and cardiac output increase during pregnancy. This can be observed as a heart rate increase of 10–15 beats per minute, translating into 14 000–21 000 extra beats per day (Osol et al. 2019). Changes to blood distribution during pregnancy occur with increased blood flow to the uterus, kidneys, intestines and skin, while perfusion of other organs such as the brain, skeletal muscle and liver is not measurably different to the non-pregnant state (Osol et al. 2019; Mushambi 2016).

Fetal circulation develops from around 22 days (Remien and Majmundar 2022) and permits the exchange of nutrients and waste materials between mother and fetus through the placenta via the umbilical vessels. Blood volume increases considerably throughout pregnancy, reaching approximately 45–50% more than non-pregnant values by term, with increased uterine blood flow from 50 ml/minute in non-pregnant women to approximately 700–1000 ml/minute (over 10% of cardiac output) at term (Osol et al. 2019; Sutton and Mann 2021).

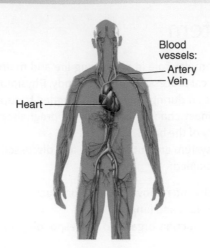

FIGURE 9.1   The circulatory system. Source: Peate and Evans (2020), p. 240/John Wiley & Sons.

Vasodilation of the blood vessels occurs, facilitated primarily by the hormone progesterone, accommodating the increased blood volume occurring during pregnancy. Despite the significant increase in cardiac output and total blood volume apparent in healthy pregnancies, systemic vascular resistance decreases during pregnancy through vasodilation. The impact of these physiological adaptations can be observed through a slight drop in maternal blood pressure, which reaches a nadir during the second trimester, increasing gradually towards term.

In addition to vasodilation, the uterus increases approximately 20-fold during pregnancy, preparing for birth initially through hyperplasia and then hypertrophy of myometrial smooth muscle (Osol et al. 2019). To accomplish this, circulation supplying the uterus undergoes angiogenesis and extensive remodelling as myometrial smooth muscle, uterine arteries and veins increase to sustain placental perfusion and fetal development (Osol et al. 2019).

Reflective Learning Activity

Prepare a diagrammatic representation of the heart and trace the flow of oxygenated blood away from the heart and deoxygenated blood back to the heart.

Red Flag Alert: Supine Hypotensive Syndrome

Avoiding the supine position for pregnant women is important. It may initiate supine hypotensive syndrome, caused by the gravid uterus compressing the inferior vena cava.

Coronary Circulation

The coronary circulation is part of the systemic circulation, transporting oxygenated blood from the ascending aorta to heart muscle (myocardium), ensuring that the heart receives a constant supply of nutrients essential for its function. Deoxygenated blood is then returned to the right side of the heart and once again begins the pulmonary circuit.

Hepatic Portal Circulation

The hepatic portal circulation refers to the circulation of blood from the gastrointestinal organs via the hepatic portal vein into the liver. It is then returned via the hepatic veins and inferior vena cava to the systemic circulation, resuming its journey to the heart.

Entering the liver, blood is filtered and processed as capillaries of the intestines and other digestive organs are connected to specialised capillaries (hepatic sinusoids; Ferng 2022). This permits the regulation, modification and storage of vitamins, glucose, amino acids and lipids, as well as removal of bacteria entering blood via the intestinal capillaries (Shier et al. 2016). Through this process, nutrients absorbed from digestion are effectively processed and stored and bacteria and toxins removed before the blood is distributed to the rest of the cells.

The Fetal Circulation

The developing fetus does not use its lungs for oxygenation, having its own distinctive circulation, enabling the exchange of nutrients and waste materials with its mother through the placenta via the umbilical vessels. The umbilical vein delivers oxygenated blood from the placenta to the fetus, providing oxygen and nutrients. The umbilical arteries transport deoxygenated blood away from the fetal cells and back towards the placenta for reoxygenation.

The developing fetal heart and brain means that the fetus has high energy demands requiring the fetal circulation to direct blood away from non-functional organs to ensure that growing tissues receive enough oxygen to meet their developmental requirements. Because the placenta is not as efficient at gaseous exchange as mature lungs, increased fetal cardiac output, higher concentration of fetal haemoglobin, together with the increased oxygen-carrying capacity of fetal haemoglobin, facilitate adequate fetal tissue oxygenation (Ross and Ervin 2017).

Four temporary structures are located within the fetal circulation, enabling blood to bypass the fetal lungs, redirecting blood instead through the umbilical cord to the placenta where the exchange of oxygen, nutrients and waste materials occurs. Oxygen diffuses from the maternal blood through the chorionic villi into the umbilical vein in the placenta. The umbilical vein carries oxygenated blood from the placenta to the fetus via the umbilical cord towards the inferior cava in the fetal abdomen. The ductus venosus, a temporary structure, directs most of the blood into the inferior vena cava while the remaining blood travels to the liver via the portal vein. Here, the blood is processed for nutrients and oxygen, following which the deoxygenated blood travels from the hepatic artery to the vena cava (Remien and Majmundar 2022).

Blood from the vena cava enters the right atrium of the fetal heart, where most of the blood is directed through the foramen ovale, an opening in the septum. Thus, the foramen ovale creates a shunt between the right atrium and the left atrium so oxygenated blood can pass through the left ventricle and into the ascending aorta, oxygenating the developing fetal brain. Blood travels from the left atrium to the left ventricle and into the aorta. The foramen ovale ensures that most of the blood does not travel in the pulmonary circulation to the non-functioning fetal lungs.

The ductus arteriosus, another temporary structure, prevents most of the blood from reaching the lungs by directing any blood entering the pulmonary arteries via the right atrium into the aorta and back into systemic circulation. The blood flowing through the fetal aorta is a mixture of oxygenated and non-oxygenated blood. Hypogastric arteries branch from the fetal iliac arteries and return blood via the umbilical arteries of the umbilical cord to the placenta (Table 9.1).

TABLE 9.1 **Overview of temporary structure required for fetal circulation.**

Temporary structure	Function
Ductus venosus	Directs oxygenated blood from the umbilical vein directly to the inferior vena cava, enabling blood from the placenta to bypass the highly demanding, but relatively inactive liver
Foramen ovale	Blood is directed through this to bypass the fetal lungs and pulmonary circulation
Ductus arteriosus	Lies between the pulmonary arteries and aorta and permits blood to pass straight from the right ventricle into the aorta bypassing pulmonary circulation
Hypogastric arteries	Direct most of the deoxygenated blood back through the umbilical arteries to the placenta

Medications Management: Non-steroidal Anti-inflammatory Drugs

Non-steroidal anti-inflammatory drugs should be avoided during the third trimester of pregnancy because of associated risk of closure of the fetal ductus arteriosus in utero and possibly persistent pulmonary hypertension of the newborn.

Adaptation of the Fetal Circulation to Extrauterine Life

Following birth, the infant takes their first breath and a series of changes occur, establishing the pulmonary circulation and effective oxygenation using the lungs. The newborn infant is stimulated to take their first breath, causing a rise in the partial pressure of oxygen and resulting in pulmonary vasodilation.

Pulmonary vasodilation causes a drop in the right atrium. This, combined with the cessation of the placental circulation, results an increase in pressure in the left atrium. The change in pressure causes a tissue flap on the left side of the foramen ovale to close over this structure (Wylie 2005).

As pulmonary and systemic circulations separate, blood can no longer divert through the foramen ovale and is directed instead into the right ventricle and pulmonary circulation. The ductus arteriosus is also bypassed in this process and the direction of fetal blood flow is reversed as blood pressure in the pulmonary artery falls while systemic blood pressure rises. Higher oxygen levels cause the ductus arteriosus to constrict over the two to three days after birth as they close, forming one of the heart ligaments (Wylie 2005).

The structural remnants of the fetal circulatory structures are referred to as the fossa ovalis (foramen ovale), the ligamentum arteriosum (ductus arteriosus) and the ligamentum venosum (ductus venosus).

Structure of the Vessels Supporting the Circulatory System

A blood vessel is a tube-like structure inside of which blood circulates. The blood vessels form a closed-circuit network enabling blood to flow from the heart to cells within the body and back to the heart (Peate 2017). The three major types of blood vessels are summarised in Table 9.2 and described in more detail below.

The heart is anchored to the diaphragm, to the back of the sternum and to the great blood vessels, the aorta, pulmonary arteries and veins and venae cavae by its outer layer, the pericardium (see Chapter 10 for the functions of the heart and cardiovascular system).

Arteries are strong elastic vessels capable of transporting oxygenated blood away from the heart under high pressure, dividing into thinner tubes branching into finer arterioles leading to capillaries. Capillaries come into close contact with tissue cells and the thin capillary walls allow for most gaseous exchanges between the blood and tissue cells. When

TABLE 9.2 Arteries, veins and arterioles.

Vessels	Description
Arteries	Arteries and arterioles transport oxygenated blood away from the ventricles of the heart at high pressure leading to capillaries where substances are exchanged between blood and body cells. Arteries have thicker walls than veins as they have more muscle tissue
Veins	Veins and venules return deoxygenated blood at a lower pressure from the capillaries to the atria. Vein walls are thinner because there is less muscle and elastic tissue. Some veins have valves preventing backflow
Capillaries	Tiny thin-walled vessels forming the point of connection in the tissues between the arteries and veins. Nutrients and waste are exchanged between blood and the body's cells through the thin walls of capillaries

oxygenated blood leaves the alveolar capillaries, it enters venules that eventually unite forming larger blood vessels transporting blood to the pulmonary veins and back to the heart (Moini 2016).

The venous system acts as an important reservoir for blood, with most of the circulating blood (65–70%) found within the venous system due to the increased compliance of veins, meaning that they are more easily able to accommodate changes in blood volume (Gelman et al. 2008). This is of particular significance to pregnancy as the circulating volume of blood increases substantially meeting the requirements of the maternal, fetal and placental circulation and birth.

Walls of arteries and veins consist of three layers:

1. Inner endothelium
2. Middle layer consisting of smooth muscle and elastic tissue
3. Outer layer consisting of connective tissue.

Arteries have thicker smooth muscle and connective tissue layers to support the higher pressure of blood contained within arteries and explained further below.

Arteries

Artery walls comprise three distinct layers, surrounding the lumen or central cavity where blood is contained (Figure 9.2). The outer layer, the tunica externa (also called tunica adventitia), is thinner and consists mainly of connective tissue. This layer is attached to surrounding tissues, containing nerve fibres and lymphatic vessels. The middle layer, known as tunica media, encompasses most of the artery wall and includes smooth muscle fibres and a thick elastic connective tissue layer. The smooth muscle fibre activity is controlled by the autonomic systems vasomotor nerve fibres and many other chemicals. The inner layer is the tunica intima, made up of a layer of simple squamous epithelium known as the endothelium.

The endothelium within the inner layer provides a smooth surface to facilitate the flow of blood cells and platelets and may help prevent blood clotting by secreting chemicals inhibiting platelet aggregation (Shier et al. 2016). It may also assist with regulating the flow of blood by secreting substances that dilate or constrict blood vessels such as nitric oxide, which relaxes smooth muscle (Moini 2016; Shier et al. 2016).

Arteries are elastic or muscular. Elastic arteries (also known as conducting arteries) are located near the heart and include the aorta and its primary branches. The largest artery, the aorta, receives oxygenated blood pumped via the left ventricle of the heart, transporting it around the body. Blood pressure is strongest when blood leaves the heart via the left ventricle and becomes weaker as the distance from the heart increases because of the peripheral resistance between

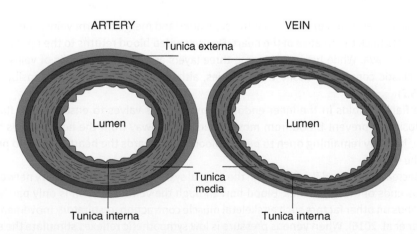

FIGURE 9.2   An artery and vein. Source: Peate (2011), p. 388/John Wiley & Sons.

the blood and the vessel walls. Elastic arteries contain more elastin than other types of artery and have the biggest lumens, ranging between 2.5 and 1 cm (Moini 2016). Because the lumens are large, they act as low-resistance pathways for blood as it moves from the heart to the medium sized arteries.

Muscular arteries (also known as distributary arteries) are smaller than elastic arteries and located distally (further from the heart). Muscular arteries have the thickest tunica media (middle layer) of all blood vessels in proportion to their size and have relatively more smooth muscle and less elastic tissue in comparison with elastic arteries. Because of this, they have more vasoconstrictive properties but are less able to stretch (Moini 2016).

In uncomplicated pregnancy, the maternal vascular endothelium has many important functions, including control of smooth muscle tone through release of vasoconstrictor and vasodilatory substances and regulation of anticoagulation, antiplatelet and fibrinolytic functions via the release of different soluble factors. The vasodilators include agents such as nitric oxide and prostacyclin, levels increase considerably in pregnancy accommodating the increased blood volume through vasodilation (Rankin 2017). In pathological conditions such as pre-eclampsia, there is an abnormal shift towards vasoconstriction, which may be a consequence of generalised dysfunction of the endothelium, and an increased production of vasoconstrictors, which influence the tone of the underlying vascular smooth muscle (McCarthy and Kenny 2010).

Arterioles and Capillaries

Arterioles are the smallest of the arteries with the diameter of their lumens reaching approximately 0.3 mm and 10 μm. The smaller arterioles lead directly into capillaries forming a dense network of capillary beds. Capillaries are the smallest diameter blood vessels connecting the smallest arterioles to the smallest venules. Their walls are made of epithelium, forming a semipermeable layer facilitating the exchange of gases, nutrients and metabolic waste products between individual cells and the circulatory system (Rankin 2017).

Some capillaries pass directly from arterioles to venules, others have highly branched networks. The greater a tissue's rate of metabolism the denser its capillary networks; for example, muscle and nerve tissues that require large amounts of oxygen are well supplied with capillaries. Regulation of blood flow through capillaries is mainly by smooth muscle forming a precapillary sphincter encircling the capillary where it branches off from an arteriole.

Precapillary sphincters control blood distribution, responding to cellular demands by relaxing when cellular oxygen is low allowing oxygenated blood to enter cells and contracting when cellular requirements have been met (Moini 2016; Rankin 2017) The autonomic nervous system coordinates arterial and venular function in regulating capillary blood flow.

Veins, Venules and Venous Valves

Venules are microscopic vessels that continue from the capillaries and merge to form veins. Veins transport blood from the capillaries and venules back to the atria of the heart. Deoxygenated blood returns to the right atrium of the heart via the largest vein, the vena cava. While having the same three layers as arteries, the walls of veins are thinner with less smooth muscle and elastic connective tissue than arteries, although veins are more distensible with wider lumens (Rankin 2017; Figure 9.2).

Many veins have flap-like folds in the inner endothelium acting as valves to ensure blood flows in one direction towards the heart, closing to prevent blood from moving backwards away from the heart. Valves facilitate the flow of blood returning to the heart by remaining open to permit blood flow towards the heart, closing to prevent any backflow of blood away from the heart.

Blood pressure decreases as blood flows through the arterial system and into the capillary networks so little pressure remains at the venous ends of the capillaries. Blood flow through the venous system is only partly the direct result of heart action and depends on other factors such as skeletal muscle contraction, respiratory movements and vasoconstriction of the veins (Shier et al. 2016). When venous pressure is low sympathetic reflexes stimulate the smooth muscle cells in the walls of the veins to contract. The layers of a blood vessel are depicted in Figure 9.3.

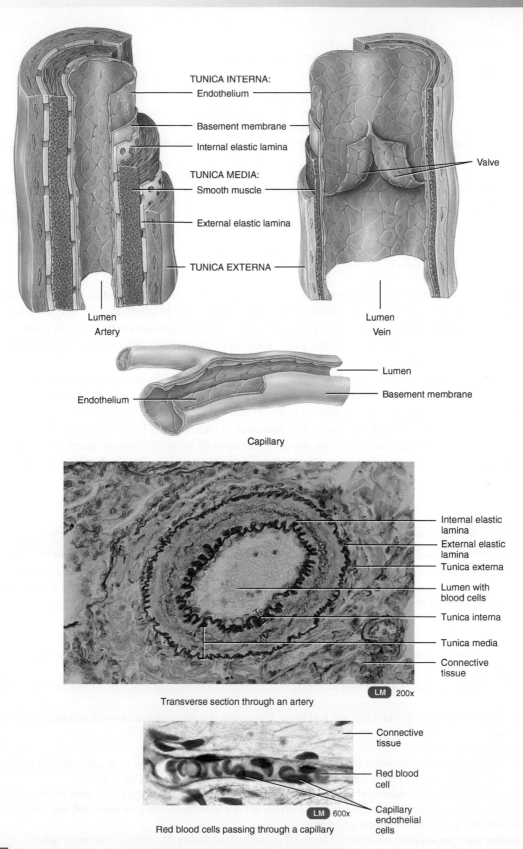

TUNICA INTERNA:
Endothelium

Basement membrane

Internal elastic lamina

TUNICA MEDIA:
Smooth muscle

External elastic lamina

TUNICA EXTERNA

Lumen
Artery

Valve

Lumen
Vein

Lumen

Basement membrane

Endothelium

Capillary

Internal elastic lamina

External elastic lamina

Tunica externa

Lumen with blood cells

Tunica interna

Tunica media

Connective tissue

LM 200x

Transverse section through an artery

Connective tissue

Red blood cell

LM 600x

Red blood cells passing through a capillary

Capillary endothelial cells

FIGURE 9.3 Layers of a blood vessel. Source: Peate (2011), p. 388/John Wiley & Sons.

BOX 9.1 | **Vein Selection for Venepuncture**

Factors to consider:

- Size of the vein and how well supported it is by surrounding tissues.
- Veins should be easy to palpate and fill quickly with blood after compression, feeling soft and bouncy.
- Avoid veins that feel hard, thin, fragile, unsupported and mobile.
- Venous valves can be observed or felt as small nodular areas on the vein, often at the intersection of two veins and should also be avoided.
- Check skin integrity and avoid broken, bruised, scarred, inflamed and previously punctured skin.
- Ensuring the angle of needle insertion is within 10–30 degrees will reduce the risk of nerve damage and also prevent inadvertently striking an artery.

Varicosities of Pregnancy

The development of varicosities or varicose veins is a common minor complication of pregnancy (NICE 2020) and can develop in around 40% of pregnant women (Rankin 2017), being estimated to affect at least one-third of the general population (NICE 2013). Varicosities are dilated, often palpable subcutaneous veins with reversed blood flow, mainly occurring in the legs but may also occur within the pelvic vessels, vulval and anal area where they present as haemorrhoids (Blackburn 2013; NICE 2013).

The development of varicosities is exacerbated during pregnancy mainly because of progesterone-mediated smooth muscle relaxation of the veins. As the increased volume of blood moves into the veins, reduced vascular resistance causes the circulation to become sluggish leading to pooling of blood and distention of the venous blood vessels further reducing the efficiency of the venous valves. Pelvic congestion and poor venous return of blood to the heart is also exacerbated by the weight of the gravid uterus. While varicosities occur because of impaired venous return, the exact underlying pathophysiology of the condition is unclear and different theories exist to explain this (Bootun et al. 2022).

Snapshot 9.1   Varicose Veins

Omar, a 36-year-old multiparous woman, has attended her 36-week antenatal clinic with her midwife Becky, and has concerns that her legs feel heavy and ache more than usual. On visual inspection, Becky notices that Omar has varicose veins that are visible on both calves. What information should Becky provide to Omar?

Key Points to Consider

- Explain to Omar that varicose veins are common in pregnancy due to the hormonal changes, vasodilation and an increase increased venous circulation.
- Reassure Omar that varicose veins are not harmful to her or her baby and often improve after birth when hormones return to their normal levels.
- Undertake a visual inspection of Omar's legs and full clinical assessment, as well as providing verbal and written information on varicose veins.
- Offer compression stockings.
- Discuss lifestyle and day-to-day activities such as smoking cessation. Advise against sitting or standing for long periods of time, which may exacerbate her symptoms, and that she should elevate her legs where possible (NICE 2020).
- Advise Omar of the signs and symptoms of venous thromboembolism, explaining when she would need to seek urgent medical help. Symptoms such as swelling, redness, tenderness and pain in the affected area, often the lower calf, may be symptomatic of a deep vein thrombosis and require urgent attention.
- Review whether there are any other complicating factors that may prompt further treatment and obstetric referral.

The Hypercoagulable State of Pregnancy

As blood is distributed around the body via the blood vessels of the circulatory system, homeostasis is maintained through complex processes required to balance the interplay between coagulation and anticoagulation. Procoagulants, or clotting factors, produced mostly by the liver are present as proteins and inorganic ions within blood plasma and required for coagulation.

Alongside platelets, clotting factors promote coagulation and are integral to the clotting mechanisms required for repair and the cessation of blood loss when blood vessels are injured (the intrinsic clotting pathway) or surrounding tissue (the extrinsic clotting pathway). These clotting factors are involved with the coordinated enzyme reactions and platelet responses required to generate thrombin and convert soluble fibrinogen into fibrin to establish a haemostatic plug formed by platelets at sites of vessel damage. Failure of coagulation mechanisms results in excessive bleeding.

The coagulation process requires regulation to prevent continued coagulation and the development of thrombi or clots that can impair blood flow to cells and vital organs such as the heart, brain and lungs. Endogenous anticoagulants are proteins synthesised by the liver, circulating in blood plasma working to maintain haemostasis, preventing blood from clotting and maintaining effective blood distribution through the regulation and inhibition of blood clotting at different stages of the coagulation pathway.

During pregnancy, the concentration of certain clotting factors is increased and fibrinolytic activity decreased. Concentrations of endogenous anticoagulants such as antithrombin and protein S, also decrease. These changes, alongside venous stasis, present in the lower limbs associated with vasodilation, decreased blood flow and the weight of the gravid uterus, predispose pregnant women to venous thromboembolism.

> ### Medications Management: Low Molecular Weight Heparins
>
> Low molecular weight heparins (LMWHs), such as dalteparin, are anticoagulant drugs used in the prophylaxis and treatment of venous thromboembolic disease during and following pregnancy. LMWH works by inhibiting the conversion of prothrombin into thrombin, an action required to convert fibrinogen into fibrin for the formation of a clot.

Blood Constituents

Blood is a liquid connective tissue composed of living cells suspended within an extracellular matrix known as plasma (Rankin 2017; Figure 9.4). Blood can be described as a dense, viscous fluid compared with water. It is bright red in colour when oxygenated within the arteries and appears a darker red when deoxygenated within the veins. The pH of blood is close to neutral, ranging from 7.35 to 7.45, and its temperature is slightly higher than that of the rest of the body, at 38°C (Dooley et al. 2021).

Blood contains red and white cells and cellular fragments known as platelets. These cells and platelets are known as the formed elements of blood, in contrast to the liquid part, plasma (Shier et al. 2016). The process by which formed elements of blood develop is known as haematopoiesis. In the final three months of gestation and throughout extrauterine life, the red bone marrow is the primary centre for haematopoiesis (Peate 2017).

Blood plasma makes up approximately 55% (between 46% and 63%) of the total blood volume and the formed elements of blood make up approximately 37–54% of total blood volume (Wylie 2005; Rankin 2017). The major types of cells circulating in the blood are red blood cells (erythrocytes), white blood cells (leucocytes) and platelets (thrombocytes). Most blood samples are about 45% red blood cells by volume, a percentage known as haematocrit or packed cell volume. White blood cells and platelets account for less than 1% of the formed elements (Shier et al. 2016). The distribution of blood around the body is a principal function of the circulatory system and the many complex functions of blood include the transportation of oxygen and nutrients, removal of waste, protection of the body through the immune system and maintaining a stable internal environment (homeostasis).

Among the significant haematological changes that occur during pregnancy are increases in blood volume, changes in volume beginning at six to eight weeks gestation, peaking during the second trimester with values up to 1600 ml higher

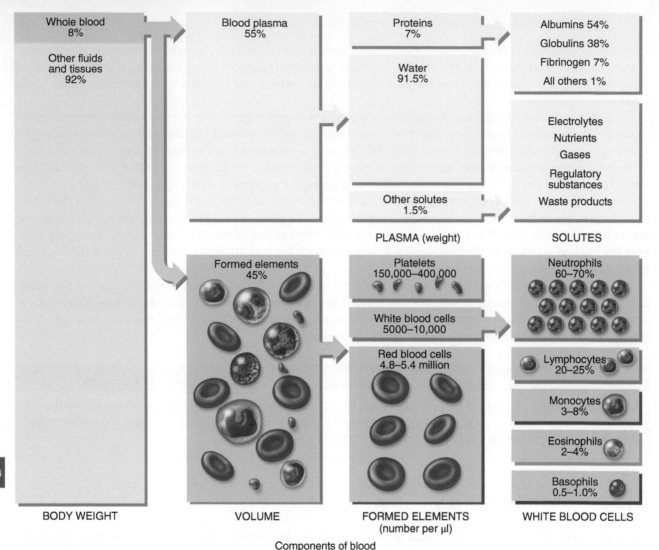

Whole blood
8%

Other fluids
and tissues
92%

Blood plasma
55%

Proteins
7%

Water
91.5%

Other solutes
1.5%

Albumins 54%

Globulins 38%

Fibrinogen 7%

All others 1%

Electrolytes

Nutrients

Gases

Regulatory
substances

Waste products

PLASMA (weight)

SOLUTES

Formed elements
45%

Platelets
150,000–400,000

White blood cells
5000–10,000

Red blood cells
4.8–5.4 million

Neutrophils
60–70%

Lymphocytes
20–25%

Monocytes
3–8%

Eosinophils
2–4%

Basophils
0.5–1.0%

BODY WEIGHT

VOLUME

FORMED ELEMENTS
(number per µl)

WHITE BLOOD CELLS

Components of blood

FIGURE 9.4   Blood cells. Source: Peate (2011), p. 369/John Wiley & Sons.

than in non-pregnant women. This volume has a protective function for maintaining maternal haemostasis and helping to protect the mother against the effects of blood loss during the third stage of labour. This results in a hypervolaemia of pregnancy, which has an impact upon blood cellular volume and plasma constituents and is discussed further below.

Erythrocytes

Erythrocytes are the most abundant blood cells, accounting for over 99% of the formed elements within blood. This equates to approximately 45% of blood volume. Red blood cells provide blood with its red colour and are the main cellular contributor to blood viscosity (Rankin 2017). They are especially adapted to suit their primary function of transporting oxygen and removing carbon dioxide from all living cells as oxygen is carried in red blood cells bound to the molecule haemoglobin.

Red blood cells appear as tiny biconcave discs, thinner in the centre than the rim, whose pliant membrane and large surface area to volume ratio permits rapid exchange of gases and the flexibility to squeeze through small arterioles and capillaries, ensuring a smooth flow through vessels without restriction (Wylie and Bryce 2016; Figure 9.5).

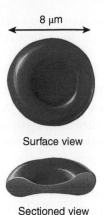

Surface view

Sectioned view

RBC shape

FIGURE 9.5 Red blood cells. Source: Peate (2011), p. 375/John Wiley & Sons.

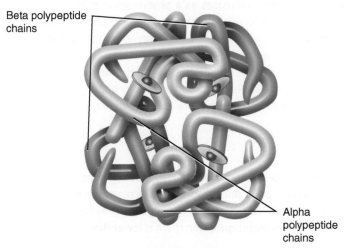

Beta polypeptide chains

Alpha polypeptide chains

Haemoglobin molecule

FIGURE 9.6 Haemoglobin molecule. Source: Peate (2011), p. 376/John Wiley & Sons.

Erythropoiesis is the method by which red blood cells are manufactured, new red blood cells are produced in the bone marrow of the sternum, vertebrae, ribs, base of the skull, and the proximal ends of the long bones in adults. Red blood cells circulate for approximately 120 days before removal from the circulatory system due to being damaged or worn. Whereas young red blood cells contain a nucleus, mature red blood cells do not, increasing their capacity to carry oxygen. Mature red blood cells are unable to repair themselves and so are ingested by macrophages and their constituent minerals and proteins recycled within the spleen and liver. Erythropoiesis is stimulated by the hormone erythropoietin, a glycoprotein produced in the kidney.

Haemoglobin is an oxygen-carrying pigment in red blood cells enabling red blood cells to transport oxygen (Moini 2016). Haemoglobin consists of haem, an iron-containing pigment binding to oxygen, and globin, a protein consisting of two pairs of polypeptide chains, holding the haem and influencing how easily it stores and releases oxygen. As red blood cells pass through the capillaries of the lungs within the pulmonary circulation, oxygen diffuses through the cell walls and attaches to the haemoglobin molecules to form oxyhaemoglobin (Figure 9.6). Oxygenated red blood cells are distributed back through the systemic circulation (Wylie 2005; Rankin 2017).

Haem is recycled as part of the red blood cell recycling process and decomposes into iron and biliverdin. This decomposed iron, combined with a protein transferrin, is transported to the bone marrow and reused in the production of new haemoglobin (Shier et al. 2016). About 80% of iron is stored in the hepatocytes in the form of an iron-protein complex called ferritin. Iron is vital for the synthesis of haemoglobin, and iron released during the destruction of red blood cells is available for reuse (Shier et al. 2016).

Physiological Changes and Haemodilution of Red Blood Cells During Pregnancy

Red blood cells increase during pregnancy and there is an overall increase in total red blood cell volume of 20–30% (Blackburn 2013). This is caused by an increase in circulating erythropoietin promoting erythropoiesis and increasing production of red blood cells (Letsky 2002). The increase in erythropoiesis and red blood cell volume begins slowly during the first trimester, accelerating during the third trimester.

Red cell mass increases by 20–30% and plasma volume increases by 45%. This discrepancy between the increases in red cell mass and plasma volume results in the physiological anaemia of pregnancy, otherwise known as the haemodilutional effect of pregnancy. Haemodilution reaches a peak at 28–34 weeks of gestation, resulting in a lower haemoglobin, haematocrit (percentage of the blood sample that is made up of red cells) and red blood cell count. The haemoglobin concentration falls from a typical prepregnancy concentration of 150 g/l to around 120 g/l at term and haematocrit falls to around 0.35 (Chambers et al. 2019). A lower haematocrit decreases the blood viscosity and lowers the resistance to blood flow in the placental circulation (Bhatia and Chhabra 2018).

Mean corpuscular volume (MCV) slightly increases as a physiological response during pregnancy and, for milder cases of iron deficiency, MCV may not fall below the normal range (NICE 2023). Changes in MCV and mean corpuscular haemoglobin volume are related to iron status and for women with adequate iron, levels remain relatively stable while they decrease in women who are iron deficient (Blackburn 2013).

These physiological changes may contribute to variations in thresholds when defining iron deficiency in pregnancy (Daru et al. 2017). While iron deficiency anaemia is a common pathology of pregnancy, not all women present with symptoms. The physiological haemodilutional effect of pregnancy makes it appear that haemoglobin is lower, leading to challenges with diagnosis (Rankin 2017).

Anaemia During Pregnancy

The fetal requirement for iron and enhanced maternal red cell production considerably increases iron requirements and the risk of iron deficiency anaemia during pregnancy, particularly as many women of childbearing age commence pregnancy with reduced iron stores. The World Health Organization (2023) defines anaemia as a condition where the number of red blood cells or the haemoglobin concentration within them is lower than normal.

Red Flag Alert: Iron Depletion
Untreated antenatal iron depletion may lead to postpartum anaemia, which can also be caused by increased blood loss at birth (Blackburn 2013).

Interpreting a Full Blood Count in a Pregnant Woman

During pregnancy, a full blood count (FBC) is a laboratory test undertaken routinely, with informed consent, at the antenatal booking interview and again at 28 weeks of gestation (NICE 2021). The results provide an overview of red and white blood cells and platelets (Table 9.3).

Serum ferritin level is the biochemical test which most reliably correlates with relative total body iron stores (in the absence of infection or inflammation). In women with adequate iron stores at conception, the serum ferritin concentration initially rises, followed by a progressive fall by 32 weeks to about 50% of prepregnancy levels. This is due to haemodilution and iron use. Levels increase slightly in the third trimester (NICE 2023).

A serum ferritin concentration less than 15 µg/l indicates iron depletion in all stages of pregnancy. Current national guidance advises that treatment should be considered when levels fall below 30 µg/l (NICE 2023). Serum ferritin analysis may also be requested to confirm iron deficiency anaemia when haemoglobin and MCV is low.

TABLE 9.3 Overview of red blood cells as analysed by full blood count testing.

Blood cells	Measure	Non-pregnant	Pregnant
Haemoglobin	Concentration of haemoglobin within blood	120–160 g/l	110–140 g/l
Haematocrit	Percentage of the blood sample made up of red cells	35–44%	28–41%
Mean corpuscular volume	Average size of red cells present in the blood sample	80–100 fl	70–90 fl
Red cell count	Number of red cells present per unit volume of blood	4.0–5.2	2.72–4.55
Reticulocyte count	Number of reticulocytes (immature red cells)	0.5–1%	1–2%
Mean corpuscular haemoglobin	Mean quantity of haemoglobin within red bloods cells	27–34 fl	23–32 fl
Mean corpuscular haemoglobin concentrate	Mean concentration of haemoglobin within red bloods cells.	32–35 fl	32–35 fl

Source: Adapted from Abbassi-Ghanavati et al. (2009) and Blackburn (2013).

Snapshot 9.2   Anaemia

Jemma is a 24-year-old multiparous woman who gave birth spontaneously to her son Ray 10 days ago. Rashida, a community midwife visits Jemma at home. During the postnatal check Jemma complains of feeling tired, and occasionally dizzy and breathless. What are and discussions that Rashida should have with Jemma? What care shoud she give?

Key Points to Consider

- Gather a full clinical history from Jemma, which involves assessing medical and obstetric history, the presence of complicating factors, vital signs, blood loss at birth, FBC, current vaginal blood loss.
- Refer Jemma immediately to the maternity assessment unit or hospital emergency department there are any concerns about Jemma's immediate wellbeing.
- Exclude other causes such as sepsis, chest infection, exacerbation of asthma or pulmonary embolism.
- In iron deficiency anaemia, a FBC, taken with consent, may demonstrate low haemoglobin, MCV, mean cell haemoglobin and mean cell haemoglobin concentration. Signs of anaemia can occur in the absence of a low haemoglobin, and a ferritin check may also be required to check Jemma's iron stores.
- Discuss diet and the appropriateness of iron supplementation.
- Advise Jemma about possible dose-related effects from iron supplementation, which include gastrointestinal disturbances and the passing of black stools.
- Advise Jemma to take iron before food to facilitate absorption while avoiding tannin-containing drinks such as tea, which inhibit absorption. The presence of vitamin C can increase absorption and taking supplementation on alternative days has also been found to be beneficial in reducing adverse effects.
- Plan with Jemma to follow up any blood results and exclude any other causes. Assess Jemma's emotional and mental health and wellbeing and signpost Jemma for further support.

White Blood Cells

Leucocytes are specialised for defence and are critical to the immune system. There are approximately 5000–11 000 white blood cells/mm³ of blood, compared with 4–6 million red blood cells/mm³. White blood cells develop from haemocytoblasts in the red bone marrow in response to hormones (Moini 2016). Leukopoiesis is the process by which white blood cells develop from stem cells in red bone marrow. Once mature, white blood cells are released into the bloodstream to protect the body from disease-causing micro-organisms such as bacteria and viruses, and to respond to any tissue damage or foreign objects. Whereas erythrocytes circulate within the blood vessels, white blood cells routinely leave the bloodstream to perform their defensive functions in the body's tissues (Dooley et al. 2021).

There are five types of white blood cells circulating in the blood, each having a different role to play. Leucocytes with granular cytoplasm are called granulocytes. Granulocytes are about twice as large as red blood cells, consisting of eosinophils, basophils and neutrophils. These cells develop in the red bone marrow, similarly to red blood cells, but only live for about 12 hours. White blood cells without granular cytoplasm are referred to as agranulocytes, consisting of lymphocytes and monocytes. The proportions of white blood cells remain constant in a healthy individual, with neutrophils making up the majority of circulating white blood cells and lymphocytes a close second. Monocytes are the third most common white blood cell.

The proportions of leucocytes remain constant in a healthy pregnant individual, although total white blood cell volume increases slightly in the first trimester, levelling off during the second and third trimester. The total white blood cell count in pregnancy varies on an individual basis ranging from 5000 to 12 000/mm³ (Blackburn 2013).

Platelets

Platelets are incomplete disc-shaped cells arising from the cytoplasm of stem cells within the red bone marrow known as megakaryocytes that have become fragmented (Moini 2016). The formation of platelets is known as thrombocytopoiesis, and platelets are formed under the influence of the hormone thrombopoietin. Platelets are approximately 2–4 μm in diameter and are numerous, with approximately 150 000–160 000/μl blood (Dooley et al. 2021).

After entering the circulation, approximately one-third of platelets travel to the spleen to be stored for later release in response to ruptured blood vessels. Platelets have a primary role in blood clotting and are activated to form a temporary platelet plug to seal broken blood vessels (Dooley et al. 2021). Platelets remain in the circulation for approximately seven days and are then ingested by macrophages (Chambers et al. 2019). Platelets also secrete a variety of growth factors essential for growth and repair of tissue, particularly connective tissue (Dooley et al. 2021).

Pregnancy is associated with enhanced platelet turnover, clotting and fibrinolysis, although in general, platelet levels do not change significantly during pregnancy. The platelet count tends to fall progressively during normal pregnancy because of the haemodilutional effects of pregnancy, although it generally remains within normal limits. In fewer than 10% of women, platelet levels reduce to $100–150 \times 10^9$ cells/l by term and this occurs in the absence of any pathological process. A woman is not considered to be thrombocytopenic in pregnancy until the platelet count is less than 100×10^9 cells/l (Soma-Pillay et al. 2016; Mushambi 2016).

Plasma

Blood plasma is a pale, straw-coloured fluid acting as the transport medium for substances carried within the blood, making up approximately 55% (between 46% and 63%) of the total blood volume (Wylie 2005; Rankin 2017). Plasma consists mostly of water (approximately 90%), the remainder containing solutes, most of which are proteins such as albumin, fibrinogen, globulins and enzymes, as well as electrolytes such as sodium and potassium; both are important ions for cell function.

Plasma proteins have a key role to play in blood clotting (fibrinogen), transportation of fat-soluble vitamins, lipids and iron, and contributing to the body's immunological response. In addition, enzymes contained within the plasma are involved with the catalyst of chemical reactions within the body and plasma proteins help maintain the blood's osmotic pressure, enabling water to remain inside the blood vessels instead of diffusing into the interstitial fluid.

The protein albumin is especially important in maintaining osmotic pressure. If albumin levels drop, osmotic pressure of the blood shifts, forcing water from blood into tissues and causing oedema. Albumin also binds with several drugs, including penicillin, helping with the transport of those drugs. Fibrinogen makes up around 4% of the plasma proteins and is important for blood coagulation. Under the influence of fibrinogen, molecules interact to form large insoluble strands of fibrin, providing the basis for blood clot formation.

Plasma volume increases by approximately 45–50% during pregnancy, which is about 1200–1600 ml above non-pregnant values (Rankin 2017). Plasma volume returns to non-pregnant levels by 6 days after birth, although there is often a sudden rise of up to 1 l in plasma volume 24 hours after birth, which may predispose women with existing cardiac disease to pulmonary oedema; careful monitoring post birth is required (Blackburn 2013).

Plasma volume correlates positively with placental mass and birth weight and fetal growth correlates more closely with plasma volume increases than with changes in red blood cell volume (Blackburn 2013).

Take Home Points

- Significant increase in blood volume is a healthy adaptation of pregnancy and has a protective function to protect the mother against the effects of blood loss during the third stage of labour.
- Erythrocyte increase is less than plasma increase resulting in a physiological anaemia of pregnancy.
- A FBC is routinely taken during pregnancy, with informed consent, at the antenatal booking interview and again at 28 weeks gestation, to provide an overview of red and white blood cells and platelets.
- During pregnancy, the concentration of certain clotting factors is increased and fibrinolytic activity decreased. These changes, alongside venous stasis present in the lower limbs associated with vasodilation, decreased blood flow and the weight of the gravid uterus, predispose pregnant women to venous thromboembolism.

Summary

This chapter has described the various components and functions of the circulatory system. The physiological adaptation that occurs in response to pregnancy is explained and the midwife's role discussed in relation to two case studies.

References

Abbassi-Ghanavati, M., Greer, L.G., and Cunningham, F.G. (2009). Pregnancy and laboratory studies: a reference table for clinicians. *Obstetrics & Gynecology* 114: 1326–1331. Erratum in *Obstetrics & Gynecology* 115: 387.

Bhatia, P. and Chhabra, S. (2018). Physiological and anatomical changes of pregnancy: implications for anaesthesia. *Indian Journal of Anaesthesia* 62 (9): 651–657. https://doi.org/10.4103/ija.IJA_458_18.

Blackburn, S.T. (2013). *Maternal, Fetal and Neonatal Physiology – A Clinical Perspective*, 4e. Philadelphia, PA: Elsevier Saunders.

Bootun, R., Onida, S., Lane, T., and Davies, A. (2022). Varicose veins. *Surgery* 40 (7): 411–419. https://doi.org/10.1016/j.mpsur.2022.05.010.

Chambers, D., Huang, C., and Matthews, G. (2019). *Basic Physiology for Anaesthetists*. Cambridge: Cambridge University Press.

Daru, J., Allotey, J., Peña-Rosas, J.P., and Khan, K.S. (2017). Serum ferritin thresholds for the diagnosis of iron deficiency in pregnancy: a systematic review. *Transfusion Medicine* 27: 167–174. https://doi.org/10.1111/tme.12408.

Dooley, L., Chrusik, A., Kauter, K. et al. (2021). Blood. In: *Fundamentals of Anatomy and Physiology*, 248. Toowoomba, Australia: University of Southern Queensland, Part v.

Ross, M.G. and Ervin, M.G. (2017). Fetal development and Physiology. In: *Obstetrics: Normal and Problem Pregnancies*, 8e, 26–37. Philadelphia, PA: Elsevier.

Ferng, A. (2022). Hepatic portal vein Leipzig: Kenhub. https://www.kenhub.com/en/library/anatomy/hepatic-portal-vein (accessed 28 October 2023).

Gelman, S., Warner, S., and Warner, M. (2008). Venous function and central venous pressure: a physiologic story. *Anesthesiology* 108: 735–748. https://doi.org/10.1097/ALN.0b013e3181672607.

Letsky, E.A. (2002). Coagulation defects. In: *Medical Disorders in Obstetric Practice*, 4e (ed. M. de Swiet), 61–96. Oxford: Blackwell.

McCarthy, F. and Kenny, L. (2010). Adaptations of maternal cardiovascular and renal physiology to pregnancy. In: *Hypertension in Pregnancy (Cambridge Clinical Guides)* (ed. A. Heazell, E. Norwitz, L. Kenny, and P. Baker), 1–18. Cambridge: Cambridge University Press https://doi.org/10.1017/CBO9780511902529.003.

Moini, J. (2016). *Anatomy and Physiology for Health Professionals*, 2e. Burlington MA: Jones and Bartlett Learning.

Mushambi, M. (2016). Physiology of pregnancy. In: *Fundamentals of Anaesthesia* (ed. C. Mowatt, T. Lin, T. Smith, and C. Pinnock), 512–530. Cambridge: Cambridge University Press https://doi.org/10.1017/9781139626798.027.

NICE (2013). *Varicose Veins: Diagnosis and Management*. Clinical Guideline CG168. London: National Institute for Health and Care Excellence.

NICE (2020). Scenario: varicose veins. Clinical Knowledge Summaries. https://cks.nice.org.uk/topics/varicose-veins/management/varicose-veins (accessed 28 October 2023).

NICE (2021). *Antenatal Care*. NICE Guideline NG201. London: National Institute for Health and Care Excellence.

NICE (2023). Anaemia – iron deficiency: What investigations should I arrange to confirm iron deficiency anaemia? https://cks.nice.org.uk/topics/anaemia-iron-deficiency/diagnosis/investigations/#basis-for-recommendation-648 (accessed 28 October 2023).

Osol, G., Ko, N.L., and Mandalà, M. (2019). Plasticity of the maternal vasculature during pregnancy. *Annual Review of Physiology* 81: 89–111. https://doi.org/10.1146/annurev-physiol-020518-114435.

Peate, I. (2017). *Fundamentals of Anatomy and Physiology Workbook – A Study Guide for Nursing and Healthcare Students*. Oxford: Wiley Blackwell.

Peate, I. and Evans, S. (2020). *Fundamentals of Anatomy & Physiology*, 3e. Oxford: Wiley-Blackwell.

Rankin, J. (2017). *Physiology in Childbearing with Anatomy and Related Biosciences*, 4e. Edinburgh: Elsevier.

Remien, K. and Majmundar, S.H. (2022). *Physiology, Fetal Circulation*. Treasure Island, FL: StatPearls Publishing https://www.ncbi.nlm.nih.gov/books/NBK539710.

Shier, D., Butler, J., and Lewis, R. (2016). *Holes Human Anatomy and Physiology*, 14e. New York: McGraw-Hill Education.

Soma-Pillay, P., Nelson-Piercy, C., Tolppanen, H., and Mebazaa, A. (2016). Physiological changes in pregnancy. *Cardiovascular Journal of Africa* 27 (2): 89–94. https://doi.org/10.5830/CVJA-2016-021.

Sutton, C. and Mann, D. (2021). Physiology of pregnancy. In: *Anesthesia for Maternal-Fetal Surgery: Concepts and Clinical Practice* (ed. O. Olutoye), 1–16. Cambridge: Cambridge University Press https://doi.org/10.1017/9781108297899.002.

World Health Organization. (2023) Anaemia. https://www.who.int/health-topics/anaemia#tab=tab_1 (accessed 28 October 2023).

Wylie, L. (2005). *Essential Anatomy and Physiology in Maternity Care*, 2e. London: Elsevier.

Wylie, B. and Bryce, H. (2016). *The Midwives' Guide to Key Medical Conditions*, 2e. Edinburgh: Elsevier.

Further Reading

RCOG (2015). *Reducing the Risk of Thrombosis and Embolism during Pregnancy and the Puerperium*. Green-top Guideline No. 37b. London: Royal College of Obstetricians and Gynaecologists.

RCOG (2015). *Thromboembolic Disease in Pregnancy and the Puerperium: Acute Management*. Green-top Guideline No. 37b. London: Royal College of Obstetricians and Gynaecologists.

Auerbach, M. and Georgieff, M.K. (2020). Guidelines for iron deficiency in pregnancy: hope abounds. *British Journal of Haematology* 188: 814–816. https://doi.org/10.1111/bjh.16220.

Bisson, D.L., Newell, S.D., and Laxton, C. on behalf of the Royal College of Obstetricians and Gynaecologists(2019). Antenatal and postnatal analgesia. Scientific Impact Paper No. 59. *BJOG* 126: e115–e124. https://doi.org/10.1111/1471-0528.15510.

Bowen, R. and Taylor, W. (2022). *Skills for Midwifery Practice*, 5e. London: Elsevier.

Creasy, R.K., Resnik, R., Iams, J.D. et al. (2014). *Creasy and Resnik's Maternal-Fetal Medicine: Principles and Practice*. Philadelphia, PA: Elsevier Saunders.

Dathe, K., Hultzsch, S., Pritchard, L.W., and Schaefer, C. (2019). Risk estimation of fetal adverse effects after short-term second trimester exposure to non-steroidal anti-inflammatory drugs: a literature review. *European Journal of Clinical Pharmacology* 75 (10): 1347–1353. https://doi.org/10.1007/s00228-019-02712-2.

Georgieff, M., Krebs, N., and Cusick, S. (2019). The benefits and risks of iron supplementation in pregnancy. *Annual Review of Nutrition* 39: 7.1–7.26.

Humphries, A., Thompson, J.M.D., Stone, P., and Mirjalili, S.A. (2020). The effect of positioning on maternal anatomy and hemodynamics during late pregnancy. *Clinical Anatomy* 33: 943–949. https://doi-org.ezproxy.uwe.ac.uk/10.1002/ca.23614.

Jarvis, S. and Nelson-Piercy, C. (2014). Common symptoms and signs during pregnancy. *Obstetrics, Gynaecology and Reproductive Medicine* 24: 245–249.

Kazma, J., Anker, J., Allegaert, K. et al. (2020). Anatomical and physiological alterations of pregnancy. *Journal of Pharmacokinetics and Pharmacodynamics* 47 (4): : 271–285.

Knight, M., Bunch, K., Tuffnell, D. et al. (ed.) on behalf of MBRRACE-UK(2021). *Saving Lives, Improving Mothers' Care - Lessons Learned to Inform Maternity Care from the UK and Ireland Confidential Enquiries into Maternal Deaths and Morbidity 2017–19*. Oxford: National Perinatal Epidemiology Unit, University of Oxford.

Kwak, D.W., Kim, S., Lee, S.Y. et al. (2022). Maternal anemia during the first trimester and its association with psychological health. *Nutrients* 14 (17): 3505. https://doi.org/10.3390/nu14173505.

Kang, S.Y., Kim, H.B., and Sunwoo, S. (2020). Association between anemia and maternal depression: a systematic review and meta-analysis. *Journal of Psychiatric Research* 122: 88–96. https://doi.org/10.1016/j.jpsychires.2020.01.00.

Lindqvist, P.G., Bremme, K., and Hellgren, M. (2011). Swedish Society of Obstetrics and Gynecology (SFOG) Working Group on Hemostatic Disorders (Hem-ARG). Efficacy of obstetric thromboprophylaxis and long-term risk of recurrence of venous thromboembolism. *Acta Obstetricia et Gynecologica Scandinavica* 90: 648–653.

Monteiro, R., Salman, M., Malhotra, S., and Yentis, S. (2019). Physiology of pregnancy. In: *Analgesia, Anaesthesia and Pregnancy: A Practical Guide*, 31–35. Cambridge: Cambridge University Press https://doi.org/10.1017/9781108684729.012.

Nursing and Midwifery Council (NMC) (2019). *Standards of Proficiency for Midwives*. London: Nursing and Midwifery Council.

Pasricha, S.R., Colman, K., Centeno-Tablante, E. et al. (2018). Revisiting WHO haemoglobin thresholds to define anaemia in clinical medicine and public health. *Lancet Haematology* 5: e60–e62.

Pavord, S., Daru, J., Prasannan, N. et al. (2020). UK guidelines on the management of iron deficiency in pregnancy. *British Journal of Haematology* 188: 819–830. https://doi.org/10.1111/bjh.16221.

Prodger, C., Jafaar, S., and Lacey, R., Pavord, S (2021). Anaemia in pregnancy and the postpartum period. *Bulletin of the Royal College of Pathologists*. (195): https://www.rcpath.org/profession/publications/college-bulletin/july-2021/anaemia-in-pregnancy-and-the-postpartum-period.html (accessed 28 October 2023).

Ronkainen, J., Lowry, E., Heiskala, A. et al. (2019). Maternal hemoglobin associates with preterm delivery and small for gestational age in two Finnish birth cohorts. *European Journal of Obstetrics, Gynecology, and Reproductive Biology* 238: 44–48. https://doi.org/10.1016/j.ejogrb.2019.04.045.

Sukrat, B., Wilasrusmee, C., Siribumrungwong, B. et al. (2013). Hemoglobin concentration and pregnancy outcomes: a systematic review and meta-analysis. *BioMed Research International* 2013: 769057. https://doi.org/10.1155/2013/769057.

Turetz, M., Sideris, A.T., Friedman, O.A. et al. (2018). Epidemiology, pathophysiology, and natural history of pulmonary embolism. *Seminars in Interventional Radiology* 35 (2): 92–98. https://doi.org/10.1055/s-0038-1642036.

Yamada, K., Yamada, K., Katsuda, I., and Hida, T. (2008). Cubital fossa venipuncture sites based on anatomical variations and relationships of cutaneous veins and nerves. *Clinical Anatomy* 21 (4): 307–313. https://doi.org/10.1002/ca.20622.

Online Resources

British National Formulary: https://bnf.nice.org.uk
Provides key information on the selection, prescribing, dispensing and administration of medicines,

Glossary

Angiogenesis	Development of new blood vessels.
Antecubital fossa	Also called the cubital fossa; a depression on the anterior surface of the elbow joint commonly selected for accessibility for venepuncture.
Cardiac output	Amount of blood pumped from the ventricles of the heart each minute, which is affected by stroke volume and heart rate.
Deoxygenated blood	Blood that has a lower oxygen saturation when compared with oxygenated blood. Deoxygenated blood has less oxygen and more carbon dioxide than oxygenated blood. It contains fewer nutrients and more metabolic waste when compared with oxygenated blood.
Ductus arteriosus	A temporary structure within the fetal circulation that lies between the pulmonary arteries and aorta and permits blood to pass straight from the right ventricle into the aorta, bypassing the fetal pulmonary circulation.
Ductus venosus	A temporary structure within fetal circulation directing blood into the inferior vena cava.

Foramen ovale	A temporary structure existing as an opening in the septum between the atria into the left atrium within fetal circulation.
Hyperplasia	Enlargement of an organ or tissue caused by an increase in the reproduction rate of its cells.
Hypertrophy	Enlargement of an organ or tissue caused by an increase in size of its cells.
Hypogastric arteries	Within fetal circulation, these arteries direct most of the deoxygenated blood back through the umbilical arteries to the placenta.
Median cubital vein	A superficial vein forming a connection point between the cephalic and basilic veins; generally the preferred vein for selection for venepuncture.
Stroke volume	The amount of blood pumped from the ventricles at each contraction.
Supine hypotensive syndrome	When a pregnant woman is in a supine position, the gravid uterus compresses the inferior vena cava, leading to decreased venous return centrally.
Systemic vascular resistance	The resistance the heart must overcome to circulate blood within the vasculature.
Venous return	The blood returned to the heart.
Vasoconstriction	A reduction or constriction in the blood vessel diameter which increases blood pressure.
Vasodilation	Dilation of blood vessels; decreases blood pressure.

Multiple Choice Questions

1. Which of these is not a temporary structure that is an integral part of fetal circulation?
   a. Vascular endothelium
   b. Foramen ovale
   c. Ductus venosus
   d. Hypogastric arteries

2. What is another name for red blood cells?
   a. Leucocytes
   b. Erythrocytes
   c. Neutrophils
   d. Fibrinogen

3. Which of the following blood cells has a key role in fighting infection?
   a. Platelets
   b. Erythrocytes
   c. Leucocytes
   d. Plasma

4. Which formed element of blood is an integral part of the clotting process and clot formation?
   a. Plasma
   b. Neutrophils
   c. Platelets
   d. Leucocytes

5. What blood test is used to detect iron deficiency anaemia?
   a. Urea and electrolytes
   b. Blood group and antibody check
   c. Full blood count and ferritin
   d. C-reactive protein

6. What dietary advice would you provide to increase iron absorption during pregnancy?
   a. Ingest on an empty stomach, increase foods containing vitamin C and avoid tannin containing drinks
   b. Ingest after food and avoid tea
   c. Take with orange juice and/or tea at breakfast and avoid ingesting late at night
   d. Avoid alcohol

7. What is a common symptom of anaemia?
   a. Fatigue
   b. Dyspepsia
   c. Venous thromboembolism
   d. Weight gain

8. Why should pregnant women avoid the supine position from 28 weeks gestation?
   a. It causes nausea and vomiting
   b. It causes supine hypotensive syndrome
   c. It causes vasodilation and is associated with anaemia
   d. It causes dyspepsia

9. What predisposes women to varicosities of pregnancy:
   a. Vasodilation
   b. Increased volume of blood circulating in the veins
   c. Weight of the pregnant uterus
   d. All of the above

10. Which of these factors must be considered when selecting the most appropriate vein for venepuncture?
    a. The vein should feel soft and bouncy, and should be well supported by surrounding tissues; the skin should be intact
    b. Valves should be present, the vein feels hard and fills quickly when compressed
    c. The skin should be previously punctured and the vein should feel warm and elastic
    d. The vein should feel hard, thin and mobile

CHAPTER 10

The Cardiac System

Mel Cameron-Radford

AIM

This chapter provides the reader with a fundamental understanding of the cardiac system when applied to women throughout the differing stages of childbirth, giving the reader an opportunity to situate themselves in the clinician's role and apply the knowledge in everyday clinical encounters.

LEARNING OUTCOMES

On completion of this chapter, you will be able to:

- Describe the structures and functions of the heart.
- Describe the conducting system and nerve supply of the heart.
- Describe physiological changes in pregnancy.
- Understand midwifery care within the context multidisciplinary care.
- Identify risk factors.

Test Your Prior Knowledge

1. Name the four chambers of the heart
2. Where is the septum located?
3. What kind of muscle is cardiac muscle?
4. What is the bundle of His?
5. What do you understand by sinus arrhythmia?

Introduction

The heart is an organ that functions to pump blood throughout the body. It has its own circulation system. The heart has a cardiac cycle; it continuously contracts and relaxes in synchronicity to circulate oxygenated, nutrient-rich blood to the cells of the body, returning deoxygenated blood and metabolic waste to be processed through other systems including the renal, hepatic and pulmonary systems.

Fundamentals of Maternal Anatomy and Physiology, First Edition. Edited by Ian Peate and Claire Leader.
© 2024 John Wiley & Sons Ltd. Published 2024 by John Wiley & Sons Ltd.

This chapter discusses the structure of the heart, its conduction system, the blood flow through the heart and the returning blood circulation. We also consider the cardiac system in pregnancy, including changes in pregnancy and childbirth and commonly encountered maternal cardiac disease that midwives may encounter. The role and remit is of clinicians in maternity services when caring for mothers throughout their pregnancy and childbirth is described in relation to screening for cardiac function and caring for those with impaired or suspected impaired cardiac function.

The terms 'woman' and 'women' are used throughout this chapter; however, we know that not all natal women identify with their biological sex and care givers should use appropriate individualised language that is sensitive to an individual's needs.

Location of the Heart

The heart is contained within the thoracic cavity above the diaphragm. The thoracic cavity's three spaces are lined with mesothelium separating the organs within it. The pericardial cavity encloses the heart, which is positioned between the left and right lungs in the mediastinum. The heart sits in a slightly left position. The apex of the organ is in a lower-left position in comparison with the base of the heart at an upper-central position (Figure 10.1).

Structures and Blood Flow of the Heart

The heart is a hollow muscled organ. The specialised cardiac muscle consists of three layers:

1. The pericardium
2. The myocardium
3. The endocardium.

Figure 10.2 depicts the three layers of the heart.

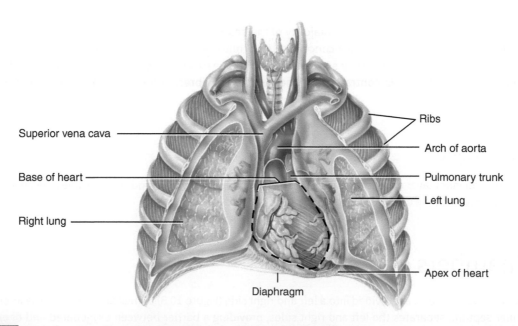

FIGURE 10.1 The thoracic cavity. Source: Peate (2017). p. 187/John Wiley & Sons.

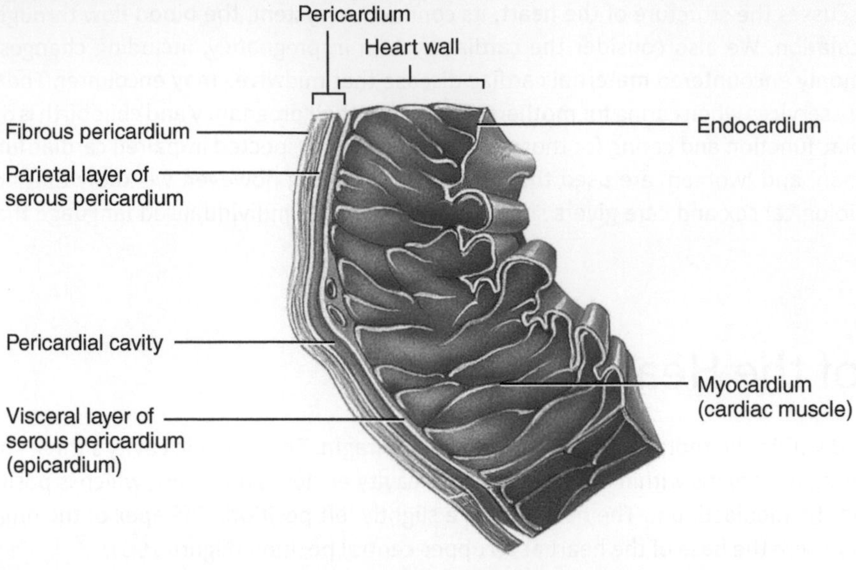

Pericardium

Heart wall

Fibrous pericardium

Parietal layer of
serous pericardium

Endocardium

Pericardial cavity

Myocardium
(cardiac muscle)

Visceral layer of
serous pericardium
(epicardium)

FIGURE 10.2   The heart wall. Source: Peate and Evans (2020)/John Wiley & Sons.

The Pericardium

The outer layer, the pericardium, is a thin fibrous sheath surrounding the heart, protecting it from enlargement. Its rigidity and non-distensible function protects the heart from overfilling. It anchors the organ to the mediastinum. The pericardial space is lubricated through interstitial fluid. Pericardial fluid protects the constantly moving heart from friction and facilitates the movement of the heart.

The Myocardium

The myocardium, the middle layer, forms the majority of the heart muscle. It has muscle cells (myocytes) of an elongated striated structure, which have a higher concentration of mitochondria. The cells are specialised, enabling them to work as a single unit while retaining their separate states. The heart's electrical impulses run through the myocardium. Its unique formation allows contraction of the myocardial fibres, collectively forming the contractions of the heart.

The Endocardium

The endocardium, an inner layer of cells (notably similar to the endothelium of blood vessels), lines the heart chambers. Its function is to assist with the unhindered flow of blood.

The Chambers of the Heart

The four chambers of the heart are divided into a left and right side (Figure 10.3). A muscular septum, the interatrial and interventricular septum, separates the left and right sides, providing a barrier between oxygenated and deoxygenated circulating blood as it flows through the heart. Oxygenated blood does not mix with deoxygenated blood.

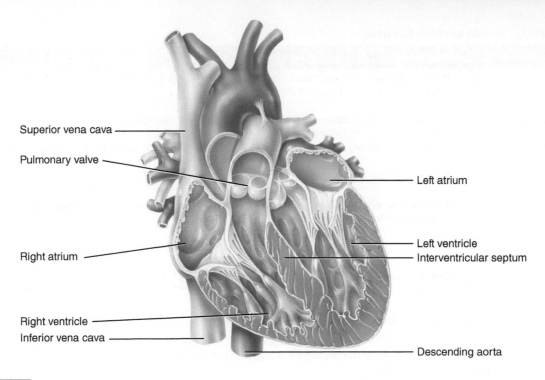

Superior vena cava

Pulmonary valve

Left atrium

Right atrium

Left ventricle
Interventricular septum

Right ventricle
Inferior vena cava

Descending aorta

FIGURE 10.3   The chambers of the heart. Source: Peate and Evans (2020)/John Wiley & Sons.

The Atria and Ventricles

The ventricles have thicker muscular walls than the atria. The left ventricle is thicker than the right; its powerful higher pressure pumps oxygenated blood into the aortic arch to supply the body with oxygenated blood. The right ventricle has a thinner muscular wall, which pumps deoxygenated blood through the pulmonary circuit to the pulmonary artery and to the lungs for reoxygenation of the circulating blood through the pulmonary veins returning to the left atria.

The direction of blood flow is assisted by valves that direct blood flow and suppress the flow from moving in the wrong direction through the heart. They are divided into two categories, the atrioventricular valves and the semilunar valves. Atrioventricular valves include the tricuspid and mitral valve, and the semilunar valves include the pulmonary valve and the aortic valve.

The atrioventricular valves sit between the atria and the ventricles. The atria act as reservoirs to fill the ventricles. The left bicuspid/mitral valve has two cusps. The right tricuspid valve has three cusps. Both bi- and tricuspid valves direct blood flow into the ventricles, preventing backflow of blood. The pulmonary artery's valve allows blood flow from the right ventricle to flow into the pulmonary artery and to the lungs. The aortic valve allows high pressure blood flow from the left ventricle into the aorta to oxygenate the whole of the body. When the ventricles relax, the mitral and tricuspid valves open and blood flows into them in preparation for the next contraction.

The chordae tendineae are tendinous string-like fibrous connective tissue. They connect the atrioventricular tricuspid and mitral valves to the heart's papillary muscle. They maintain the position and tension on the valves.

The Great Vessels of the Heart

The five great vessels are large vessels that enter and exit the heart: the superior and inferior vena cava, the pulmonary artery, the pulmonary vein and the aorta. Table 10.1 describes the vessels and their functions. The aorta has three layers: the intima, media and externa (inner, middle and external). Deoxygenated blood flows into the heart through the superior

197

TABLE 10.1   Vessels and their functions.

Vessel	Function
Superior vena cava	Returns circulating deoxygenated blood from the arms, head, neck, thoracic organs (main organs of respiration and circulation) into the right atrium
Inferior vena cava	Returns circulating deoxygenated blood from the body into the right atrium
Pulmonary artery	Divides to the left and right, taking deoxygenated blood from right ventricle to the lungs
Pulmonary vein	Returns oxygenated blood from lungs to the left atrium
Aorta	Three-layered vessel: intima, media and externa. Oxygenated blood circulates from the left ventricle through aorta to supply the whole body
Coronary arteries	Circulate oxygenated blood to the tissues of the heart
Coronary veins	Returns deoxygenated blood from the heart tissues to the right atrium

vena cava and the inferior vena cava into the right atrium, then on to the right ventricle, which in turn takes the deoxygenated blood to the pulmonary artery and to the lungs for reoxygenation. The oxygen-rich blood returns through the pulmonary veins and into the left atrium through to the left ventricle and into the aorta.

The aortic arch has three large vessels:

1. The brachiocephalic artery, which branches into the right subclavian artery and the right common carotid artery
2. The left common carotid artery
3. The left subclavian artery.

The heart has its own blood supply, coronary arteries and coronary veins (Figure 10.4).

Cardiac Conducting System

The heart's conducting system has electrical impulses which run through the myocardium. Its unique formation allows contraction of the myocardial fibres, collectively forming the contractions of the heart. Four chambers contract rhythmically. The heartbeat initiates at the sinoatrial node, situated at the top of the right atrium, which sets the rate of contraction. The electrical impulse travels to the atrioventricular node within the bundle of His. The bundle of His is a fibrous branch within the intraventricular septum. It divides into two bundle branches to the left and right within the muscular interventricular septum. These branches supply electrical activity to the left and right ventricles. The electrical impulses are distributed through the Purkinje fibres, located beneath the endocardium. They quickly conduct impulses, to enable synchronised contractions of the ventricles. The cardiac conduction system is outlined in Figure 10.5.

Nerve Supply

The heart's conducting system ensures that the contractions of the heart are continuous, irrespective of the nerve supply. Contraction rates, however, are influenced by the nerve supply. The autonomic nerve supply unconsciously regulates heart rate and begins within the brain stem. It is divided into sympathetic and parasympathetic nerves (Figure 10.6). The sympathetic nerves arise from the superior, middle and inferior cervical ganglia. They prepare the body for a 'fight or flight' response by increasing heart rate. The parasympathetic nerve originates in the medulla oblongata and through the vagus nerve system. The parasympathetic system works when the body is at rest and slows down the heart rate.

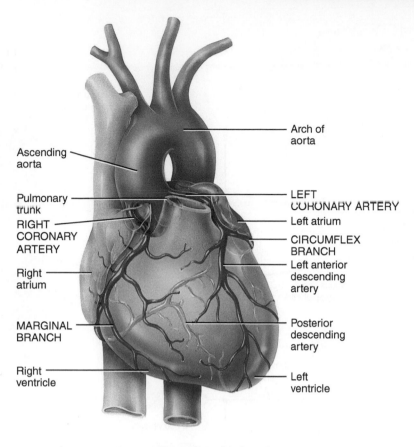

Arch of
aorta

Ascending
aorta

Pulmonary
trunk

LEFT
CORONARY ARTERY

RIGHT
CORONARY
ARTERY

Left atrium

CIRCUMFLEX
BRANCH

Right
atrium

Left anterior
descending
artery

MARGINAL
BRANCH

Posterior
descending
artery

Right
ventricle

Left
ventricle

FIGURE 10.4   The coronary arteries. Source: Peate and Evans (2020)/John Wiley & Sons.

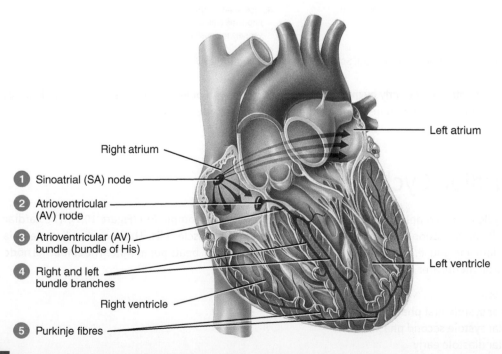

Left atrium

Right atrium

1 Sinoatrial (SA) node

2 Atrioventricular
(AV) node

3 Atrioventricular (AV)
bundle (bundle of His)

4 Right and left
bundle branches

Left ventricle

Right ventricle

5 Purkinje fibres

FIGURE 10.5   The conduction system of the heart. Source: Peate and Evans (2020)/John Wiley & Sons.

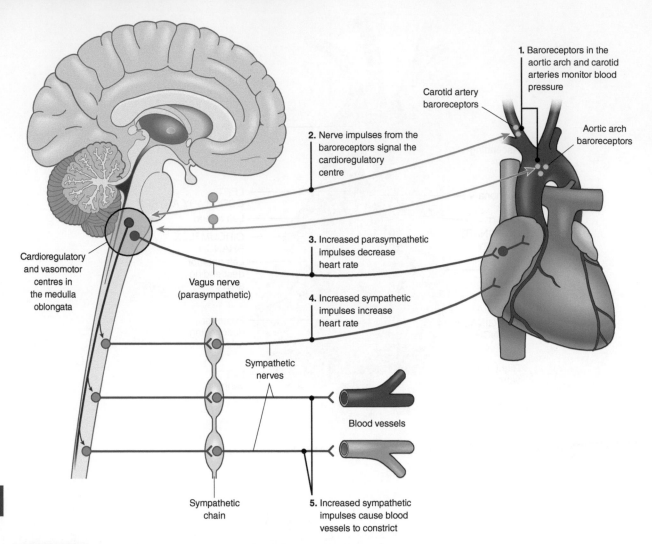

FIGURE 10.6   The cardioregulatory centre. Source: Peate (2022)/John Wiley & Sons.

Heart rates are affected directly by internal and external factors. For women during pregnancy, these factors include maternal age, circulating blood volume, pre-existing heart disease, medications, stress, smoking, recreational drug use and exercise.

The Cardiac Cycle

The cardiac cycle is one completed heartbeat from its initiation to its completion (Figure 10.7). The cardiac muscle can depolarise (cellular excitation), which leads to a contraction of the muscle cells. This includes diastole (relaxation), systole, (contraction) and pause. The frequency of the cycle is measured in beats per minute. The sinoatrial node initiates the heartbeat; the elements are:

- Atrial systole
- Ventricular systole first phase
- Ventricular systole second phase
- Ventricular diastole early
- Ventricular diastole late.

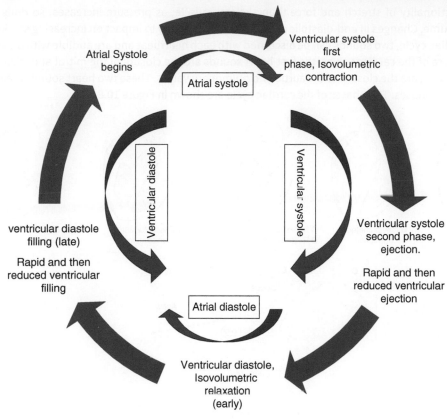

Atrial Systole begins

Atrial systole

Ventricular systole first phase, Isovolumetric contraction

Ventricular diastole

Ventricular systole

Ventricular systole second phase, ejection.

Rapid and then reduced ventricular ejection

ventricular diastole filling (late)

Rapid and then reduced ventricular filling

Atrial diastole

Ventricular diastole, Isovolumetric relaxation (early)

FIGURE 10.7 The cardiac cycle.

The isovolumetric period occurs between the time of aortic valve closure and mitral valve opening at this point ventricular muscle tension is decreased, but ventricular volume remains unchanged.

- The *atrial systole* contraction forces the preload blood into and fills the ventricles. Ventricular volume post filling is known as end-diastolic volume (EDV); the pressures at EDV are higher in the left ventricle because of its increased musculature. The EDV determines the strength of the subsequent contraction (Starling's law). Atrial depolarisation occurs. In an echocardiogram (ECG) report, this is illustrated as the P wave.
- In *ventricular systole,* first phase, with the increased ventricular pressure, the valves close. Ventricular depolarisation occurs. ECG illustrated this as the QRS wave.
- In *ventricular systole,* second phase, the semilunar valves open, ejection occurs. Repolarisation occurs In an ECG this is illustrated as the T wave.
- In *ventricular diastole,* early, semilunar valves close and blood flows into the atria.
- In *ventricular diastole,* late, relaxation occurs and blood flows into the ventricles.

Starling's Law

Starling's law explains the heart's ability to respond to increases in blood volume. The stroke volume in the ventricles increases in response to their preload; the force of the contraction is proportionate to the degree to which it is stretched. The amount of preload dictates the volume of blood leaving the heart, which is the cardiac output. Increased cardiac output is a direct response to the stretch of the muscle fibres in relation to the increased pressure within the ventricles. Right ventricle end-diastolic pressure is determined from the right atrium, which is determined from the central venous pressure. The left ventricle end-diastolic pressure is determined by the pulmonary venous pressure. Cardiac muscle has more effective functionality of stretch and force than skeletal muscle; as pressure increases, so does volume, which results in stroke volume. Changes in end-diastolic pressure have the ability to impact on increasing stroke volume.

During the cardiac cycle, two sounds can be discerned with each heartbeat and are audible with a stethoscope. Both occur with the closure of the cardiac valves: the first heart sounds are the closure of the mitral and tricuspid valves, and the second heart sounds are the closure of the aortic and pulmonary valves. These two heart sounds create the 'lub-dup' sound heard between pauses. The phases of the cardiac cycle are shown in Figure 10.8.

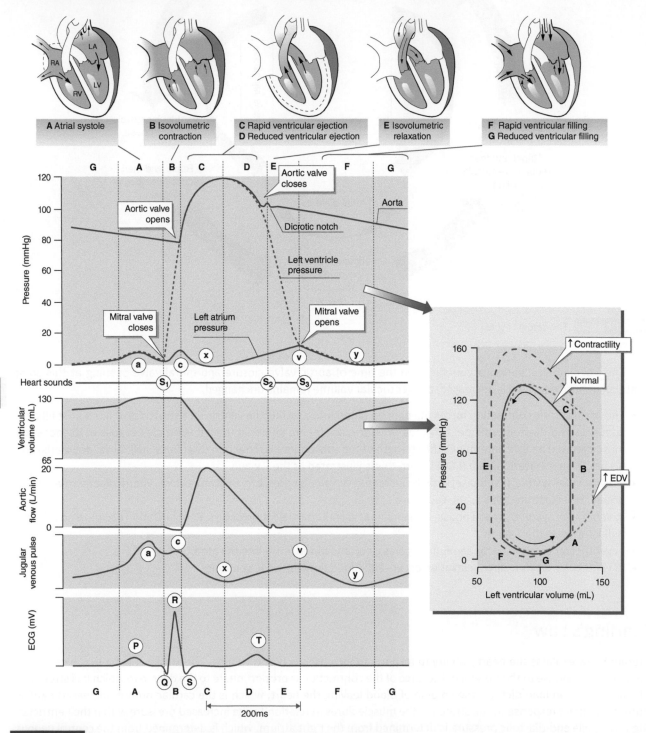

FIGURE 10.8 Phases of the cardiac cycle. Source: Peate (2022)/John Wiley & Sons.

Pregnancy and Childbirth and Maternal Cardiac System

Every mother, regardless of her risk factors, will receive care from a midwife at some point in her pregnancy and childbirth journey, it is vital that clinical care is in collaboration with the mother, and is holistic and multidisciplinary (Ockenden 2022). Having a sound understanding of normal cardiac functioning will assist in the recognition of deviations from the norm.

Pregnancy and childbirth have a profound effect upon every woman's body. Outcomes for those mothers who have increased risk factors can be improved through equitable personalised safer provision (NHS England 2016). There are more women in the United Kingdom having babies when they are older or of an increased body mass index (BMI) and/or have underlying health conditions than previously recorded (Webster 2021). Maternity services are evolving to provide safer care for all women and the understanding of the effects of inequality on outcomes is a national driver to improve service delivery and improve perinatal outcomes, through a single delivery plan for maternity and neonatal services.

Stark inequalities in outcomes are experienced by those mothers from black, Asian and mixed ethnic groups and women who live in the most deprived areas (Knight et al. 2022). Maternal mortality rates from indirect cardiac disease per 100 000 maternities, accounts for 1.62 per 100 000 maternities. Cardiac disease is the largest single cause of indirect maternal deaths (Knight et al. 2022). The evidence of poorer outcomes for those mothers who are at a disadvantage is shaping maternity care going forwards. Accurate data collection for this cohort of women contributes to national safer care planning (NMPA 2022). All health professionals caring for women throughout the perinatal period should be aware of common risk factors for heart disease. Taking into account individualised known maternal or familial risk factors, mothers should be counselled to be aware of the signs and symptoms of heart disease.

Changes in Pregnancy

In a normal pregnancy of a healthy mother, the circulating volume of blood increases up to around the 34th week of pregnancy, and the heart responds to the increase in workload. The left ventricle hypertrophies and the heart enlarges. As the growing uterus' fundal height increases, the mother's heart is slightly repositioned upwards and further left.

The blood volume rises from 65 ml/kg prepregnancy to 100 ml/kg in pregnancy (Vricella 2017), and requires greater cardiac output. The demands on the heart are proportionate to the pregnancy progression. Cardiac output increases to 50% by 34 weeks of gestation to around 7 l/minute by the end of pregnancy. The woman's heart rate increases in pregnancy by 10–20 beats/minute, reaching maximum heart rate in the third trimester (Long et al. 2021). It is not uncommon to auscultate maternal heart murmurs during pregnancy (Marshall and Raynor 2020).

Postnatal cardiac output and plasma volumes change rapidly in the immediate postnatal period and continue two weeks postpartum; thereafter, changes to the prepregnancy state are incremental and can take up to six months (McLean et al. 2013).

Within maternity services, there are a number of clinicians who frequently work within the speciality: midwives, obstetricians, maternity support workers, maternity nurses, general practitioners, anaesthesia and neonatal clinicians; all come into regular contact with mothers and neonates. Understanding anatomy and physiology of the cardiac system during contact with mothers and babies will improve safety. Knowing to whom and when to refer is an essential element of safer care. When midwives identify mothers or babies with signs and symptoms of cardiac impairment or deterioration of existing conditions, their professional responsibility is to refer to a medical doctor (obstetrician, anaesthetist or neonatologist; Nursing and Midwifery Council 2019).

Interdisciplinary working to support mothers where cardiac disease is known or suspected would ideally include preconceptual care and early referral into specialist services at tertiary referral centres. Combined obstetric and cardiac clinics and specialist maternal medicine input is recommended for women with suspected or continuing cardiac concerns or who have comorbidities. Midwifery input for these women will be alongside the obstetric and cardiology specialists. Each woman requires an individualised risk assessment. Known risk factors of extreme obesity, lifestyle, deprivation indices score, ethnicity and familial cardiac history are fundamental to forming a holistic overview.

Women attending appointments who present with symptoms of raised respiratory rates, chest pain, persistent tachycardia and orthopnoea, may be displaying signs and symptoms of cardiac disease and should be fully investigated. Persistent sinus tachycardia should always be investigated, particularly when there is accompanying breathlessness (Jarvis and Saman 2017, Knight et al. 2019).

Changes in Pregnancy for Women with Known Cardiac Impairment

For mothers who have known cardiac impairment, their consultant-led care is shared in a combined cardiac and obstetric clinic, run from either obstetric or cardiothoracic centres. Midwifery input in these clinics varies across the UK. Many maternity units have specialist maternal medicine midwife and consultant midwife posts, which ensures that the midwifery input for these mothers is included.

Many women with medical complexities or comorbidities who are categorised as high risk attend specialist hospital clinics and may not see a midwife as often as a low-risk mother. Ensuring that these mothers have access to midwifery advice and guidance is an essential element of holistic care. For mothers with existing cardiac disease, their knowledge and understanding of their condition and how it affects their daily living activities may well exceed that of their caregiver. It is important to recognise the mother's autonomy and ownership of her condition.

Congenital heart disease is the most common cardiovascular disease in pregnancy (Siu et al. 2001). Some 0.8% of pregnant women have congenital heart disease (Khairy et al. 2010), whereas acquired heart disease is responsible for the majority of women who die. A mother with a family history or confirmation of genetic aortopathy or cardiac channelopathy should be referred for cardiac assessment before pregnancy (Knight et al. 2022).

Those pregnant mothers who have congenital cardiac abnormalities require information with which to make informed decisions about their care. The recommendation of continuing surveillance and individualised care planning forms a plan for antenatal, intrapartum and postnatal care offer, providing a comprehensive care package for women.

Mothers with existing congenital heart defects will be offered a fetal ultrasound scan to screen for fetal cardiac structural abnormalities. Use of prophylactic antibiotics where endocarditis for cardiac defects (which are not fully closed) may be considered for the intrapartum period.

Medications Management

Many women with congenital heart defects are treated with prophylactic anticoagulation therapy (heparin/warfarin). An accurate maternal weight for dosage is required and mothers require continuing obstetric and cardiology review throughout pregnancy and in the postnatal period. Routine care within the midwifery setting will be complimentary to maternal medicine/ combined cardiac and obstetric clinic appointments, depending on a woman's needs, and will be individualised.

Monitoring mother's vital signs, regardless of where they present (e.g. maternity services, general practitioner, emergency care) requires a Modified Early Obstetric Warning Score (MEOWS) to be used (RCOG 2012, 2016; NICE 2007).

This tool identifies deviations from the norm specifically for pregnant and postnatal women. It is recommended that all clinicians who take maternal observations should have annual training in the use of MEOWS. MEOWS are now extensively used throughout maternity services (Appendix); however, there is no national standardised MEOWS tool, and slight variations in the reference ranges are currently seen across healthcare providers.

Clinical Assessment

Where a mother presents with symptoms of breathlessness, nocturnal cough, palpitations, heart murmurs, extreme lethargy, ankle oedema, and where there is not another likely cause for a mother's displayed symptoms, the clinician should take a cardiac history and should suspect heart failure. If of any of the following apply, clinicians should escalate clinical concerns:

- A familial history or sudden death of a young relative (less than 40 years) where indication of potential inherited cardiac conditions are present.
- Breathlessness when lying down or at rest (orthopnea), paroxysmal nocturnal dyspnoea or breathlessness when in a left-lateral position (exclude aortocaval compression).
- An unexplained cough when lying down, which may produce frothy pink sputum (improved on moving to an upright position).
- A persistent wheezing which does not respond to routine asthma management.
- Palpitations, persistent elevated heart rate when at rest.

Recognition of Deviations from the Norm

When clinicians care for mothers who have known cardiac risk factors, clinical assessment of these mothers' conditions requires a working knowledge of what is normal physiology and what is normal physiology for that individual. Knowledge of the most common pathophysiology and diseases will assist in providing individualised care to the woman. Clinicians recording in or accessing these mother's maternal medical history records should become familiar with commonly found cardiac diseases and their presentations.

Congenital Heart Disease

A woman may present for maternity care having had a congenital heart defect corrected. Common congenital heart defects include:

- Atrial septal defect: a hole between the two atrial chambers.
- Ventricular septal defect: a hole between the two ventricular chambers.
- Transposition of the great arteries (repaired in childhood): the pulmonary artery arises from left ventricle and the aorta arises from the right ventricle.
- Tetralogy of Fallot: a combination of four defects – ventricular septal defect, overriding aorta, pulmonary stenosis and right ventricular hypertrophy.
- Patent ductus arteriosus (in babies): the fetal ductus arteriosus vessel fails to close after their birth.
- Coarctation of the aorta: a narrowing of the aorta below the left subclavian artery.
- Pulmonary atresia: a closed or malformed valve.
- Stenosis: narrowing of the valves.

Complex Heart Defects

Many heart defects are associated with each other (e.g. transposition of the great arteries and pulmonary atresia, ventricular septal defect, valve regurgitation; Nair and Peate 2017). Mothers may have a mechanical valve or conduits supporting their cardiac function; their ventricle function may be impaired.

For women who have complex severe heart disease, where pregnancy is contraindicated, close supervision is required. These conditions include single ventricle function, corrected complex congenital heart disease, cardiomyopathy, cyanotic congenital heart disease, Marfan syndrome, Eisenmenger syndrome. Marfan syndrome is associated with aortic dissection, aortic aneurysm, dilatation of aortic root, aortic or mitral valve regurgitation, heart murmurs, cardiomyopathy and arrhythmias (McLean et al. 2013).

Rheumatic and Valvular Heart Disease

Rheumatic and valvular heart disease is a complication of rheumatic fever that causes permanent damage to the aortic mitral valve, with regurgitation of blood flow. Prosthetic heart valves are bioprosthetic valves; they can develop structural deterioration over a long time. Mechanical valves carry a known risk of developing thrombosis.

Cardiomyopathy

Cardiomyopathy is a term used to cover five potential presentations of the disease: dilated, hypertrophic, restrictive, arrhythmogenic and peripartum.

Snapshot 10.1   Impaired Cardiac Function

Background

Amita Begum is a 26 year old Asian mother who was booked for maternity care in her first pregnancy at 12 weeks and 0 days (12^{+0} weeks) gestation. During a telephone booking appointment, her medical, obstetric and social history was obtained. She was placed on a high-risk consultant-led pathway with referral into the raised BMI obstetric-led hospital-based clinic. Amita's schedule of care included routine primigravida schedule of midwifery appointments in a community setting.

History

Amita has a familial history of congenital heart disease. She was noted to have a BMI of 36.7 kg/m^2 above the expected range. Her haemoglobin was 120 g/l at booking. She was advised to take 150 mg aspirin daily, as of her two moderate risk factors were a high BMI and nulliparity. Because of these factors, she was advised to take vitamin D due to her ethnicity and was offered and accepted gestational diabetes screening. Baseline observations were found to be within the expected range. All further antenatal observations have been within the expected ranges. Ms Begum attended for routine antenatal ultrasound appointments where findings were within expected ranges. The baby is plotting on the 50th centile of the customised growth chart.

Ms Begum works as a nurse in a district general hospital. At 35^{+4} weeks, she attended a community midwife appointment, where she reported that she has had heartburn, frequent dizzy spells and has fainted when on a busy shift at work. She says that she is able to take regular breaks, to eat and drink to thirst and hunger when at work. She states she feels breathless when walking upstairs.

Amita indicates she is continuing to work a mixture of day and night shifts, but is finding this difficult as her sleep was broken by being woken with coughing and breathlessness. She is due to take maternity leave at 36 weeks.

Observations

The midwife recorded Amita's observations in the community setting using the Modified Early Obstetric Warning Score (MEOWS; Box 10.1) and took a blood test. The results are as follows.

MEOWS

Vital sign	Observations (MEOWS)
Temperature (°C)	36.9
Pulse (beats/min)	122
Respiratory rate (breaths/min)	23
Blood pressure systolic (mmHg)	130
Blood pressure diastolic (mmHg)	65
O_2 saturations (% air/O_2)	Not performed
Consciousness (AVPU)	Alert

Blood Tests

Full blood count	Result	Normal range
Haemoglobin (g/l)	109	110–140
White cell count ($\times 10^9$/l)	10	6–16
Platelets ($\times 10^9$/l)	170	150–400
Mean cell volume (fl)	80	80–100
C-reactive protein (g/l)	6	0–7
Sodium (mmol/l)	134	130–140
Potassium (mmol/l)	4	3.3–4.1
Urea (mmol/l)	4	<4.5
Creatinine (μmol/l)	35	<75

Reflective Learning Activity

Review the information in Snapshot 10.1. Consider what actions should be undertaken. Consideration should be given to:

- Risk assessment
- Accumulative risk factors
- Health promotion
- MEOWS
- Escalation
- Place of care
- Further investigations
- Explanations for findings out of the expected ranges
- What concerning features constitutes a red flag alert.

BOX 10.1   Modified Early Warning Score

Vital sign	Reference ranges				
	2	1	0	1	2
Temperature (°C)	<35.0	35.1–35.9	36.0–37.4	37.5–37.9	>38.0
Pulse (beats/min)	<50	50–60	60–100	100–120	120–160
Respiratory rate (breaths/min)	<10		10–20	21–26	>26
Blood pressure systolic (mmHg)	50–80	80–100	100–140	40–160	160–180
Blood pressure diastolic (mmHg)	<40		40–90	90–110	110–140
O_2 saturations (% Air/O_2)	<94		95–100		
Consciousness (AVPU)			A	V	U, P

A, alert; P, pain; U, unresponsive; V, voice.

- If MEOWS = 1–3, escalate: inform midwife and for obstetric review within four hours.
- If MEOWS = 4, escalate: inform senior midwife and for obstetric review within one hour.
- If MEOWs = 5 or above, escalate: for immediate review by obstetric team and obstetric anaesthetic team.

Clinicians create a MEOWS according to the number of triggers. Measurements that fall within the green parameters are within the expected ranges. Amber and red measurements are out of an expected range and a clinician will be prompted to increase observations and alert the obstetricians and/or anaesthetists.

It is the responsibility of the person carrying out the observations to alert a midwife if the MEOWS is 1 or more. If the MEOWS is 1–3, it is the responsibility of the midwife to decide whether increased frequency of observations or a medical review is needed. If the MEOWS is 4 or above, or 3 in any single parameter, the midwife should escalate to the obstetric team.

Appendix shows the obstetric early warning chart from the Royal College of Obstetricians and Gynaecologists (RCOG 2016).

Orange Flag Alert: Concerns

Clinicians must retain a holistic overview of mothers in their care. Regardless of MEOWS, if a clinician has concerns about a woman's condition advice should be sought.

Ms Begum's Assessment

- MEOWS 3: the clinician should consider that the assessment occurred in a community setting; this may influence a clinician to liaise with the obstetric team sooner and refer a mother into the obstetric unit rather than wait and repeat all observations.
- A holistic overview will include maternal perception of wellbeing.
- Revisiting local and national guidelines will assist in recognition of the abnormal.
- The mother's accumulative risks included a known raised BMI, ethnicity, familial cardiac history. Her emergent risk factors include persistent tachycardia, bouts of syncope, low haemoglobin, being woken with coughing and breathlessness.

Red Flag Alert: Persistent Sinus Tachycardia

A persistent sinus tachycardia is a red flag; maternal heartrate will vary throughout a 24-hour period but a persistent tachycardia at rest is a red flag. Mothers who are anaemic may have a tachycardia; a haemoglobin level blood test is indicated.

Red Flag: Syncope on Exertion

Amita reports bouts of syncope when at work. Her diastolic blood pressure is within the expected range; she reports that she gets regular breaks and is able to hydrate and eat when at work. She reports that her sleep is being broken by being woken with coughing and breathlessness. Indicators of potential impaired cardiac function require immediate referral to the obstetric team.

Reflective Learning Activity

It is important that midwives recognise conditions outside of the scope and practice of midwifery and refer appropriately. Through routine assessments, deviations from the norm are found and addressed. Consider what the following list of actions may prompt you to discover and how that impacts on the immediate and planned clinical care for the mother.

- Early booking.
- Thorough history taking.
- Referral to obstetric care.
- Vital signs baseline assessment including maternal weight, blood pressure, full blood count and coagulation.
- Dietary advice.
- Continuing observations alert to signs of respiratory rates, breathlessness, cough, wheezing, syncope on exertion, pulse oximetry deviations from the expected range.
- Recognition of cyanosis; use of saturation monitor.
- Capillary refill times.
- Consideration of an intrapartum left lateral position.
- Second-stage length planning in collaboration with mother and obstetrician.
- Consideration of episiotomy to expedite birth to shorten second stage, avoiding using the Valsalva manoeuvre. Avoiding a supine or lithotomy position may be advised.
- For mothers with moderate heart disease, developing a postnatal care plan.
- For mothers with complex cardiac disease, bespoke care will be designed around their individual needs and midwifery care may be required on an intensive care unit.

Snapshot 10.2

Background

Neema Addo, A 41-year-old black African mother was booked for obstetric-led care at 16 weeks and 3 days' gestation (16^{+3} weeks) in her third pregnancy. Her medical, obstetric and social history was obtained. Neema has previously had two uncomplicated vaginal deliveries. She was noted to have a BMI of 23.1 kg/m^2, within the expected range, and her haemoglobin was 130 g/l at booking. Neema's risk assessment indicated a recommendation of high-dose vitamin D 20 µg supplements and a gestational diabetes screening test because of her ethnicity.

At a routine ultrasound dating scan, Neema's pregnancy was confirmed to be a twin pregnancy; her baseline observations were found to be within the expected range. At subsequent ultrasound scan, the pregnancy was found to be dichorionic diamniotic.

All further antenatal observations have been within the expected ranges. Neema attended for routine antenatal ultrasound appointments for multiple pregnancies, where findings were within expected ranges. She had an obstetric review at 28^{+0} weeks, which detected a heart murmur. Her antenatal care included regular ultrasound scans and antenatal clinic appointments, and a planned caesarean section was booked for 37^{+4} weeks. She received regular obstetric surveillance throughout her pregnancy.

At 36^{+2} weeks, Neema highlighted to her caregivers that she was experiencing tiredness and oedema of her ankles. Her blood pressure was taken and was found to be 120/70 mmHg. She had been struggling to sleep and felt that her heart had been racing when she had been working (she works part time from home as a data annalist).

Neema had a planned caesarean section with no complications. She remained in hospital while her babies received support, and at postnatal day 5 she felt unwell, feeling dizzy and breathless, reporting being unable to get out of a chair to mobilise to care for her babies.

Reflective Learning Activity

Review Neema's antenatal history:

- What commonly experienced symptoms of pregnancy can indicate potential heart failure?
- What are Neema's risk factors, innate and modifiable?
- What investigations may be required to form a working diagnosis?

review her postnatal history:

- What commonly experienced symptoms in the postnatal period can indicate potential heart failure or commonly experienced symptoms of a postnatal mother?
- Who would Neema's condition need to be escalated to?
- What investigations may be required to form a working diagnosis?

Observations

The midwife recorded Neema's observations using the Modified Early Obstetric Warning Score (MEOWS; Box 10.1) at postnatal day 5. The results are as follows.

Vital sign	Observation
Temperature (°C)	36.5
Pulse (beats/minute)	140
Respiratory rate (breaths/minute)	25
Blood pressure systolic (mmHg)	82
Blood pressure diastolic (mmHg)	39
O2 saturations (% air/O$_2$)	95
Consciousness (AVPU)	Voice

Neema's MEOWS = 7.

Further investigations that may be ordered include:

- Physical examination
- ECG (12 lead)
- Chest x-ray
- Blood tests: full blood chemistry, troponin
- ECG
- Transoesophageal echocardiogram
- Medications review.

MBRRACE-UK (Knight et al. 2022) and the Royal College of Physicians (2019), recommend using the Acute Care Toolkit 15: Managing Acute Medical Problems in Pregnancy, which facilitates recognition of 'red flag' symptoms. It fosters interdisciplinary collaborative working between acute medicine physicians, obstetricians, midwives, interventionists and other clinicians involved in a multidisciplinary care pathway of the acutely ill mother.

Orange Flag Alert: Ethnicity

MBRACE-UK warns that black women are 3.7 times more likely to die than white women (34 women per 100 000 giving birth). Asian women are 1.8 times more likely to die than white women (16 women per 100 000 giving birth; Knight et al. 2019).

Red Flag Alert: Wheeze

Wheeze can be caused by pulmonary oedema. A wheeze that does not respond to standard asthma management requires investigation.

Red Flag: Exertional Syncope

Exertional syncope can be a symptom of cardiovascular disease in addition to orthopnoea and chest pain.

Take Home Points

- The cardiac system adapts to multiple changes throughout pregnancy and the immediate period after birth.
- Identification and understanding of the expected ranges facilitates recognition of any deviations from the norm.
- Black and Asian women have a higher risk of mortality in pregnancy: white women, 9 in 100,000; women of mixed ethnicity, 12 in 100,000 (1.3 times); Asian women, 16 in 100,000 (1.8 times); black women 34 in 100,000 (3.7 times).
- Increasing numbers of women book for pregnancy care with risk factors for heart disease. A wide range of factors are readily screened for during routine maternity care.
- Identified risk factors and symptoms of heart disease in pregnancy or immediately after birth should be escalated to the wider multidisciplinary team involved in a woman's care.

211

Summary

An overview of the anatomy and physiology of the cardiac system and the changes that occur in pregnancy and the post-natal period have been explored. Some of the main diseases of the cardiac system in relation to pregnancy have been visited. Healthcare professionals who provide services for women during pregnancy and in the immediate period afterwards require a working knowledge of the cardiac system to assist them in identifying deviations from the norm. All women who access maternity services are screened through routine observations and risk analysis at each episode of care; thus, the caregiver who understands the combined physiological, socioeconomic and cultural factors that contribute to the overall wellbeing of the woman will be better able to act on their findings and will provide safer care. Holistic care is the tenet of maternity provision, with an onus on the provider to give accessible information to women for them to be able to make informed decisions.

References

Jarvis, S. and Saman, S. (2017). Heart failure 1: pathogenesis, presentation and diagnosis. *Nursing Times* 113 (9): 49–53.

Khairy, P., Ionescu-Ittu, R., Mackie, A. et al. (2010). Changing mortality in congenital heart disease. *Journal of American College Cardiology* 56: 1149–1157.

Knight, M., Bunch, K., Tufnell, D. et al. (2019). *Saving Lives, Improving Mothers' Care - Lessons Learned to Inform Maternity Care from the UK and Ireland Confidential Enquiries into Maternal Deaths and Morbidity 2015–17.* Oxford: National Perinatal Epidemiology Unit, University of Oxford.

Knight, M., Bunch, K., Patel, R. et al. (ed.) (2022). *MBRRACE-UK. Saving Lives, Improving Mothers' Care Core Report – Lessons Learned to Inform Maternity Care from the UK and Ireland Confidential Enquiries into Maternal Deaths and Morbidity 2018–20.* Oxford: National Perinatal Epidemiology Unit, University of Oxford.

Long, V., Mathieu, S., and Fiset, C. (2021). *Heart Rhythm* 2 (2): 168–173. https://doi.org/10.1016/j.hroo.2021.03.001.

Marshall, J. and Raynor, M. (2020). *Myles Textbook for Midwives*, 17e. New York, NY: Elsevier.

McLean, M., Frances, A.B.'L., and Robson, S. (2013). Heart disease. In: *Medical Disorders in Pregnancy: A Manual for Midwives*, 2e (ed. S.W. Robson), 43–72. Chichester: Wiley.

Nair, M. and Peate, I. (2017). *Fundamentals of Applied Pathophysiology: An Essential Guide for Nursing and Healthcare: An essential guide for nursing and healthcare strudents*, 3e. Chichester: Wiley.

National Maternity and Perinatal Audit. (2022). *National Maternity and Perinatal Audit: Clinical Report 2022. Based on births in NHS maternity services in England and Wales between 1 April 2018 and 31 March 2019.* London: RCOG.

NHS England (2016). *Better Births: Improving Outcomes of Maternity Services in Engl and A Five Year Forward View for Maternity Care.* London: NHS England.

NICE (2007). *Acutely Ill Patients in Hospital: Recognition of and Response to Acute Illness in Adults in Hospital.* Clinical Guideline CG50. London: National institute of Health and Care Excellence.

Nursing and Midwifery Council (2019). *Standards of Proficiency for Midwives.* London: Nursing and Midwifery Council.

Ockenden, D. (2022). *Ockenden Report – Final: Findings, Conclusions and Essential Actions from the Independent Review of Maternity Services and the Shrewsbury and Telford Hospital NHS Trust.* HC 1219. London: HMSO.

Peate, I. (ed.) (2017). *Fundamentals of Applied Pathophysiology: An essential guide for nursing and healthcare students.* Chichester: Wiley.

Peate, I. (2022). *Anatomy and Physiology for Nursing and Healthcare Students at a Glance*, 2e. Chichester: Wiley.

Peate, I. and Evans, S. (2020). *Fundamentals of Anatomy and Physiology*, 3e. Oxford: Wiley-Blackwell.

RCOG (2012). *Bacterial Sepsis in Pregnancy.* Green-top Guideline No. 64b. London: Royal College of Obstetrics and Gynaecology.

RCOG (2016). *Prevention and Management of Postpartum Haemorrhage.* Green-top Guideline No. 52. London: Royal College of Obstetrics and Gynaecology.

Royal College of Physicians (2019). *Acute Care Toolkit 15 Managing Acute Medical Problems in Pregnancy.* London: Royal College of Physicians. https://obgyn.onlinelibrary.wiley.com/doi/epdf/10.1111/1471-0528.14178 www.rcplondon.ac.uk/guidelines-policy/acute-care-toolkit-15-managing-acute-medical-problems-pregnancy (accessed 30 October 2023).

Siu, S., Sermer, M., Colman, J. et al. (2001). Prospective multicentre study of pregnancy outcomes in women with heart disease. *Circulation* 104: 515–521.

Vricella, L.K. (2017). Emerging understanding and measurement of plasma volume expansion in pregnancy. *American Journal Clinical Nutrition* 106 (Suppl 6): 1620S–1625S. https://doi.org/10.3945/ajcn.117.155903.

Webster, K. (2021). NMPA Project Team. Ethnic and Socio-economic Inequalities in NHS Maternity and Perinatal Care for Women and their Babies: Assessing care using data from births between 1 April 2015 and 31 March 2018 across England, Scotland and Wales. London: RCOG. Available at:www.maternityaudit.org.uk/pages/sprintpub.

Reflective Learning Activity

Conditions Associated with the Cardiac System

Below is a list of conditions that are associated with the cardiac system. Take some time and write notes about each of the conditions. Think about the medications that may be used to treat these conditions and be specific about the pharmacokinetics and pharmacodynamics. Remember to include aspects of patient care. If you are making notes about people you have offered care and support to you must ensure that you have adhered to the rules of confidentiality.

The condition	Your notes
Arrhythmia	
Congenital heart disease	
Heart failure	
Valve disease	
Heart muscle disease	

Appendix: Obstetric Early Warning Chart

OBSTETRIC EARLY WARNING CHART.   **FOR MATERNITY USE ONLY**

NAME: _____   DOB: _____

CHI: _____   WARD: _____

CONTACT DOCTOR FOR EARLY INTERVENTION IF PATIENT TRIGGERS ONE RED OR TWO YELLOW SCORES AT ANY ONE TIME

Date :																	
Time :																	
RESP (write rate in corresp. box) >30																	>30
21-30																	21-30
11-20																	11-20
0-10																	0-10
Saturations 90-100%																	90-100%
<90%																	<90%
O2 Conc. %																	%
Temp 39 38 37 36 35																	39 38 37 36 35
HEART RATE 170 160 150 140 130 120 110 100 90 80 70 60 50 40																	170 160 150 140 130 120 110 100 90 80 70 60 50 40
Systolic blood pressure 200 190 180 170 160 150 140 130 120 110 100 90 80 70 60 50																	200 190 180 170 160 150 140 130 120 110 100 90 80 70 60 50
Diastolic blood pressure 130 120 110 100 90 80 70 60 50 40																	130 120 110 100 90 80 70 60 50 40
Passed Urine Y or N																	Y or N
Lochia Normal																	Normal
Heavy / Foul																	Heavy / Foul
Proteinuria 2+																	2+
> 2+																	>2+
Liquor Clear / Pink																	Clear/Pink
Green																	Green
NEURO RESPONSE (√) Alert																	Alert
Voice																	Voice
Pain / Unresponsive																	Pain /Unresponsive
Pain Score (no.) 2-3																	2-3
0-1																	0-1
Nausea (√) YES (√)																	YES (√)
NO (√)																	NO (√)
Looks unwell YES (√)																	YES (√)
Looks unwell NO (√)																	NO (√)
Total Yellow Scores																	
Total Red Scores																	

Royal College of Obstetricians and Gynaecologists RCOG (2016 / John Wiley & Sons).

Glossary

Aortopathy	Disease of the aorta; includes aortic aneurysms, aortic dissection and aortic enlargement.
Artery	Blood vessel carrying blood away from the heart.
Atria	The two upper chambers of the heart.
Atrioventricular valves	Connect the atrium to the ventricles; comprise the bicuspid valve (left atrioventricular valve) and tricuspid valve (right atrioventricular valve).
Atrioventricular node	A component of electrical conduction which connects the atria and ventricles.
Bicuspid valve	Also known as the mitral valve; the left atrioventricular valve.
Cardiac channelopathy	Disruption of cardiac ion channel function, resulting in altered electrical function and dysrhythmia.
Cardiac output	Amount of blood the heart pumps over one minute, calculated by multiplying heart rate and stroke volume.
Coronary arteries	Supply the heart muscles with oxygenated blood.
Dyspnoea	Shortness of breath.
Echocardiogram	Structure and function ultrasound scan of heart.
Electrocardiogram (ECG)	Records the heart's rhythm and electrical activity.
Endocardium	Endothelial membrane of the inner heart.
Hypertrophy	Muscle mass increase.
Inferior vena cava	Vein returns deoxygenated blood to the heart from the body, into the right atrium.
Medulla oblongata	Area of brain for organ control.
Mitral valve	Left atrioventricular or bicuspid valve.
Myocardium	Middle layer of heart.
Orthopnoea	Shortness of breath (dyspnoea) that occurs when lying flat.
Parasympathetic nerve	Division of the autonomic nervous system which regulates resting and relaxation.
Paroxysmal nocturnal dyspnoea	Being woken from sleep by severe breathlessness and coughing, with accompanying pink frothy sputum (improved by moving to an upright position).
Pericardium	Double-layered sac that encloses the heart.
Pulmonary artery	Takes deoxygenated blood from right ventricle to the lungs.
Pulmonary vein	Takes reoxygenated blood from lungs to left atrium.
Semilunar valve	Prevents blood flowing back into the ventricles after a contraction.
Septum	A partition dividing a body space or cavity.
Sinoatrial node	Initiates the heartbeat; the heart's natural pacemaker.
Sinus tachycardia	A regular cardiac rhythm where the heart beats faster than normal, resulting in an increased cardiac output.
Superior vena cava	Vein that returns deoxygenated blood to the heart from above the diaphragm into the right atrium.
Sympathetic nerve	A division of the autonomic nervous system.
Transoesophageal echocardiogram	Ultrasound scan of heart via the oesophagus.
Tricuspid valve	Right atrioventricular valve.
Ventricle	The two lower chambers of the heart.

Multiple Choice Questions

1. The pericardial cavity encloses which organ(s)?
   a. Lungs
   b. Heart
   c. Lungs and heart
   d. Lungs, heart and diaphragm

2. Which of these is not a heart muscle layer?
   a. Smooth muscle
   b. Pericardium
   c. Myocardium
   d. Endocardium

3. The heart has two ventricles which are separated by what?
   a. Inferior vena cava
   b. Aortic arch
   c. Interventricular septum
   d. Pericardium

4. The left side of the heart receives oxygenated blood from where?
   a. Superior vena cava
   b. Inferior vena cava
   c. Subclavian artery
   d. Pulmonary veins

5. The mitral and tricuspid valves ensure that directional blood flow into what?
   a. The atrium
   b. The ventricles
   c. The lungs

6. Where is the heart beat is initiated?
   a. Atrioventricular node
   b. The bundle of His
   c. Sinoatrial node
   d. Purkinje fibres

7. Which statement describes the cardiac cycle?
   a. Ventricular diastole early, ventricular diastole late, ventricular systole first phase ventricular systole second phase, atrial systole
   b. Atrial systole, ventricular systole first phase, ventricular systole second phase, Ventricular diastole early, ventricular diastole late
   c. Atrial systole, Ventricular diastole early, ventricular diastole late, ventricular systole first phase ventricular systole second phase
   d. Ventricular diastole early, ventricular systole first phase ventricular diastole late, ventricular systole second phase, atrial systole

8. Cardiac output increases in pregnancy up to 50% to around 7 l/minute by how many weeks of gestation?
   a. 30 weeks
   b. 38 weeks
   c. 34 weeks
   d. 28 weeks

9. What heart disease in pregnancy is responsible for the majority of cardiovascular mortality?
   a. Acquired heart disease
   b. Congenital heart disease
   c. Subarachnoid haemorrhage
   d. Cardiac valve disease

10. Shortness of breath when lying down is what condition?
    a. Paroxysmal nocturnal dyspnoea
    b. Orthopnoea
    c. Apnoea
    d. Central and obstructive apnoea

CHAPTER 11

The Digestive System

Clare Gordon

AIM

This chapter provides the reader with insight into the digestive system, its function and some of the adaptations women may experience during pregnancy.

LEARNING OUTCOMES

On completion of this chapter, you will be able to:

- Identify the anatomical structures of the digestive system.
- Describe the function of the digestive system and function of each of the organs.
- Explain the hormones and enzymes used in digestion.
- Describe the adaptations to pregnancy that affect the digestive system.

Test Your Prior Knowledge
1. What is the main function of the digestive system?
2. List the main structures of the digestive system.
3. Name the hormones and enzymes involved in digestion.
4. Name the adaptations to the digestive system in pregnancy.

Introduction

The digestive system is also referred to as the gastrointestinal (GI) tract/system or alimentary canal; these terms are interchangeable. See Figure 11.1 for an overview of the digestive system. The digestive system plays an essential role in the digestion of food and the absorption of nutrients. It is also responsible for removing waste products from the body.

The GI tract is a long muscular tube. Food passes through from the point at which it is ingested in the mouth, then through several different organs with different functions, which breakdown the food ready for absorption into nutrient molecules and where any remaining matter, usually fibre and waste, is finally eliminated or egested through the anus as faeces. The constituents of digestion are amino acids, mineral salts, fats and vitamins. Enzymes within the digestive

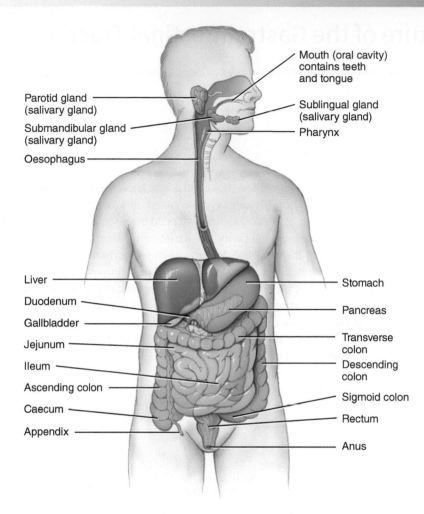

Parotid gland
(salivary gland)

Submandibular gland
(salivary gland)

Oesophagus

Mouth (oral cavity)
contains teeth
and tongue

Sublingual gland
(salivary gland)

Pharynx

Liver

Duodenum

Gallbladder

Jejunum

Ileum

Ascending colon

Caecum

Appendix

Stomach

Pancreas

Transverse
colon

Descending
colon

Sigmoid colon

Rectum

Anus

FIGURE 11.1 Diagram of the digestive system. Source: Peate and Evans (2020)/John Wiley & Sons.

system are responsible for this process and are also created in the GI tract by specialist glands. The GI tract is around 5 m in length from the mouth, where it starts, to the anus where it finishes. There are various organs that play a vital role in the digestion process along the length of the tract. These consist of:

- The mouth
- The pharynx
- Upper GI tract
- The oesophagus
- The stomach
- The small intestine
- The large intestine
- Lower GI tract
- The rectum and anal canal.

There are two additional accessory organs that play a major part in the digestive process: the pancreas and the liver. Ingestion, propulsion, digestion, absorption and elimination are the key activities that take place in the digestive system.

There are two mechanisms of digestion: mechanical, which uses movement or a mechanism; and chemical, which is a result of the action of enzymes and secretions in the digestive tract.

The Structure of the Gastrointestinal Tract

The structure of the GI tract, from the oesophagus to the anus, is composed of four layers (Figure 11.2):

1. The serosa/adventitia or outer covering
2. The muscularis (muscle) layer
3. The submucosa
4. The mucosa.

The serosa is the outermost protective layer of the GI tract and is also known as the adventitia. It consists of connective tissue and squamous and serous epithelium. The serosa is also called the visceral peritoneum as it forms part of the peritoneum. The parietal layer lines the walls of the abdominal cavity and the visceral layer covers the external surface of the digestive organs and supports their position in the cavity. The parietal and visceral layers make up the peritoneal cavity, which contains serous fluid and enables the two layers to slide over one another without any friction.

The muscularis layer is formed of smooth involuntary muscle. There is an inner layer of circular fibres and an outer layer of longitudinal cells. The stomach has an additional oblique layer containing nerve fibres called the plexus of Auerbach or mesenteric plexus. The smooth muscle fibres contract and relax in waves, pushing the contents of the tract onwards in a process known as peristalsis. The onward movement of the contents of the tract is controlled at various points by thick rings of circular muscle known as sphincters. The sphincters play an important role in allowing time for digestion and absorption to take place in the GI tract.

220

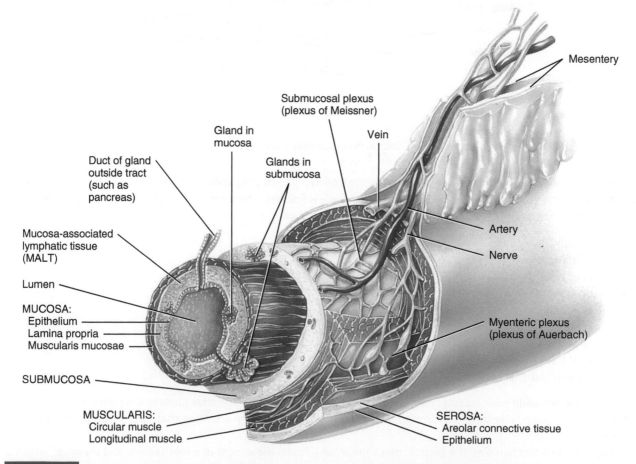

FIGURE 11.2   Structure of the gastrointestinal tract. Source: Peate and Evans (2020), p. 240/John Wiley & Sons.

The submucosa is formed of connective tissue and contains blood vessels, nerves and lymphoid tissue. The submucosal nerve plexus, or Meissner's plexus, is located in this layer. It contains sympathetic and parasympathetic nerves, which supply the mucosal lining. Meissner's plexus plays an important role in the release of gastric secretions.

The mucosa is the inner layer of the digestive tract. It contains a layer of epithelium supported by connective tissue and a layer of smooth muscle. The stratified squamous epithelial cells line the lumen and contain mucus-secreting glands that have a protective function in areas such as the oesophagus and anal canal. Where the secretion of digestive juices and absorption occurs, the mucosa consists of columnar epithelial cells that contain mucus-secreting goblet cells, which lubricate the walls of the GI tract, providing a barrier against the effects of the digestive enzymes. The connective tissue layer contains blood vessels, nerve cells and lymph vessels. The lymph cells defend the GI tract against microorganisms.

The Mouth

The mouth or the oral cavity is made up of muscular cheeks (at the sides), the hard and soft palates (the roof) and the tongue and soft tissues (floor of the mouth). The entrance to the mouth is surrounded by the lips. Behind the lips are the ridges of the maxilla and mandible, which are covered with a mucous membrane called the gingiva or gum (Figure 11.3).

Teeth

Teeth form part of the oral cavity and are embedded into the ridges of the mandible and maxilla. Babies are born with two sets of teeth. These teeth develop in the maxilla and mandible. They are known as deciduous (temporary or baby teeth) and permanent teeth. There are usually 20 deciduous teeth, 10 in each jaw. The deciduous teeth erupt through the gum

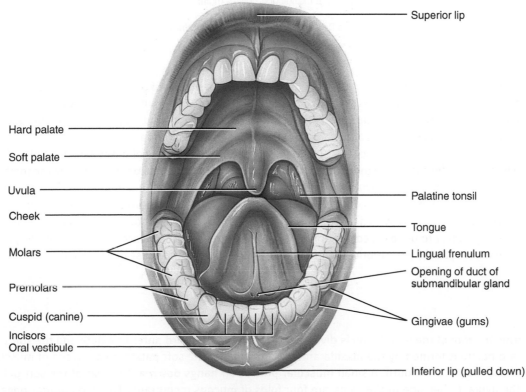

FIGURE 11.3 The oral cavity. Source: Tortora and Derrickson (2017) p. 789/John Wiley & Sons.

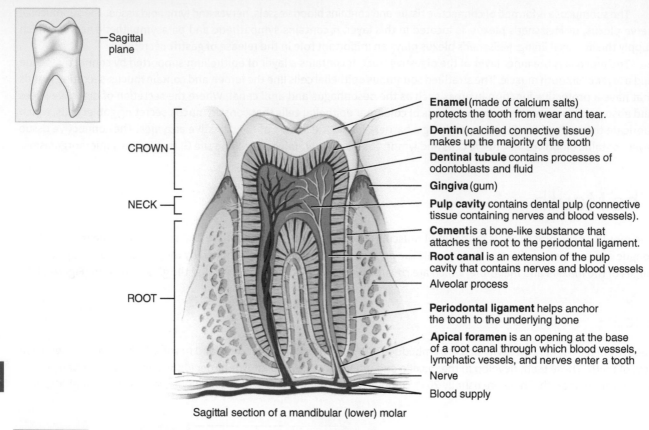

Sagittal plane

CROWN

NECK

ROOT

Enamel (made of calcium salts) protects the tooth from wear and tear.

Dentin (calcified connective tissue) makes up the majority of the tooth

Dentinal tubule contains processes of odontoblasts and fluid

Gingiva (gum)

Pulp cavity contains dental pulp (connective tissue containing nerves and blood vessels).

Cement is a bone-like substance that attaches the root to the periodontal ligament.

Root canal is an extension of the pulp cavity that contains nerves and blood vessels

Alveolar process

Periodontal ligament helps anchor the tooth to the underlying bone

Apical foramen is an opening at the base of a root canal through which blood vessels, lymphatic vessels, and nerves enter a tooth

Nerve

Blood supply

Sagittal section of a mandibular (lower) molar

FIGURE 11.4   Tooth structure. Source: Tortora and Derrickson (2017) p. 897/John Wiley & Sons.

222

into the oral cavity from around the sixth month of life. The permanent teeth begin to replace the deciduous teeth from around the age of 6 years and this process is usually complete by the age of 13 years. In an adult, the dentition consists of 32 teeth, with the wisdom teeth (third molars) being the last to erupt. There are two types of teeth: incisors and canines, used for cutting and biting, and premolars and molars, used for grinding and chewing.

While the shapes of the teeth differ, the structure remains the same and consists of the crown, the root and the neck (Figure 11.4). The crown is the part of the tooth that protrudes from the gum and the root is the part of the tooth embedded into the gum. The neck is the slightly narrow part where the crown and the root are merged. Within the tooth, there is a pulp cavity that contains blood vessels, lymph vessels and nerve cells. A dense hard substance called dentine is surrounded by the crown. The crown is covered by a thin layer of a very hard substance known as enamel. The root is covered with a substance very similar to bone called cementum and this holds the tooth in place in its socket in the gum. Small blood vessels and nerves pass into the tooth through a small foramen (hole) at the base of each root.

Palate

The palate forms the roof of the mouth and is divided into two parts: the hard anterior palate and the soft posterior palate. The hard palate is formed by the maxilla and palatine bones. The soft palate is composed of muscle and is at the back of the roof of the mouth. A small muscular protrusion hangs down at the rear of the soft palate; this is known as the uvula. Either side of the uvula are four folds of mucous membrane. The two anterior ones are the palatoglossal arches and the two posterior ones are the palatopharyngeal arches. There is a collection of lymphoid tissue on each side, which is known as the palatine tonsils.

Tongue

The tongue is a large muscular structure attached to the floor of the mouth. It is attached to the hyoid bone at the posterior and by a mucous membrane called the frenulum to the floor of the mouth. The surface of the tongue is covered in stratified epithelium with lots of tiny projections known as papillae, some of which contain taste-sensitive nerve endings that stimulate the sense of taste in taste buds. Glands are also found on the surface of the tongue which secrete digestive enzymes. The muscular action of the tongue plays an important role in chewing (mastication), swallowing, speech and taste.

Salivary Glands

Saliva is produced by three pairs of salivary glands (Figure 11.5) that release their digestive enzymes into the ducts that lead into the mouth: the parotid glands, the submandibular glands and the sublingual glands. These glands contain clusters of cells known as acini. Saliva is made up of a combination of secretions from the six saliva glands and the many small mucus secretin glands that are found in the mouth in the oral mucosa.

Approximately 1–1.5 l of saliva is produced daily. It is made up mainly of water (99.5%), mineral salts, salivary amylase, mucus and antimicrobial substances such as immunoglobulins and the enzyme lysozyme. Saliva has several functions including keeping the mouth clean and moist, mixing with foods to stimulate the sense of taste, lubricating food for easier swallowing; the presence of lysozyme and immunoglobulins helps to combat infection in the mucous membranes and helps to prevent tooth decay and in starting the chemical breaking down of food. The salivary amylase starts the breakdown of complex sugars including starches. The pH range for salivary amylase is between 5.8 and 7.4, and the optimum level for salivary action is around a pH of 6.8.

223

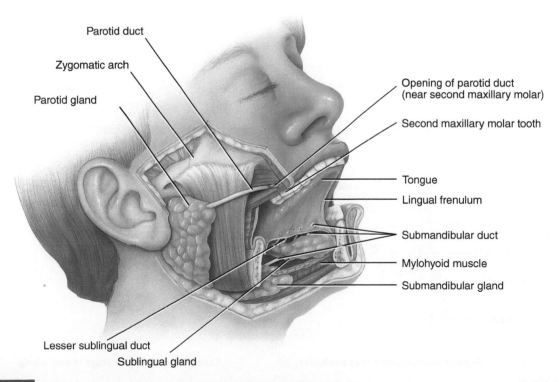

FIGURE 11.5 Salivary glands. Source: Peate and Evans (2020)/John Wiley & Sons.

Pharynx

The pharynx is described in three parts. The nasopharynx, which is involved in respiration (see Chapter 13), the oropharynx and the laryngopharynx, which are associated with the GI tract. Food passes from the mouth to the pharynx and through the oesophagus in a continuous process.

Swallowing happens in three phases once chewing is complete and a bolus is formed: the oral, pharyngeal and oesophageal phases (Figure 11.6)

Oral Phase
The voluntary action of the tongue and cheek muscles pushes the food bolus to the rear of the mouth towards the pharynx. Food is taken into the mouth then chewed (masticated) by the teeth, mixed with saliva and formed into a bolus (small mass) in preparation for swallowing (deglutition). The saliva coats the bolus to provide a slippery surface to make the passage of the bolus smoother. The tongue and cheeks help to move the food into position.

Pharyngeal Phase
The nasopharynx is occluded as the soft palate rises upwards. The tongue and pharyngeal folds block the bolus from coming back into the mouth. The larynx is moved upwards and forwards, occluding the epiglottis, thus preventing the food bolus from entering the trachea. This action is a reflex that is stimulated by the deglutition centre in the medulla. The swallowing reflex is initiated as the bolus reaches the posterior pharyngeal wall. These coordinated actions ensure that the bolus of food moves into the correct tube.

Oesophageal Phase
The action of peristalsis moves the food bolus through the oesophagus and into the stomach.

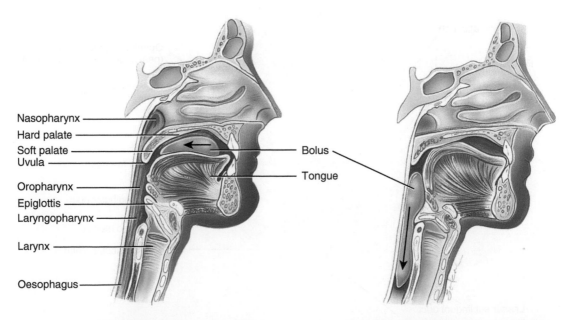

Position of structures before swallowing   During the pharyngeal stage of swallowing

FIGURE 11.6   Swallowing. Source: Peate and Evans (2020)/John Wiley & Sons.

Oesophagus

The oesophagus runs continuously from the pharynx to the stomach and is approximately 25 cm long. It passes through the muscle fibres of the diaphragm and then curves sharply upwards before joining the stomach. This anatomical feature is thought to be one of the factors that prevents the regurgitation of gastric contents into the oesophagus. There are also two sphincters at either end of the oesophagus. The cricopharyngeal sphincter or upper oesophageal sphincter prevents air passing into the oesophagus during inspiration, and the cardiac sphincter or lower oesophageal sphincter prevents the regurgitation or reflux of gastric contents into the oesophagus. The food bolus passes through the oesophagus by the process of peristalsis (Figure 11.7).

Snapshot 11.1:   Heartburn

Vanessa is currently 28 weeks pregnant in her first pregnancy. She attends a routine antenatal appointment with the community midwife. She mentions that she is experiencing discomfort after she has eaten. She describes her symptoms as an uncomfortable burning sensation under her breastbone. She has never experienced this feeling before and it is worrying her. She is concerned that it may affect the wellbeing of her baby. Vanessa is otherwise well and her pregnancy is progressing as expected. It appears that Vanessa is experiencing heartburn (acid reflux).

- What symptoms would you expect Vanessa to be reporting to you?
- What information would you give to reassure Vanessa?
- Consider the anatomical structures and physiology that could result in causing the symptoms of acid reflux.

Reflective Learning Activity

Explore what non-pharmacological and pharmacological advice could you give to a pregnant woman to alleviate symptoms of heartburn.

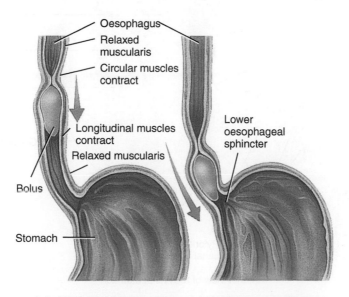

Anterior view of frontal sections of peristalsis in oesophagus

FIGURE 11.7   Peristalsis in the oesophagus. Source: Peate and Evans (2020)/John Wiley & Sons.

Adaptations in Pregnancy

Approximately 60–75% of pregnant women can experience gingivitis in pregnancy and this is when the gums become swollen and spongy. Women may experience bleeding gums when brushing their teeth due to the elevation of progesterone and oestrogen levels, which results in increased vascular permeability.

Some women experience an increase in salivation, also known as ptyalism. There is little evidence to support the notion that there is an increase in the production of saliva, but it is thought that ptyalism is the inability of women experiencing nausea to swallow normal amounts of saliva.

During pregnancy, many women experience a change in their appetite. They may find that their appetite increases or they can experience specific cravings or dislikes for certain types of food. Some women can experience a phenomenon known as pica. This is when a pregnant woman has a craving for non-food substances. It is also reported that women experience changes to their sense of smell and taste.

Stomach

The stomach is a J-shaped portion of the GI tract and it is continuous with the oesophagus at the lower oesophageal sphincter and with the duodenum at the pyloric sphincter (Figure 11.8). The stomach is made up of the four basic layers of tissue that are seen in the GI tract. However, the muscle layer consists of three layers of smooth muscle fibres, whereas elsewhere in the GI tract there are only two layers. There is an outer layer of longitudinal fibres, a middle layer of circular fibres and an inner layer of oblique fibres. This additional layer of muscle allows for the churning action that is required for digestion.

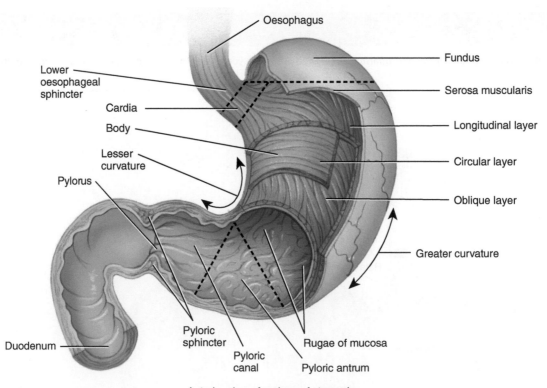

Anterior view of regions of stomach

FIGURE 11.8   The stomach. Source: Peate and Evans (2020)/John Wiley & Sons.

The functions of the stomach are:

- A reservoir for food.
- Mechanical digestion – churning up food to mix with gastric juices, facilitated by the strong muscular contractions of the smooth muscle. The mixed contents are liquefied to chyme.
- Defence against microbes and other harmful microorganisms – provided by hydrochloric acid in the gastric juice.
- Chemical digestion – pepsins breaking proteins into polypeptides.
- Production and secretion of intrinsic factor required for the absorption of vitamin B12.
- Secretion of gastrin.
- Regulation of the passage of gastric contents into the duodenum.

The stomach has three main regions:

1. The fundus, which is above the cardiac sphincter.
2. The body, which makes up the main part of the stomach.
3. The pylorus, at the lower end of the stomach, leading to the duodenum.

The mucosa in the stomach is arranged into folds, known as rugae, when the stomach is empty. These folds provide a large surface area for absorption to take place. The rugae enable the stomach to distend according to the amount of food present. The surface appears smooth in appearance. The shape and size of the stomach will depend on the quantity of food stored and it will also vary from person to person. It can contain anything between 1.5 and 4 l in an adult. The mucosa also contains gastric glands just beneath the surface that secrete many different substances that are required in the process of digestion.

When food enters the stomach, it is broken down by a wave-like muscle action, churned and mixed with gastric secretions. As it reduces to a more fluid-like substance, it becomes known as chyme. The action of peristalsis moves the contents towards the pylorus. This rhythmical contraction of smooth muscle is responsible for motility and is under the influence of the sympathetic and parasympathetic nerves. The pyloric sphincter between the stomach and the duodenum is relaxed and open when the stomach is inactive. When the stomach contains food, the sphincter is closed.

About 2 l of gastric juices are secreted daily by specialist gastric glands in the epithelium (Figure 11.9). The gastric juices are made up of water, mucus and hydrochloric acid, which makes the stomach contents highly acidic, helping to protect against any ingested harmful microorganisms. It also enables enzymes to begin the process of protein digestion. Pepsinogen, which is the precursor of pepsin responsible for the breakdown of proteins and intrinsic factor, is required for the absorption of vitamin B12.

227

Red Flag Alert: Hyperemesis Gravidarum

Hyperemesis gravidarum is excessive vomiting that continues through the day from the first trimester and can continue up to birth. When a woman presents with nausea and vomiting and is unable to retain food or fluid, there is a risk of dehydration and metabolic imbalance. On urine analysis, signs of oliguria, where the urine is dark in colour, ketones, glucose, protein and bile may be present. Weight loss and offensive smelling breath may also be noticeable. It is important to take a full set of observations including blood pressure, pulse, temperature and respiration rate. The mother's pulse is likely to be rapid (tachycardic) and her blood pressure low (hypotensive). She is likely to look pale (it may be more difficult to identify with women of colour – you may need to consider observing the palms of the hand or inside the lower eyelid). She may be very lethargic. On most occasions, a woman would be admitted to hospital for further investigations and treatment. This would include the administration of antiemetics and intravenous fluid. Close observation and strict fluid balance must occur until the women is safely rehydrated.

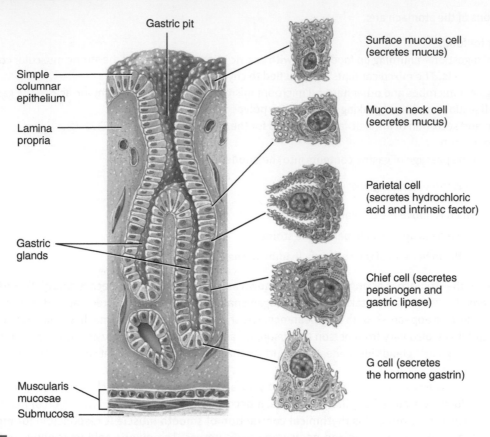

Gastric pit

Simple columnar epithelium

Lamina propria

Gastric glands

Muscularis mucosae

Submucosa

Surface mucous cell (secretes mucus)

Mucous neck cell (secretes mucus)

Parietal cell (secretes hydrochloric acid and intrinsic factor)

Chief cell (secretes pepsinogen and gastric lipase)

G cell (secretes the hormone gastrin)

FIGURE 11.9   Gastric glands and cells. Source: Peate and Evans (2020)/John Wiley & Sons.

Medications Management: Cyclizine Hydrochloride

Women may often experience periods of nausea and vomiting during pregnancy and labour. An antiemetic drug such as cyclizine hydrochloride block the receptors histamine (H_1) and acetylcholine (muscarinic) in the emetic centre.

- Route of administration: oral, intramuscular (IM), intravenous (IV).
- The standard dose is 50 mg orally eight-hourly, with a maximum of three doses per day (tablet form).
- 50 mg IM or IV eight-hourly, three times daily.
- Postoperatively – slow IV injection 20 minutes before the end of surgery.
- Cyclizine hydrochloride is a prescription-only medication (POM) and a Midwives' Exemptions (NMC 2021). Midwives' exemptions are a specific list of substances that midwives can supply or administer at the point of registration under specific legislation.
- Women should be advised that cyclizine is generally an effective drug but, in some women, it may not work and an alternative can be prescribed.
- The most common adverse effects are dryness of the mouth, fall in cardiac output, urticaria, rash, drowsiness, tachycardia, blurred vision, urinary retention, constipation.
- There is no evidence of teratogenicity and the drug is commonly used in pregnancy. It is considered as moderately safe with breastfeeding; however, there are few data from studies in breastfeeding women.

There are three phases to gastric juice secretion (Figure 11.10): the cephalic phase, the gastric phase and the intestinal phase.

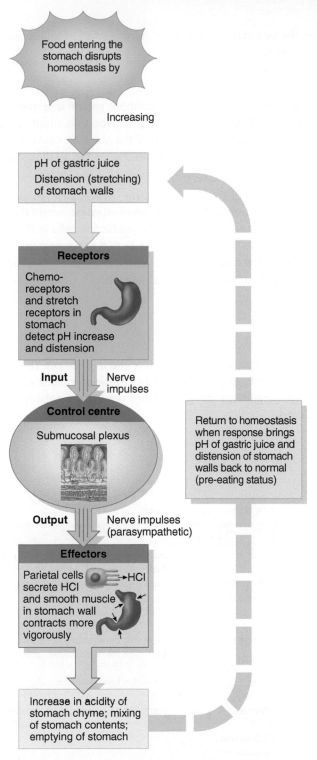

Food entering the stomach disrupts homeostasis by

Increasing

pH of gastric juice
Distension (stretching) of stomach walls

Receptors

Chemo-receptors and stretch receptors in stomach detect pH increase and distension

Input   Nerve impulses

Control centre

Submucosal plexus

Output   Nerve impulses (parasympathetic)

Effectors

Parietal cells secrete HCl and smooth muscle in stomach wall contracts more vigorously → HCl

Increase in acidity of stomach chyme; mixing of stomach contents; emptying of stomach

Return to homeostasis when response brings pH of gastric juice and distension of stomach walls back to normal (pre-eating status)

FIGURE 11.10   Phases of gastric secretion. Source: Peate and Evans (2020)/John Wiley & Sons.

The Cephalic Phase

The cephalic phase begins before the ingestion of food. The sight and smell of food stimulates the autonomic nervous system and the secretion of gastric juices.

The Gastric Phase

The gastric phase occurs when food reaches the stomach. The hormone gastrin is secreted into the bloodstream and this stimulates the secretion of gastric juices. Gastrin circulates in the blood that supplies the stomach, stimulates more gastric juices to be produced from the gastric glands. The pH of the stomach contents is reduced by the secretion of hydrochloric acid. The secretion of gastrin in the pylorus is inhibited when the pH drops to below 2.

The Intestinal Phase

The acidic partially digested contents of the stomach enter the small intestine, where the hormones secretin and cholecystokinin (CCK) are secreted. These hormones are produced by endocrine cells in the intestinal mucosa. They act to reduce the secretion of gastric juice and gastric motility (Table 11.1). CCK prevents overdistension of the duodenum and allows greater time for gastric digestion. The rate of gastric emptying depends on the size and type of meal; it can take between two and six hours after ingestion for food to leave the stomach.

Adaptations in Pregnancy

Around two-thirds of pregnant women will suffer with acid reflux and indigestion. This is thought to be caused by the relaxation of the tone of the lower oesophageal sphincter. This relaxation causes acid reflux from the stomach into the oesophagus. In addition, the growing uterus compresses and upwardly displaces the stomach, which causes the capacity of the stomach to be reduced.

TABLE 11.1   Summary of the role of the digestive hormones.

Hormone	Origin	Target	Action	Stimulus
Gastrin	Stomach	Stomach	Increases gastric gland secretion of hydrochloric acid; gastric emptying	Presence of protein in the stomach
Secretin	Duodenum	Stomach	Inhibits gastric gland secretion; inhibits gastric motility	Acidic and fatty chyme in the duodenum
		Pancreas	Increases pancreatic juice secretion; promotes cholecystokinin action	
		Liver	Increases bile secretion	
Cholecystokinin	Duodenum	Pancreas	Increases pancreatic juice secretion	Chyme in the duodenum
	Gallbladder	Stimulates contraction		
	Hepatopancreatic sphincter	Relaxes – entry to duodenum open		

Source: McErlean (2017) p. 281/John Wiley & Sons.

The Small Intestine

The small intestine is continuous with the stomach from the pyloric sphincter and is approximately 6 m in length. The lumen of the small intestine is approximately 2.5 cm in diameter. It is situated in the abdominal cavity and opens into the large intestine (Figure 11.11).

There are four layers to the small intestine; however, the mucosa and submucosa layers are modified to facilitate digestion and absorption. The surface area of the mucosal layer is increased by circular folds called plicae circulars, with further folding of the epithelial cells that produce villi and hair-like projections known as microvilli. Microvilli form what is known as a brush border (Figure 11.12).

There are four types of cell types within the mucosa of the small intestine:

- Absorptive cells absorb nutrients.
- Goblet cells are found throughout the epithelial cells; they secrete mucus. As chyme is acidic, the mucus helps to protect the intestine from damage.
- Enteroendocrine cells secrete the hormones secretin and CCK. These hormones are secreted into the bloodstream and act on their target organs to release pancreatic juice and bile.
- Paneth cells secrete lysozyme. This helps to protect the small intestine from pathogens. Lymphatic tissue within the small intestine (Peyer's patches) also protect the small intestine.

The small intestine is supplied by a network of blood vessels. A network of capillaries and lymph vessels are present in each of the villi. The arterial blood supply is received via the superior mesenteric artery and the superior mesenteric vein drains away nutrient rich blood towards the hepatic portal vein.

The functions of the small intestine are:

231

- The completion of chemical digestion of carbohydrates proteins and fats.
- The absorption of nutrients.
- Mechanical digestion by the process of segmentation and peristalsis.
- The continued onward movement of the contents of the small intestine by the action of peristalsis.
- The secretion of intestinal juices and pancreatic juices from the pancreas increasing the pH of chyme, which facilitates the action of the enzymes.
- Secretion of secretin and CCK.

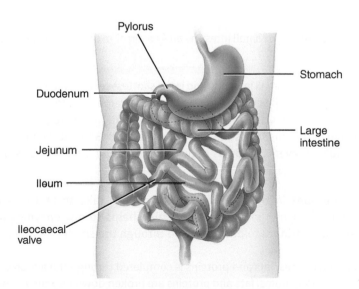

FIGURE 11.11   The small intestine. Source: Peate and Evans (2020)/John Wiley & Sons.

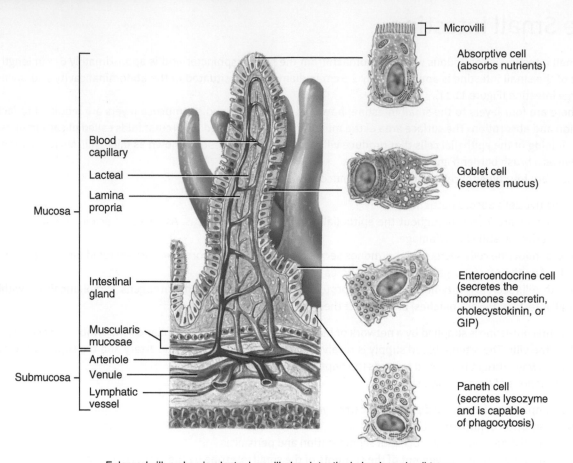

Enlarged villus showing lacteal, capillaries, intestinal glands and cell types

FIGURE 11.12   The cells within the villi of the small intestine. Source: Peate and Evans (2020)/John Wiley & Sons.

The digestion of food is completed in the small intestine and absorption of most nutrients takes place here. The small intestine is divided into three parts:

- The duodenum is the entrance to the small intestine and is the shortest section, measuring around 25 cm. The common bile duct and the pancreas open into the duodenum. The duodenum empties into the jejunum.
- The jejunum is the mid section of the small intestine and measures approximately 2.5 m; it empties into the ileum.
- The ileum is the last section of the small intestine and measures about 3.5 m. It is joined to the large intestine at the ileocecal sphincter. This valve prevents products of digestion from the large intestine backflowing into the small intestine.

Mechanical digestion continues in the small intestine and can take three to six hours to pass through. Segmentation (the movement of chyme) in the small intestine helps to mix enzymes with the contents of the chyme. The action of peristalsis continues to push the food through the small intestine. It also aids the mixing of chyme and enzymes.

Chemical digestion of carbohydrates, fats and proteins is completed through the action of the intestinal secretions, bile and pancreatic juices. The carbohydrates, fats and proteins are broken down into their smallest components: monosaccharides, fatty acids and glycerol and amino acids.

The Large Intestine

The large intestine is continuous from the small intestine from the ileocaecal valve to the rectum and anal canal. it is approximately 1.5 m in length. The lumen of the large intestine is approximately 6.5–7 cm in diameter (Figure 11.13). The functions of the large intestine are:

- Absorption of water by osmosis until semi-solid faeces are formed.
- The heavy colonisation of bacteria synthesises vitamin K and folic acid.
- Bacterial fermentation of unabsorbed nutrients, particularly carbohydrates, produces hydrogen carbon dioxide and methane. These gases are eliminated from the bowel in the form of flatus (wind).
- Further breakdown of bile pigment bilirubin to urobilinogen.
- Mass movement occurs through the action of peristalsis as a result of food entering the stomach.
- The process of defecation occurs by an involuntary reflex.

The large intestine is divided into the caecum, the colon, the rectum and the anal canal. The large intestine is contained within the abdominal cavity.

The caecum is the first part of the large intestine and is separated from the ileum by the ileocaecal sphincter. The vermiform appendix (more often known simply as the appendix) is a fine, narrow tube-like structure that is closed at the distal end and leads from the inferior aspect of the caecum. It is approximately 8–9 cm in length and has the same structure as the rest of the GI tract but it contains more lymphoid tissue. The appendix plays no part in digestion, but it can become problematic if it becomes inflamed.

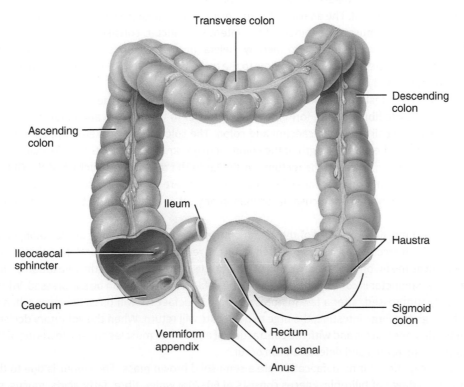

FIGURE 11.13 The large intestine. Source: Peate and Evans (2020)/John Wiley & Sons.

Red Flag Alert: Gut Microbiome

The gut microbiome consists of trillions of bacteria residing in the intestinal tract. It plays an important role in immunity, metabolism and overall health. Pregnancy is associated with a number of inflammatory, hormonal and immune changes that alter the bacterial composition and functioning of the gut. There are anti-inflammatory properties within the placental bed, which protect from rejection of the fetus. As the pregnancy advances, however, the mucosal surface of the gut and other tissues will experience a low-grade inflammation as cytokines and white blood cells increase. When conditions such as obesity and gestational diabetes are present, this causes an imbalance in the gut microbiome, which can further increase inflammation and influence obstetric outcomes, such as preterm birth, fetal growth restriction and pre-eclampsia, as well as longer-term issues for mother and baby. The impact of nutrition on health cannot be underestimated and women should be advised preconceptually and throughout pregnancy of the importance of a healthy diet, which consists predominantly of fresh whole foods and a reduction/elimination of processed foods containing high levels of trans fat, sugar and salt. This will increase the diversity of the gut microbiome, leading to improved functioning, reduced inflammation and more efficient immunological responses.

The colon has four parts:

- The ascending colon is on the right side of the abdomen and passes upwards from the caecum to just beneath the level of the liver, where it curves to the left to become the transverse colon.
- The transverse colon extends across the abdominal cavity and passes the base of the spleen and in front of the duodenum to the left side of the abdomen, where it bends downwards to form the descending colon.
- The descending colon is on the left side of the abdomen and then curves towards the midline until it enters the pelvis, where it is then known as the sigmoid colon.
- The sigmoid colon is S-shaped and continues downwards to join the rectum.

The rectum is the final part of the digestive tract and is approximately 13 cm in length. It leads directly from the sigmoid colon and leads to the anal canal. The anal canal is approximately 4 cm long and leads from the rectum to the exterior of the body. It contains two muscular sphincters: the internal sphincter, consisting of smooth muscle and under involuntary control, and the external sphincter, formed by skeletal muscle, which is under voluntary control. Both the rectum and the anus are constructed of similar structures to the rest of the GI tract. The sphincters are responsible for the elimination of faeces from the body.

The structure of the large intestine is similar to the rest of the GI tract, although the structure of the muscularis layer differs. The longitudinal muscle fibres do not form a continuous layer in the caecum and colon but are thickened into three strips called the taeniae coli along the caecum and colon. The colon has a puckered appearance, as the muscle strips are slightly shorter than the overall length of the colon. Pouches known as haustra are formed in the walls of the large intestine. The longitudinal muscles in the rectum are similar to the rest of the structure of the GI tract and form a complete layer around the rectum and anal canal. The anal sphincters are formed by a thickened circular muscle layer. There is more lymphoid tissue in the submucosal layer than in any other part of the GI tract and this protects against infection.

The rectum is usually empty but because of the action of mass movement of chyme in the colon, faeces are moved into it. Stretch receptors in the rectal walls are stimulated when the rectum is distended and this initiates the defaecation reflex. Defaecation involves the involuntary contraction of the muscle of the rectum and the relaxation of the internal anal sphincter. As the external sphincter is controlled voluntarily, the defaecation reflex can be suppressed. When the defaecation reflex is voluntarily suppressed, after a few minutes the urge to defaecate will pass; however, when the next mass movement occurs through the large intestine, the urge to defaecate will return. When the voluntary decision to defecate is made, the external sphincter relaxes and with the contraction of abdominal muscles and the lowering of the diaphragm, intra-abdominal pressure increases and defecation can occur.

The faeces that are expelled during defaecation are a semi-solid brown mass. The colour is due to the presence of stercobilin from the breakdown of bilirubin. Faeces consists of 60–70% water, fibre, fatty acids, mucus, shed epithelial cells, dead and live microbes. The mucus from the anal sinuses lubricates the faeces and dietary roughage helps to bulk out the contents of the large intestine and stimulate defaecation. An excess of water in faeces results in diarrhoea.

This usually occurs when food residue has passed through the large intestine too quickly. However, if food spends too long in the large intestine, constipation can occur.

Adaptation to Pregnancy

The increase in the hormone progesterone during pregnancy causes smooth muscle in the body to relax. In the stomach, this decreases motility and prolongs gastric emptying time. In the small and large intestine, the action of progesterone continues to have an effect on the tone of the smooth muscle and continues to prolong transit time. Owing to the prolonged transit time, there is an increase in water absorption in the colon and this can result in constipation. An increase in flatulence may also be experienced. As the fetus grows and the uterus increases in size during pregnancy, there is an increase in intra-abdominal pressure and venous congestion. When combined with the straining in constipation caused by the high levels of progesterone, some women develop haemorrhoids.

Snapshot 11.2   Constipation

Shawna is 34 weeks pregnant and has arrived for her antenatal appointment with her midwife. In conversation with the midwife, Shawna mentions that she is having difficulty opening her bowels and thinks she could be constipated. The midwife asks Shawna about her dietary habits and Shawna gives her a breakdown of an average day's food intake.
Breakfast: cereal with sugar and milk, white bread toast, butter and jam. Cup of coffee with milk and sugar.
Lunch: wholemeal bread sandwich, butter, ham and cheese, packet of crisps, a drink of water and an apple.
Dinner: chicken, new potatoes and green beans.
Snacks: chocolate bar, mid morning cup of coffee with biscuits, a small glass of water in the afternoon with a peach.

- What advice could you give Shawna to help her alleviate her symptoms? Think about her nutritional intake, are there any changes that she could make to her diet?

Reflective Learning Activity

What causes constipation? Think about the related anatomical GI structures and hormones.

Medications Management: Lactulose

Constipation and/or faecal impaction can be experienced by pregnant women. Gut motility and gastric emptying slow down due to action of progesterone on the smooth muscle causes difficulty in passes faeces. Lactulose contains osmotically absorbent substances that are not digested or absorbed by the body but remain in the lumen of the gut. They act by retaining water in the stool therefore maintaining its volume and this stimulates the action of peristalsis. Lactulose softens the stool and makes it easier to pass.

- Route of administration: oral.
- The standard dose is starting dose of 15 ml twice daily. Can be taken with or without food.
- It is a P type drug – a pharmacy-only medication.
- Women should also be encouraged to drink plenty of water, around 1.5–2 l/day – this may vary according to how active a woman is; some consideration should also be given to the environmental temperature. As the temperature increases so should the amount of fluids a woman should consume.
- The most common adverse effects are stomach cramps and flatulence.
- There is no reported teratogenicity to the fetus and it is not contraindicated with breastfeeding.

Accessory Structures

There are three accessory structures associated with the GI tract (Figure 11.14).

The Pancreas

The pancreas is a soft pinkish coloured gland approximately 12–15 cm in length. It consists of a head body and tail. It is situated across the posterior abdominal wall behind the stomach with the head tucked into the curve of the duodenum the body and the tail lying behind the stomach (Figure 11.14). The abdominal aorta and inferior vena cava lie behind the pancreas. The pancreas is supplied by the splenic and mesenteric arteries. The splenic and mesenteric veins provide venous drainage and join other veins to form the portal vein. The pancreas is an exocrine and an endocrine organ.

The exocrine tissue forms the majority of the pancreas and is made up of lobules containing alveoli lined with secretory cells. The exocrine tissues produce pancreatic juice containing enzymes, which further aid the digestion of carbohydrates proteins and fats. Each lobule is drained by a tiny duct, which eventually join together to form the pancreatic duct and the accessory duct. The pancreatic duct joins with the common bile duct before entering the duodenum with the accessory duct entering directly into the duodenum.

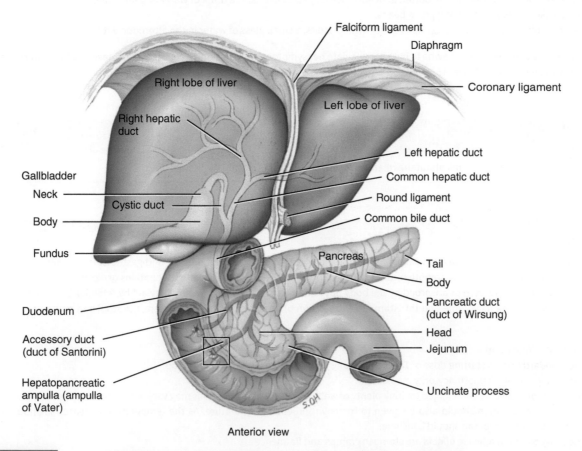

Anterior view

FIGURE 11.14   The liver, gallbladder and pancreas. Source: Peate and Evans (2020)/John Wiley & Sons.

Endocrine tissue is found throughout the tissue in groups of specialised cells called the pancreatic islets (islets of Langerhans). These produce endocrine hormones insulin and glucagon, which control blood glucose levels. Blood glucose levels are maintained by a balance of both insulin and glucagon. Insulin lowers blood glucose levels by stimulating the conversion of glucose to glycogen that can be stored. Glucagon has the opposite effect and stimulates the conversion of glycogen to glucose to raise blood glucose levels.

The Liver

The liver is a large gland in the body and is reddish brown in colour and weighs between 1 and 2 kg. It lies in the upper part of the abdominal cavity under the diaphragm, protected by the ribs. The upper and anterior surfaces of the liver are smooth and curved. The posterior surface is irregular. The liver has four unequal sized lobes. The right and left lobes are separated by a deep fissure and by the falciform ligament. The ligamentum teres, the fibrous remanent of the left umbilical vein, runs alongside the free edge of the falciform ligament (Figure 11.14).

The lobes of the liver are made up of small units known as lobules (Figure 11.15). The lobules are hexagonal in shape and contain hepatocytes. At each corner of the lobule is a portal triad (portal canal). This contains a branch of the hepatic artery, hepatic portal vein and a bile duct. The hepatic artery supplies oxygenated arterial blood to the liver, and the hepatic portal vein carries nutrient-rich deoxygenated blood from the digestive tract. Each hepatocyte

237

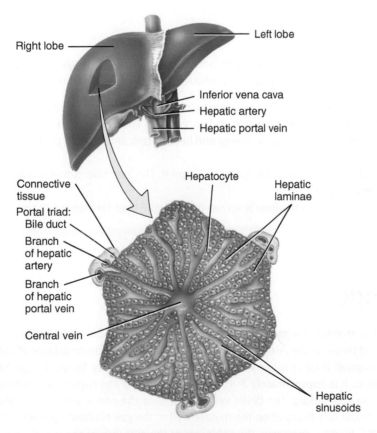

Overview of histological components of liver

FIGURE 11.15 Liver lobule. Source: Peate and Evans (2020)/John Wiley & Sons.

contains a central sinusoid (enlarged capillary) that contains a mixture of venous and arterial blood from tiny branches of the portal vein and hepatic artery. Around the walls of the sinusoids are specialised cells called Kupffer cells, which are hepatic macrophages that ingest and destroy any foreign particles and worn-out blood cells in the blood flowing through the liver. The functions of the hepatocytes are to produce bile, filter and detoxify and process nutrients from the digestive tract.

Bile

Bile is produced by the hepatocytes and flows into channels called bile canaliculi. The canaliculi form larger canals and become the left and right hepatic ducts. This is where bile is drained from the liver. Approximately 1 l of bile is produced daily and is stored in the gall bladder which is situated beneath the liver. Bile is alkaline greenish yellow substance made up of water, bile salts, bile pigments and cholesterol. Bile pigments are derived from haemoglobin from old red blood cells that are excreted through the liver. Bile salts are formed in the liver from cholesterol. Bile salts deodorise faeces, activate enzymes in the duodenum and helps to emulsify fats. It also helps to stimulate the peristaltic action of the intestine. Where bile salts are absent, approximately 25% of fat ingested in food will be eliminated in the faeces. The fats remain in the intestine, coat other foods and restrict digestion and absorption. As a result, fats are found in the faeces and, due to the bacteria and the decomposition of undigested proteins, an excess of hydrogen sulphide is produced and the faecal matter takes on an abnormal rotten egg smell.

Urea

Urea is a substance that is transported in the blood stream from the liver to the kidneys, where it is excreted from the body in the urine. Urea is a product of protein metabolism in the liver. The functions of the liver include:

- Metabolism – blood sugar is regulated by converting glucose to glycogen as a response to insulin. Glycogen is converted back to glucose when glucagon is present and as required. The liver uses fatty acids and glycerol that are the products of the breakdown of fats to provide energy and heat. Excess amino acids are broken down and converted to urea and uric acid.
- Storage – the liver acts as a store for vitamin A, B12, D, E and K. The liver also stores glucose in the form of glycogen, and elements of iron and copper.
- Secretion – bile that is produced by the liver is secreted by the gall bladder into the GI tract and aids the breakdown of fats.

The Gall Bladder

The gall bladder is a small pear-shaped organ that lies to the posterior of the liver. It is a reservoir for bile (Figure 11.14). It contains the same layers of tissue as the rest of the GI tract, but there is an additional layer of oblique muscle fibres and the mucous membrane has small folds or rugae when the gall bladder is empty. When the gall bladder is filled and distended these rugae disappear. It is approximately 3–4 cm long. A branch of the hepatic artery known as the cystic artery provides blood supply to the gallbladder. The cystic vein, which joins the portal vein, drains blood away from the gall bladder. Bile is excreted into the bile ducts when the muscle wall of the gall bladder contracts. This is stimulated by the hormone CCK. When the gall bladder contracts, the sphincter at the entrance of the bile duct relaxes. This sphincter is known as the hepatopancreatic sphincter (sphincter of Oddi).

> ### Take Home Points
>
> - The digestive system carries out six processes from ingestion, propulsion, mastication, digestion, absorption through to elimination.
> - The GI tract is made up of several organs that play a vital role in digestion.
> - There are a number of hormones that play a key role in the digestion process.
> - The action of progesterone on smooth muscle during pregnancy causes several adaptations to the GI tract, which can cause women to experience some common disorders of pregnancy such as delayed gastric emptying time, constipation, acid reflux and changes in appetite.

Summary

The digestive system plays a vital role for life. The GI tract extends from the mouth to the anus and is formed of several organs and enzymes that breakdown food or ingested nutrients, both chemically and mechanically, so it can be absorbed into the cells. During pregnancy, there are number of adaptations that take place due to the hormonal action on smooth muscle and this can cause women to experience a number of common disorders of pregnancy.

References

McErlean, L. (2017). The digestive system. In: *Fundamentals of Applied Pathophysiology: An essential guide for nursing and healthcare students* (ed. I. Peate and Nair), 257–298. Chichester: Wiley.

Nursing and Midwifery Council (2021). *Practising as a midwife in the UK*. London: Nursing and Midwifery Council.

Tortora, G.J. and Derrickson, B. (2017). *Principles of Anatomy and Physiology, Global Edition*. Singapore: Wiley.

Further Reading

Centers for Disease Control and Prevention (2022). Pregnancy and Oral Health. Washington, DC: National Center for Chronic Disease Prevention and Health Promotion. https://www.cdc.gov/oralhealth/publications/features/pregnancy-and-oral-health.html (accessed 1 November 2023).

Davey, L. and Houghton, D. (2021). *The Midwife's Pocket Formulary*, 4e. London: Elsevier.

NHS England (2022). Pregnancy, breastfeeding and fertility while taking cyclizine. https://www.nhs.uk/medicines/cyclizine/pregnancy-breastfeeding-and-fertility-while-taking-cyclizine (accessed 1 November 2023).

Reflective Learning Activity

Conditions Associated with the Gastrointestinal Tract

Below is a list of conditions that are associated with the gastrointestinal tract. Take some time and write notes about each of the conditions. Think about the anatomy and physiology associated these conditions. Remember to include aspects of patient care. If you are making notes about people you have offered care and support to you must ensure that you have adhered to the rules of confidentiality.

The condition	Your notes
Gastro-oesophageal reflux disease	
Haemorrhoids	
Hyperemesis gravidarum	
Constipation	
Obstetric cholestasis	
Gingivitis	

Glossary

Absorption	The uptake of digested food by the intestine into the bloodstream.
Amylase	An enzyme that digests carbohydrate.
Bile	An alkaline greenish-yellow substance made up of water, bile salts, bile pigments and cholesterol. Produced by the liver and required for the digestion of fat.
Bile duct	A small tube that carries bile from the liver.
Bilirubin	A product of the breakdown of haemoglobin excreted in bile.
Canine	A type of tooth.
Carbohydrate	One of the major food groups.
Cardiac sphincter	A circle of muscle at the lower end of the oesophagus – also known as the lower oesophageal sphincter. Prevents reflux of gastric contents into the oesophagus.
Cholecystokinin	A digestive hormone.
Cholesterol	A fat-like material present in the blood and most tissues.
Chyme	A semi-fluid mass of partially digested food mixed with gastric secretions.
Defaecation	The expulsion of faeces through the anus.
Deglutition	Swallowing.
Digestion	The chemical and mechanical breakdown of food.
Duodenum	The first part of the small intestine.
Faeces	The waste material eliminated through the anus.
Fat	A substance in which energy is stored by the body.
Fatty acids	A fundamental constituent of important lipids including triglycerides.
Flatus	Intestinal gas composed of swallowed air and bacterial fermentation from the intestinal contents.
Frenulum	The fold between the lip and the gum.
Fundus	The base of a hollow organ: the furthest part from the opening.
Gastric juices	Liquid secreted by the gastric glands containing hydrochloric acid, pepsinogen, mucin and rennin.
Gastrin	The hormone produced in the mucous membrane of the pyloric region of the stomach.
Gingivitis	Inflammation of the gums.
Glucagon	A a peptide hormone produced by the pancreas; causes an increase in blood sugar level.
Glycogen	The principal form in which carbohydrate is stored in the liver and muscles.
Heartburn	Discomfort or burning pain that is felt behind the breast bone; often caused by regurgitation of the stomach contents into the oesophagus.
Hepatocyte	Liver cell.
Hydrochloric acid	An acid produced by parietal cells in the stomach.
Hypochondriac region	The upper lateral divisions of the abdominopelvic cavity.
Ileocecal valve	The point at which the small and large intestine meet.
Ileum	The end of the small intestine.
Incisor	A type of tooth.
Insulin	A hormone produced in the pancreas and required to regulate blood sugar.
Intrinsic factor	Substance required for the absorption of vitamin B_{12}.

Jejunum	The mid part of the small intestine between the duodenum and ileum.
Kupffer cell	Hepatic macrophage.
Laryngopharynx	The point at which the larynx and pharynx meet.
Lysozyme	Antimicrobial enzyme.
Mastication	Chewing.
Meissner's plexus	Nerves of the small intestine.
Mesenteric plexus	Digestive track innervation.
Microvilli	Cytoplasmic extensions of the villi.
Molar	A type of tooth.
Monosaccharides	A simple sugar.
Mucosa	A layer of the digestive tract.
Nasopharynx	The part of the pharynx that lies above the soft palate.
Oesophagus	The muscular tube for the from laryngopharynx to the stomach.
Oral cavity	The first part of the digestive system.
Oropharynx	Part of the pharynx closest to the oral cavity.
Osmosis	The passage of water across a semipermeable membrane from a weak to a strong solution.
Parasympathetic nerves	Autonomic nervous system nerve fibres.
Pepsin	Enzyme required for the breakdown of protein.
Pepsinogen	The enzyme precursor to pepsin.
Peristalsis	Wavelike contractions that move food through the digestive tract.
Peritoneum	The serous membrane that lines the abdominal cavity.
Peyer's patches	Lymphatic tissue of the small intestine.
Plicae circulars	Folds in the small intestine.
Portal triad	Corner of a liver lobule.
Premolar	A type of tooth.
Protein	A large polypeptide.
Pyloric sphincter	The valve that controls the passage of food from the stomach to the small intestine.
Rectum	The final portion of the large intestine.
Rugae	Folds or ridges found in the digestive tract.
Saliva amylase	Carbohydrate digesting enzyme found in saliva.
Secretin	The hormone that regulates the secretion of pancreatic juice.
Segmentation	The movement of chyme in the small intestine.
Serosa	The outer layer of the digestive tract.
Stercobilin	Product of the breakdown of bilirubin.
Stomach	The reservoir where the digestion of protein begins in the digestive tract.
Sublingual glands	Saliva glands situated in the floor of the mouth.
Submandibular glands	Saliva glands situated below the jaw on both sides.
Submucosa	The connective tissue layer of the digestive tract.
Superior mesenteric artery	The blood vessel that supplies the small intestine with arterial blood.
Taeniae coli	Muscle bands in the large intestine.

Urea	The main breakdown product of protein metabolism.
Uvula	A small piece of tissue that protrudes from the soft palate.
Vermiform appendix	The blind ended tube that is connected to the caecum.
Villi	Tiny finger-like projections found on the surface of the mucosa in the small intestine.

Multiple Choice Questions

1. Which of the following organs do not belong to the digestive system?
   a. Gallbladder
   b. Ureter
   c. Stomach
   d. Salivary glands

2. Which of the following is not an effect of pregnancy on the digestive system?
   a. Constipation
   b. Vomiting
   c. Nosebleeds
   d. Haemorrhoids

3. Which of the following hormones decreases gastric motility?
   a. Oestrogen
   b. Progesterone
   c. Glycogen
   d. Insulin

4. Which of the following substances is not a constituent of saliva?
   a. Water
   b. Salivary amylase
   c. Mucus
   d. Gastric juice

5. Which sphincter prevents the regurgitation of gastric contents into the oesophagus?
   a. Cricopharyngeal sphincter
   b. Cardiac sphincter
   c. Pyloric sphincter
   d. Ileocaecal sphincter

6. Segmentation is the movement of what?
   a. Water
   b. Bile
   c. Chyme
   d. Fats

7. Which of the following is not part of the large intestine?
   a. The caecum
   b. The anus
   c. The vermiform appendix
   d. The duodenum

8. What is gingivitis?
    a. Inflammation of the gums
    b. Excretion of urea
    c. Secretion of bile
    d. Filtration of toxins

9. Which layer of the digestive tract aids peristalsis?
    a. The mucosa
    b. The submucosa
    c. The serosa
    d. The muscle layer

10. Where is the plexus of Auerbach found?
    a. The stomach
    b. The mouth
    c. The rectum
    d. The liver

CHAPTER 12

The Renal System

Ashleigh Ward and Elizabeth Routledge

AIM

The aim of this chapter is to introduce readers to the anatomy and physiology associated with the renal system.

LEARNING OUTCOMES

On completion of this chapter, you will be able to:

- Describe how the macroscopic structure of the urinary system changes during pregnancy.
- Discuss how the microscopic structures of the kidneys change during pregnancy.
- Explain key differences in substances filtered and secreted in the nephron tubules evident during pregnancy.
- Describe how the lower urinary tract changes with advancing pregnancy.

Test Your Prior Knowledge

1. What are the steps involved in producing urine?
2. Describe the common measures of kidney function and how they change during pregnancy.
3. How is the composition of urine affected by pregnancy?
4. List the hormones involved in fluid and electrolyte balance during pregnancy.

Introduction

The kidneys have many functions, including the removal of waste products through the production and excretion of urine and regulation of fluid balance in the body. To enable the kidneys to continue their important role in homeostasis during pregnancy, they undergo extensive change in both anatomy and physiology. This chapter provides an overview of the structure and function of the kidneys and how they change during pregnancy. It also includes some common disorders that can occur during pregnancy together with their related management and treatment.

Fundamentals of Maternal Anatomy and Physiology, First Edition. Edited by Ian Peate and Claire Leader.
© 2024 John Wiley & Sons Ltd. Published 2024 by John Wiley & Sons Ltd.

Renal System

As shown in Figure 12.1, the renal system (or urinary system) consists of:

- Kidneys, which filter blood to produce urine.
- Ureters, which convey urine to the bladder.
- Urinary bladder, a storage organ for urine until it is eliminated.
- Urethra, which conveys urine to the exterior.

Kidneys

External Structures

Most people have two kidneys, one on each side of the spinal column, with the right kidney sitting 1–2 cm lower than the left kidney as this kidney sits below the large right lobe of the liver. The external kidney consists of (Figure 12.2):

- Renal fascia, outermost layer consisting of a thin layer of connective tissue that anchors the kidneys to the abdominal wall and surrounding tissues.
- Adipose layer, the middle layer that cushions the kidneys from trauma.
- Renal capsule, the innermost layer, consisting of smooth connective tissue, which is continuous to the ureters and also protects the kidneys from trauma.
- Hilum, or hilus, where the renal arteries, veins, nerves and ureters enter and leave.

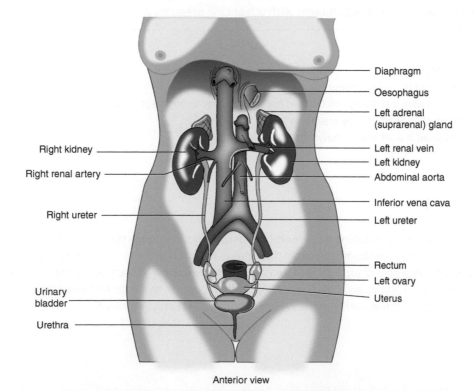

Anterior view

FIGURE 12.1   The renal system. Source: Tortora and Derrickson (2017)/John Wiley & Sons.

Before pregnancy, healthy kidneys are approximately 11 cm long, 5–6 cm wide and 3–4 cm thick. During pregnancy, the overall volume of the kidneys increases by 30%, leading to a 1- to 1.5-cm increase in kidney length. The kidneys are not thought to return their normal size until six months postpartum.

Internal Structures

Inside the kidney, there are three distinct regions or macrostructures (Figure 12.2):

- The renal cortex sits against the renal capsule and tissues from the cortex project between the renal pyramids creating 'renal columns'.
- The renal medulla consists of 8–12 cone-shaped renal pyramids surrounded by renal columns.
- The renal pelvis forms the upper end of the ureter.

The internal structures of the kidneys also consist of nephrons and a complex network of blood vessels, which together with the macrostructures, create a system for the production and excretion of urine and regulation of fluid balance in the body. An increase in size can be expected across all three structures during pregnancy.

Nephrons are microscopic structures located within the renal cortex and renal medulla (Figure 12.3). Nephrons are considered the functional units of the kidneys, as they filter blood, perform selective reabsorption and excrete unwanted waste as urine. This includes regulating the amount of water, salts, glucose, urea and other minerals in the body.

The increased volume of the kidney during pregnancy is a result of increased volume of fluid in the nephrons and not an increase in the number of nephrons. Increases in size are seen in the renal cortex and renal medulla as a result of accommodating the higher volume in nephrons and blood vessels. An increase in size also occurs in the renal pelvis to accommodate increases in volume of urine produced.

247

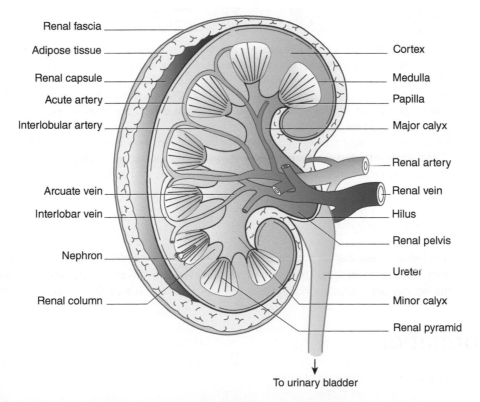

FIGURE 12.2 External layers of the kidney. Source: Tortora and Derrickson (2017)/John Wiley & Sons.

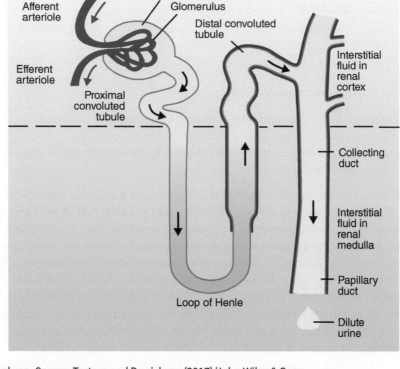

FIGURE 12.3   The nephron. Source: Tortora and Derrickson (2017)/John Wiley & Sons.

Red Flag Alert: Hydronephrosis

Hydronephrosis is the swelling of the kidney due to increased urine volume; it is most visible on ultrasound in the renal pelvis. The renal pelvis and ureters dilate as a result of the increased volume of urine within the kidneys and compression caused by the increasing size of the uterus, possibly also helped by increased level of progesterone.

While studies report varying incidence of hydronephrosis in pregnancy, all conclude that it is common. It has been found to be more common in women experiencing their first pregnancy. Hydronephrosis becomes more common and significant with advancing pregnancy and usually reaches its peak at 28 weeks.

Most women experience no symptoms as a result of hydronephrosis and do not require treatment. Hydronephrosis is thought to be the cause of abdominal pain in the first or second trimester. However, the increased urine volume within the renal pelvis can cause urinary stasis and places women at increased risk (40%) of kidney infection (pyelonephritis).

Blood Supply of the Kidney

The blood supply to the kidney is substantial and enters the kidney through the hilum (Figure 12.4). The rise in cardiac output during pregnancy leads to an increased blood flow and increased demand on the kidneys. Vasodilation occurs in the vessels entering the kidneys and within the kidneys to accommodate the increased fluid present within bloodstream.

Urine Formation

Three processes are involved in the formation of urine:

- Filtration
- Selective reabsorption
- Secretion.

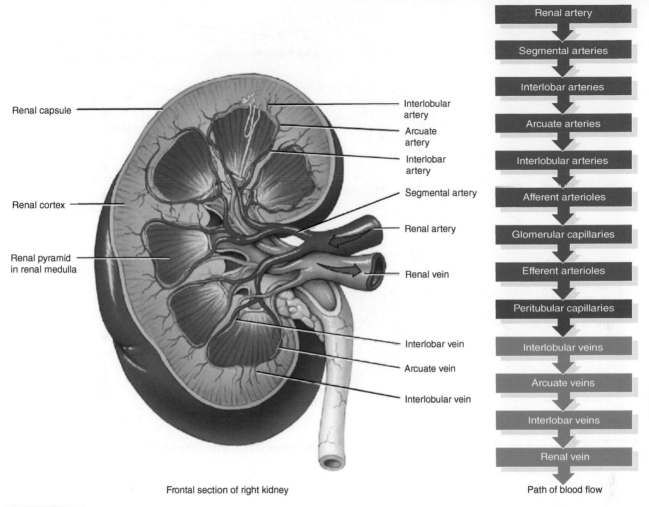

Renal capsule

Renal cortex

Renal pyramid
in renal medulla

Interlobular
artery

Arcuate
artery

Interlobar
artery

Segmental artery

Renal artery

Renal vein

Interlobar vein

Arcuate vein

Interlobular vein

Frontal section of right kidney

Renal artery

Segmental arteries

Interlobar arteries

Arcuate arteries

Interlobular arteries

Afferent arterioles

Glomerular capillaries

Efferent arterioles

Peritubular capillaries

Interlobular veins

Arcuate veins

Interlobar veins

Renal vein

Path of blood flow

FIGURE 12.4   The kidney: internal structures. Source: Tortora and Derrickson (2017)/John Wiley & Sons.

Each of these processes adapts during pregnancy as a result of increased fluid volume and changes in the nutrient requirements of the mother. Figure 12.5 shows the pathway of urine formation.

Filtration

Urine formation begins with the process of filtration, which goes on continually in the renal corpuscles. Filtration takes place in the glomerulus. which lies in the Bowman's capsule. As blood passes through the glomeruli, much of the blood's fluid filters into the Bowman's capsule. This filtrate is called glomerular filtrate. This filtrate contains water, waste products, salt, glucose and other chemicals such as urea, uric acid and creatinine.

During pregnancy, filtration increases significantly. This is known as hyperfiltration. It begins early in the luteal phase of menstruation, increasing further following conception. Hyperfiltration occurs with a considerable increase in the glomerular filtration rate (GFR) and renal plasma flow (RPF) rate and increases alongside systemic and renal vasodilation. This returns to normal one month postpartum (Cheung and Lafayette, 2013).

The increase in filtration can be measured using filtration fraction. Filtration fraction is the GFR divided by the RPF (Box 12.1). While progesterone can lead to an increase in GFR and RPF, it cannot explain the increase in filtration rates seen in pregnancy.

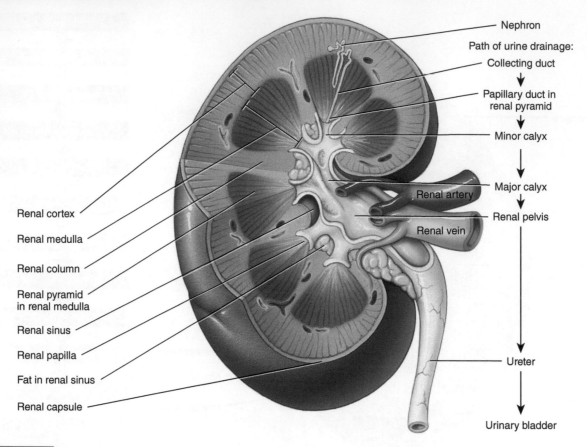

Nephron

Path of urine drainage:

Collecting duct
↓
Papillary duct in
renal pyramid
↓
Minor calyx
↓
Major calyx
↓
Renal pelvis

Renal artery

Renal vein

Renal cortex

Renal medulla

Renal column

Renal pyramid
in renal medulla

Renal sinus

Renal papilla

Fat in renal sinus

Renal capsule

Ureter
↓
Urinary bladder

FIGURE 12.5   The pathway of urine formation. Source: Tortora and Derrickson (2017)/John Wiley & Sons.

BOX 12.1   Calculation of Glomerular Filtration Rate

Glomerular filtration rate (ml/min/1.73 m²):

- If patient is white = $129.85 \times (S_{cr})^{-1.154} \times (age)^{-0.203}$
- If patient is black = $157.38 \times (S_{cr})^{-1.154} \times (age)^{-0.203}$

S_{cr} = serum creatinine level
age = age of the patient in years at time of test

Source: Adapted from NIDDK, 2010.

Glomerular Filtration Rate

GFR is an estimate of the rate that blood is filtered by the glomerulus. It is the most commonly used measure of kidney function. During pregnancy, GFR increases by 50% and this increase begins before increases in blood volume are detected. The increase in GFR occurs progressively over the course of the pregnancy and plateaus when the fetus reaches full term. Studies have yet to give clarity on the cause of increases in GFR, although it is hypothesised that this may be due to increased pressure in the glomerulus (Hussein and Lafayette, 2013). However, GFR calculations are highly sensitive to an individual's biology (Box 12.1). This has also resulted in much debate and several calculations being proposed for measuring GFR. The calculations in Box 12.1 are given for female populations and illustrate the differences in calculations for different ethnic groups.

While GFR is an excellent tool for early indication of renal impairment, its sensitivity to individual biology makes it inaccurate for use during pregnancy, so it should be used with caution as the macroscopic structure of the kidneys changes.

Renal Plasma Flow Rate

The RPF is a measure of the rate that blood enters the kidneys. More specifically, it is a measure of the clearance of para-aminohippuric acid (PAH) from the kidneys. PAH is used to measure RPF as at normal levels. PAH is cleared completely from the blood each time the bloodstream enters the kidneys, or in a single pass. Box 12.2 shows how to calculate the RPF.

It is thought that the increase in RPF may begin as early as the luteal phase of the menstrual cycle. By week 16, flow has increased by 75–80%, which remains constant until week 34, when it declines by 25%. Like GFR, the rise in RPF comes before increases in blood volume.

Selective Reabsorption and Secretion

Selective reabsorption processes ensure that any substances in the filtrate that are essential for body function are reabsorbed into the plasma. Some 99% of the glomerular filtrate is reabsorbed into the bloodstream via three processes:

- Osmosis
- Diffusion
- Active transport.

Substances not removed through filtration are then secreted into the renal tubules mainly by active transport.

Glomerular filtrate moves from the Bowman's capsule to the next part of the nephron, where selective reabsorption occurs:

1. *Proximal convoluted tubule*: sodium pumps are contained in the microvilli within this part of the tubule, and substances such as uric acid and drug metabolites are actively transferred from blood capillaries into the glomerular filtrate. Glomerular filtrate is hypertonic in this part of the nephron.

2. *Descending limb of loop of Henle*: extends from the renal cortex into the renal medulla. The descending loop has high permeability to water and low permeability to ions and urea. Glomerular filtrate becomes hypotonic in this part of the nephron.

251

BOX 12.2   Calculating the Renal Plasma Flow

$RPF = C_{PAH} = U_{PAH} \times V / P_{PAH}$

Where:

RPF = renal plasma flow
PAH = para-aminohippuric acid
C_{PAH} = clearance of PAH (ml/min)
U_{PAH} = urine concentration of PAH (mg/ml)
V = urine flow rate (ml/min)
P_{PAH} = plasma concentration of PAH (mg/ml)

Calculation

You can calculate the RPF or C_{PAH} in two steps:

1. Divide the urine flow rate (V) by the plasma concentration of PAH (PPAH). This will give you V/PPAH.
2. Then take this number (V/PPAH) and multiply this by the urine concentration of PAH (UPAH).

Source: Meltzer (2019).

3. *Ascending limb of loop of Henle*: completing the loop from the renal medulla to the renal cortex, this limb is much thicker. The ascending loop has low permeability to water and high permeability to ions and urea. Glomerular filtrate remains hypotonic in this part of the nephron.

4. *Distal convoluted tubule*: as the final part of the tubule before urine is transferred to the collecting ducts to be removed from the kidneys, this part of the tubule is highly susceptible to hormones. The following actions take place in the distal convoluted tubule:

   a. Active secretion of ions and acids.

   b. Selective reabsorption of water.

   c. Regulates pH of urine through absorption of bicarbonate and secretion of H+.

   d. Walls of tubule contain arginine vasopressin receptor 2 proteins.

   e. Excretes calcium ions when calcitonin is present.

   f. Permeable to water when antidiuretic hormone (ADH) is present, resulting in concentrated urine.

5. *Collecting duct*: urine leaves the tubule via the collecting ducts, where there is a final opportunity for sodium and water to be reabsorbed. This reabsorption occurs only when ADH is present.

Table 12.1 provide a summary of tubular reabsorption and excretion at each part of the nephron loop.

There are a number of changes in selective reabsorption that occur during pregnancy to ensure that the body has what it needs to remain healthy (Table 12.2).

Uric Acid

Increases in GFR results in increased uric acid excretion, a waste product that is completely excreted by the kidneys. It is thought that decreased tubular reabsorption may also play a role. It is thought that increased uric acid clearance is necessary, given increased uric acid levels created by placenta and fetus. In pregnancy, serum uric acid levels fall gradually until week 24, when a gradual rise to normal levels begins.

Glucose

Glucose reabsorption during pregnancy can be poor, resulting in a small amount of glucose being lost in urine. It is hypothesised that increased GFR overwhelms the capacity of the tubule to effectively reabsorb glucose combined with reduced ability to reabsorb glucose in both the proximal and distal convoluted tubule. Women who had no detectable glucosuria regained normal ability to reabsorb glucose by 12 weeks postpartum. Women with detectable levels of glucosuria continued to have some impairment following pregnancy (Cheung and Lafayette 2013).

Amino Acids and Beta-Microglobulin

Like glucose, reabsorption of amino acids and beta-microglobulin is diminished during pregnancy and small amounts are secreted in urine.

Protein and Albumin

The concentration of protein in urine usually increases by 50% during pregnancy and becomes prominent after week 20. While levels of albumin increase during pregnancy, levels remain within the normal range, which is sometimes attributed to increased GFR. However, this is not widely accepted. While proteinuria is common, it can be a sign of pre-eclampsia so, when detected, clinical guidelines should be followed.

TABLE 12.1 **Tubular reabsorption and excretion.**

Tube	Reabsorption	Excretion
Proximal convoluted tubule	Water (~ 65%)	Hydrogen ions
	Sodium and potassium (65%)	Urea
	Glucose (100%)	Creatinine
	Amino acid (100%)	Ammonium ions
	Chloride (~ 50%)	
	Bicarbonate, calcium, magnesium	
	Urea	
Loop of Henle	Water	Urea
	Sodium and potassium (~ 30%)	
	Chloride (~ 35%)	
	Bicarbonate (~ 20%)	
	Calcium and magnesium	
Distal convoluted tubule	Water (~ 15%)	Potassium, depending on serum values
	Sodium and chloride (~ 5%)	Hydrogen ions, depending on pH of blood
	Calcium	
	Urea (some)	
Collecting duct	Bicarbonate (depending on serum values)	Potassium, depending on serum values
	Urea	Hydrogen ions, depending on pH of blood
	Water (~ 9%)	
	Sodium (~ 4%)	

Source: Adapted from Tortora and Derrickson (2007)/John Wiley & Sons.

Creatinine Clearance

The equation used to estimate GFR was developed to be accurate in non-pregnant populations. As GFR rises during pregnancy, the equation used to calculate GFR becomes inaccurate and measures like creatinine clearance become preferred. Like GFR, there are many ways to measure creatinine clearance and much debate. The urine protein to creatinine ratio may be used to measure kidney function during pregnancy. You may be asked to measure the amount of creatinine excreted in urine over a 24 hour period and compare this with the serum creatinine level.

253

TABLE 12.2   Common laboratory values in pregnancy.

Test	Normal range before pregnancy	Direction of change	Normal range during pregnancy
Glomerular filtration rate	>59 ml/min	Increase	55% increase
Creatinine clearance (ml/min.1.73m²)	90–130	Increase (until 16 weeks, then stable)	120–160
Protein excretion (mg/d)	≤150	Increase (until 20 weeks, then stable)	≤300
Urea (mmol/l)	2.5–7.8	Decrease	2.0–4.5
Creatinine (μmol/l)	40–130	Decrease	25–75
Bicarbonate (mmol/l)	23–29	Decrease	18–22
Potassium (mmol/l)	3.5–5.0	Decrease (until 20 weeks, then stable)	3.5–5.0
Sodium (mmol/l)	135–145	Decrease (by 20 weeks, then stable)	130–140
Uric acid (mmol/l)	0.18–0.35	Decrease (until 27 weeks, then stable)	0.14–0.23
		Decrease at 40 weeks	0.21–0.38

Source: Adapted from Main and Main (1984) and Nelson-Piercy (2015).

Snapshot 12.1   Proteinuria

Background

Anna presented to midwifery services in the community at 12 weeks of gestation for her booking appointment. She reported three previous pregnancies, with pre-eclampsia in each pregnancy. Her youngest child had an induced delivery at 21 weeks' gestation due to severe pre-eclampsia. She also reported a history of 'kidney problems', which had been diagnosed at a different hospital. She was on no medication.

Observations

Anna had a blood pressure of 142/75 mmHg. A ward test urine was strongly positive for protein. Her blood biochemistry was normal, with a serum creatinine of 64 μmol/l.

Investigations

The community midwife referred Anna to the hospital obstetric team for further assessment. She was started on nifedipine 30 mg once daily to treat her high blood pressure. A discussion with the specialist renal team revealed that she had chronic proteinuria for many years, and that, because of this, it would not be possible to use urinary protein to assess for the development of pre-eclampsia during her pregnancy.

Monitoring

Anna was monitored during her pregnancy by midwifery staff in the day unit, with input from the obstetric team as needed. She had twice weekly blood pressure monitoring, and alternative markers for pre-eclampsia were measured regularly including kidney and liver biochemistry, fetal growth and umbilical artery Doppler.

Composition and Characteristics of Urine

Urine is a sterile and clear fluid of nitrogenous wastes and salts. Common characteristics of urine are included in Table 12.3. In healthy pregnancy, the detectable characteristics of urine change very little. The common changes are:

- *Colour*: urine can appear darker most commonly within trimesters 2 and 3. This can be a result of dehydration and non-harmful changes in urine composition. Morning sickness can present challenges in staying hydrated.
- *Smell*: urine can develop a smell during pregnancy. This should only present as a light aroma and is a result of non-harmful changes in urine composition.
- *Human chorionic gonadotrophin (hCG)* levels rise early in pregnancy and urine tests are sensitive to this from less than 20 miu/ml, making this an ideal target for pregnancy tests.
- *Urinary urgency and frequency* normally increase during pregnancy as a result of hormones irritating the bladder, such as hCG. In addition, as the fetus increases in size, the womb begins to press on the bladder, reducing the bladders ability to fill. The woman may find that this pressure causes urinary leakage when abdominal pressures increases, such as when laughing, coughing or sneezing.

TABLE 12.3   Common characteristics of urine.

Characteristic	Normal values Not pregnant	Pregnant
Colour	Amber or light-yellow colour	Can appear darker
Odour	None when fresh	Slight smell
Volume (l/24 h)	Approximately 2	Approximately 2
hCG (miu/ml)	<5	<70
pH	4.5–8.0	4.5–8.0
Specific gravity	1.003–1.032	1.003–1.032
Osmolarity (mOsmol/kg)	40–1350	40–1350
Urobilinogen (mg/100 ml)	0.2–1.0	0.2–1.0
White blood cells (HPF)	0–2	0–2
Leukocyte esterase	None	None
Protein	None or trace	None or trace
Bilirubin (mg/100 ml)	<0.3	<0.3
Ketones	None	None
Nitrites	None	None
Blood	None	None
Glucose	None	Undetectable

Source: Adapted from Nelson-Piercy (2015) and Cheung and Lafayette (2013).

255

Fluid and Electrolyte Balance

The composition of electrolytes differs between intracellular and extracellular fluid (Figure 12.6). Concentrations of electrolytes within the different parts of the body are controlled carefully by the body, often using hormones. Optimum levels of electrolytes are critical in maintaining healthy bodies and optimum levels of electrolytes are shown in Table 12.4. Irregularities in levels of electrolytes within parts of the body often result in disorders and can be caused by disorders and the treatment of disorders.

As a woman's body changes during pregnancy, the level of electrolytes needed within the body also change. As such, close attention should be paid to women with existing disorders or who are taking medication likely to affect or be affected by levels of electrolytes. The main changes in electrolytes during pregnancy are seen in sodium and potassium. During pregnancy, sodium and potassium are both retained by the body through many mechanisms, leading to increases in total body sodium and potassium, contributing to oedema later in pregnancy. However, serum levels of both sodium and potassium decline. The reasons for this are still poorly understood.

Eight hormones play a role in the regulations of fluid and electrolytes during pregnancy:

- Angiotensin II
- Aldosterone
- Oestradiol (during pregnancy only)
- Antidiuretic hormone
- Atrial natriuretic peptide (ANP)
- hCG (during pregnancy only)
- Progesterone (during pregnancy only)
- Relaxin (during pregnancy only).

256

We are still discovering the role of many of these hormones during pregnancy, and in this chapter, we provide a summary of current theories and understandings.

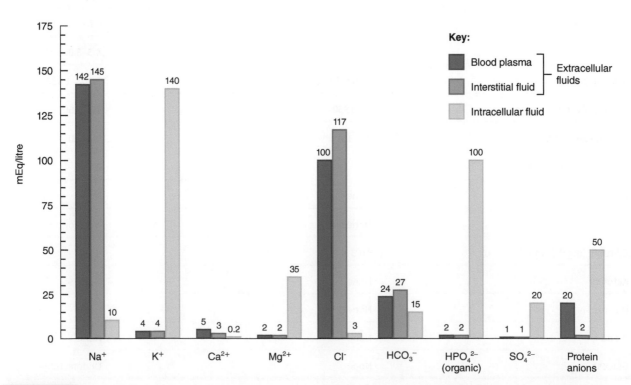

FIGURE 12.6   Electrolytes of intracellular and extracellular compartments. Source: Nair and Peate (2021)/John Wiley & Sons.

TABLE 12.4 Principle electrolytes and their functions.

Electrolytes	Normal values in extracellular fluid (mmol/l)	Function	Main distribution
Sodium (Na$^+$)	135–145	Important role in fluid and electrolyte balance. Increases plasma membrane permeability. Helps to promote skeletal muscle function. Stimulates conduction of nerve impulses. Maintains blood volume	Main cation of extracellular fluid
Potassium (K$^+$)	3.5–5	Important cation in establishing resting membrane potential. Regulates acid–base balance. Maintains intracellular fluid volume. Helps promote skeletal muscle function. Helps to promote the transmission of nerve impulses	Main cation of intracellular fluid
Calcium (Ca^{2+})	2.1–2.6	Important clotting factor. Plays a part in neurotransmitter release in neurons. Maintains muscle tone and excitability of nervous and muscle tissue. Promotes transmission of nerve impulses. Assists in the absorption of vitamin B$_{12}$	Mainly found in the extracellular fluid
Magnesium (Mg^{2+})	0.5–1.0	Helps to maintain normal nerve and muscle function; maintains regular heart rate, regulates blood glucose and blood pressure. Essential for protein synthesis	Mainly distributed in the intracellular fluid
Chloride (Cl$^-$)	98–117	Maintains a balance of anions in different fluid compartments. Combines with hydrogen in gastric mucosal glands to form hydrochloric acid. Helps to maintain fluid balance by regulating osmotic pressure	Main anion of extracellular fluid
Hydrocarbons (HCO$_3$$^-$)	24–31	Main buffer of hydrogen ions in plasma. Maintains a balance between cations and anions of intracellular and extracellular fluids	Mainly distributed in the extracellular fluid
Phosphate – organic (HCO$^{2-}_4$)	0.8–1.1	Essential for the digestion of proteins, carbohydrates and fats and absorption of calcium. Essential for bone formation	Mainly found in intracellular fluid
Sulphate (SO$^{2-}_4$)	0.5	Involved in detoxification of phenols, alcohols and amines	Mainly found in intracellular fluid

Snapshot 12.2   Hyperemesis Gravidarum

Background

Lucy presented to the early pregnancy assessment service. She had been referred by her general practitioner after she had attended the practice with significant vomiting over the previous week. She had a positive pregnancy test. Her gestation was estimated to be eight weeks by dates. She had one previous child, now three years old. She had also had two miscarriages in early pregnancy within the past year.

In the seven days before presentation, Lucy had been keeping down no food and only minimal fluid. She had no abdominal pain and no change in her bowel habits. There was no blood in her vomit. She had lost 6 kg in weight in the last 10 days.

Investigations

A ward urine test was moderately positive for ketones and negative for protein, ketones and nitrates. Her blood biochemistry showed an acute kidney injury (urea 11.4 mmol/l, creatinine 97 μmol/l), which was attributed to dehydration.

Diagnosis and Treatment

A diagnosis of hyperemesis gravidarum was made. She was started on cyclizine to control her vomiting and was admitted to the antenatal ward for intravenous fluids to treat her dehydration and acute kidney injury.

After 24 hours in hospital, Lucy's vomiting had settled and her blood biochemistry had returned to normal. Intravenous fluids were discontinued and she was able to maintain good levels of oral hydration. She was discharged from hospital with oral cyclizine and was encouraged to maintain her own fluid intake.

Reflective Learning Activity

Midwives play a key role in supporting pregnant women to maintain good levels of hydration during pregnancy. How can you support Lucy in this goal? Read Box 12.3 to help you decide.

BOX 12.3   Hydration in Pregnancy

Water constitutes 60% of total body weight in a non-pregnant woman and is needed to perform a range of functions including control of body temperature, lubrication of cells and transportation of nutrients. Dehydration can have severe effects on a woman's health including:

- Low blood pressure
- Problem with clotting of blood
- Kidney dysfunction leading to renal failure
- Severe constipation
- Multisystem failure
- Proneness to infection
- Electrolyte imbalance

Fluid Levels

During pregnancy, fluid levels within the women's body begin to increase prior to six weeks of gestation, leading to the increases in GFR that we detect. This water retention is important in supporting development and maintenance of amniotic fluid, and also later in breastfeeding. The increases in GFR which occur as a normal part of pregnancy mean that the threshold for detecting renal failure is considerably lower in pregnancy; a serum creatinine level of >77 μmol/l is considered abnormal in women who did not have renal failure prior to becoming pregnant.

Pregnancy Fluid Levels

During pregnancy, it is thought that an additional 300 ml/day is required, increasing to 700 ml after pregnancy to support women who are breastfeeding. These fluid levels are recommendations only, and a person-centred approach should be taken to support women during pregnancy.

Angiotensin, Aldosterone and Oestradiol

The renin–angiotensin–aldosterone–system (RAAS) is an important homeostatic process that activates in response to decreases in blood pressure, which changes during pregnancy. When blood pressure decreases, renin is secreted into the bloodstream by cells located near the glomerulus called juxtaglomerular cells. During pregnancy, renin is also released by the ovaries and decidua.

A hormone produced by the embryo (dehydroisoandrosterone sulfate or DHAS), is converted to oestradiol by trophoblast tissue, which enables the production of oestrogen. The level of oestradiol in the mother's blood increases steadily from 10 weeks until birth. Oestrogen increases the production of angiotensinogen by the liver.

Renin and angiotensinogen are transported to the lungs by the bloodstream where renin converts angiotensinogen to angiotensin I. Angiotensin 1 is then converted by angiotensin-converting-enzymes (ACE) to angiotensin II. Angiotensin II acts as a vasoconstrictor that acts to increase blood pressure and is present in a pregnant woman's body in much higher levels due to increased renin and angiotensinogen production. However, during the first trimester, vessels lose sensitivity to angiotensin II. This is called pregnancy-induced vascular refractoriness to angiotensin II. This refractoriness enables blood pressure to remain low when blood volume increases and causes low blood pressure during the first and second trimesters. Angiotensin II also promotes the reabsorption of sodium, chloride and water in the proximal convoluted tubule.

Angiotensin II also stimulates the adrenal glands to produce aldosterone, a hormone that stimulates the cells in the collecting ducts to reabsorb sodium and chloride and secrete potassium. Aldosterone levels rise at week 8 and increase steadily until the third trimester. This results in an increase in fluid volume of 1.1–1.6 l and 30–50% increase in blood volume.

Medications Management: Antihypertensives

The RAAS is a target for a number of common antihypertensive medications that patients may have been taking before they became pregnant. These are medications that are not recommended for use during pregnancy:

- *ACE inhibitors* (e.g. ramipril, captopril, enalapril) taken during the second and third trimesters of pregnancy can cause a number of problems. These include abnormal development of the kidneys, fetal growth restriction, reduced levels of amniotic fluid, and a problem with the neonatal circulation that occurs when the blood vessel between the aorta and the pulmonary artery is prevented from closing. There is no good evidence that ACE inhibitors taken in the first trimester cause harm.
- *Angiotensin II receptor blockers* (e.g. losartan, candesartan) taken during the second and third trimesters can cause abnormal development of the kidneys, fetal growth restriction and reduced levels of amniotic fluid.
- *Spironolactone* is a drug that acts to inhibit the effects of aldosterone. There is some evidence from animal models that spironolactone can reduce testosterone levels in the fetus, which could affect the genital development of male fetuses.

A patient who presents for their booking appointment while on any of these medications should be discussed with an obstetrician, as it is likely that they will need to be changed onto a different medication to manage their blood pressure during pregnancy.

Antidiuretic Hormone and Relaxin

The ADH is produced by the hypothalamus gland and stored by the posterior pituitary gland. ADH is released by the posterior pituitary gland when increased serum osmolality is detected. ADH then travels through the bloodstream to the kidneys resulting in increased permeability of the cells in the distal convoluted tubule and the collecting ducts. Water reabsorption is increased and urine volume is decreased.

It is thought that reduced sodium level in the blood during pregnancy results in vasodilation and ADH release. To enable fluid balance to occur considering changes in volume and sodium concentration in the blood, the threshold for stimulating ADH are reduced in pregnancy.

Further, relaxin is present within the body throughout pregnancy, but in higher levels during the first trimester. Relaxin prepares the lining of the womb for implantation and supports development of the placenta. Then relaxin helps to prevent contractions early in pregnancy and plays a significant role during birth. It is thought that relaxin also plays a role in increasing ADH secretion and thirst.

Atrial Natriuretic Peptide

The ANP is a powerful vasodilator. When blood pressure increases, ANP stimulates the kidneys to excrete sodium and water from the renal tubules, thus decreasing blood volume, and ANP inhibits the release of aldosterone and ADH. During pregnancy, increases in blood volume lead to an increase in ANP and result in increased urine volume and inhibition of sodium reabsorption in the distal convoluted tubule.

Human Chorionic Gonadotrophin and Progesterone

hCG is produced by trophoblast tissue from early embryo development. On conception, level of hCG in the blood double every 24 hours, peaking at approximately week 10 to support the secretion of progesterone while the placenta forms. Levels then decrease until week 16, where they remain constant until birth. Progesterone is secreted by the corpus luteum and then the placenta, steadily rising in the bloodstream until birth.

In pregnancy, progesterone is thought to have a role in hydronephrosis, though the exact role is unclear. It is thought that progesterone has a role in reducing muscle tone, thus enabling easier dilation of the renal pelvis and peristalsis of the ureters.

Ureters

Ureters carry urine from the kidney to the neck of the urinary bladder; they extend anatomically from the renal pelvis. Ureters are approximately 25–30 cm in length and 5 mm in diameter and transport urine by peristalsis. The frequency of the peristaltic waves are determined by the volume of urine and thereby pressure within the renal pelvis, with higher urine volume and pressure leading to more regular waves. These waves encourage urine towards the bladder.

During pregnancy, the kidney increases in size, most notably in the renal pelvis, where urine builds up. Hydronephrosis can occur, leading to widening of the ureters and lack of pressure, which hinders transportation of urine to the bladder. This is often asymptomatic, and not concerning unless the ureter extends beyond 2 cm in diameter or the woman is at increased risk of pyelonephritis.

Hydronephrosis peaks at 28 weeks of gestation and while there is still much speculation about the cause, several key factors are thought to contribute. These factors include progesterone, which may decrease muscle tone and function within the ureters, progressive dilation and increased size of the renal pelvis, and mechanical compression on the ureters.

Mechanical compression on the ureters is thought to be a primary factor in incidence of hydronephrosis. This is evidenced by the higher incidence of hydronephrosis seen in the right ureter, which passes the iliac and ovarian arteries at an acute angle before entering the bladder. Unlike the right ureter, the left ureter has a less strained journey to the bladder as it passes the ovarian vein.

Lower Urinary Tract

The lower urinary tract accepts urine from the ureters and is composed of the urinary bladder and urethra. During pregnancy, women experience significant lower urinary tract symptoms resulting from a number of anatomical and physiological changes to the bladder and urethra, which are evident in Figure 12.7.

Urinary Bladder

Urine moves through the ureters by peristalsis and falls into the bladder. The bladder undergoes several changes during pregnancy:

- The bladder is a hollow muscular organ that is spherical in shape and is easily altered by surrounding organs. As a result, the bladder changes shape significantly during pregnancy. First, the base of the bladder becomes enlarged and more convex in shape as the uterus increases in size. There is some relief from bladder changes during the second trimester as the uterus moves in the abdomen. However, in the third trimester, the bladder becomes severely compressed.

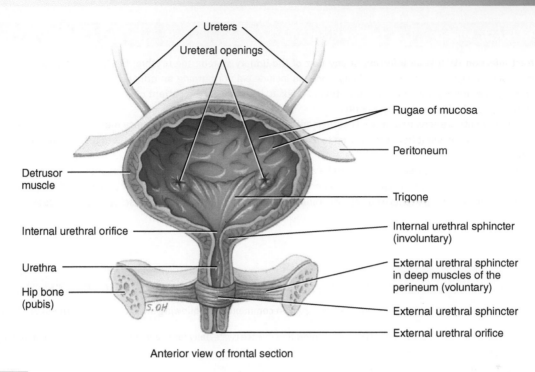

Anterior view of frontal section

FIGURE 12.7 Layers of the urinary bladder. Source: Tortora and Derrickson (2017)/John Wiley & Sons.

- The thick muscular layer of the bladder, the detrusor muscle, relaxes enabling the bladder to distend (stretch) when filling with urine and then contracts when the bladder is full to facilitate urination. In pregnancy, the detrusor muscle hypertrophies and muscle tone reduces, enabling the bladder to fill with more urine.
- While the detrusor muscle hypertrophies, other tissues thicken and surrounding blood vessels enlarge. This results in fluid collecting in the tissues within the walls of the bladder.
- The bladder is located in the pelvic cavity posterior to the symphysis pubis, anterior to the vagina and inferior to the uterus. During pregnancy, the bladder is displaced upwards and becomes more anterior to the midline of the body.

Urethra

The urethra protrudes from the floor of the bladder and is a continuation of the tissues of the bladder. In women, the urethra is a 4-cm tube that carries urine from the bladder out of the body. This is bound to the anterior vaginal wall, with the external urethral orifice is usually located anterior to the vagina and posterior to the clitoris.

Micturition (urination) is controlled by the internal and external urethral sphincter. The internal urethral sphincter is controlled by the nervous system and opens in response to the bladder stretching allowing urine to flow from the bladder into the urethra. Women can then voluntarily open their external urinary sphincter when they are ready for urine to leave the body.

In pregnancy, many women experience stress incontinence, where they urinate involuntarily when they laugh or sneeze. There are two changes to the urethra and urethral sphincters during pregnancy that cause this:

- The internal urinary sphincter is an extension of the detrusor muscle in the bladder. As it hypertrophies and loses muscle tone, this sphincter becomes less powerful weakening the internal urinary sphincter.
- During the third trimester, growth of the uterus pushes the urethra downwards. Instead of sitting against the pelvis, the urethra distends downwards past the urethra and moves more freely. This leads to poorer control over the internal and external sphincters.

Red Flag Alert: Urinary Tract Infection

A urinary tract infection (UTI) is an infection of any part of the urinary system: the urethra, bladder, ureters and/or kidneys. The symptoms of an infection in the lower urinary tract can include pain or burning on urination, pain in the lower abdomen, urinary frequency and urinary urgency. If the infection ascends to the kidneys, the patient may develop flank pain and pyrexia or may become septic. This is called pyelonephritis.

All pregnant patients are screened for a UTI at their antenatal visits. A UTI during pregnancy must always be treated, even if asymptomatic. This is to prevent it from progressing to a more serious infection, which could result in preterm labour, premature delivery or fetal loss.

A patient with an uncomplicated lower UTI can be safely managed in the community with oral antibiotics. Any patient with features concerning for sepsis (e.g. tachycardia or hypotension) or pyelonephritis (e.g. flank pain or pyrexia) and any patient who is at risk of a complicated UTI (e.g. patients who are catheterised or have pre-existing kidney disease) should be assessed in hospital.

Medications Management: Lower Urinary Tract Infection

The National Institute of Health and Care Excellence (NICE 2023) recommends the following antibiotics for treatment of a lower UTI:

- Nitrofurantoin (first line in symptomatic UTI): 100 mg modified release twice daily for seven days, usually avoided near term due to risk of neonatal anaemia.
- Cefalexin 500 mg twice daily for seven days.
- Amoxicillin 500 mg three times daily for seven days, only to be used if culture results are available.

All patients should have their clinical record checked for previous urine culture results, as some patients may have resistance to standard antibiotics. All patients should have a midstream urine sample taken and sent for urine culture and sensitivity. This result should be reviewed when results are available, and if resistance to the initial choice of antibiotic is demonstrated an alternative antibiotic should be offered. All patients who are treated for a UTI should have a further midstream urine sample sent once treatment has been completed, to confirm that the infection has cleared.

Summary

The renal system consists of the kidneys, ureters, urinary bladder and urethra. To enable the renal system to maintain its important role in homeostasis during pregnancy or to make room for the growing fetus, all structures undergo extensive change in both anatomy and physiology. These include:

- Increase in renal size, most evident in the renal pelvis, which enables the kidneys to filter increased blood volume and store greater volume of urine.
- Hydronephrosis is common the right ureter as a result of increased volume of urine stored within the renal pelvis and increased mechanical pressure on the right ureter.
- The detrusor muscle of the urinary bladder hypertrophies facilitating storage of greater volumes of urine.
- In the third trimester, the growing fetus forces the urethra below the pelvis, increasing likelihood of stress incontinence.

Blood is filtered and balanced by the kidneys through filtration, selective reabsorption and secretion. In pregnancy, urine filtration and flow is thought to be controlled by eight hormones: angiotensin II, aldosterone, and estradiol, ADH, and relaxin, ANP, hCG and progesterone. Micturition is then controlled by nervous system, though a combination of autonomic and voluntary control.

Take Home Points

- There are multiple changes to the structure and physiological function of the kidneys during pregnancy. These are driven by the effects of pregnancy hormones and, in later pregnancy, by mechanical compression from the gravid uterus.
- The changes that occur in the kidneys during pregnancy can affect fluid balance, electrolyte balance, blood pressure and susceptibility to infection.
- There is an increase in GFR during pregnancy and the equation used to calculate it becomes inaccurate. The estimated GFR, which is reported on laboratory tests as standard, is therefore not reliable and measures such as serum creatinine or creatinine clearance are preferred.
- A number of medications that are commonly used to control blood pressure and work via their actions on the kidneys are not recommended for continued use during pregnancy.
- UTIs are common in pregnant woman and must always be treated, even if asymptomatic.

References

Cheung, K.L. and Lafayette, R.A. (2013). Renal physiology of pregnancy. *Advanced Chronic Kidney Disease* 20 (3): 209–214.

Hussein, W. and Lafayette, R.A. (2013). Renal function in normal and disordered pregnancy. *Current Opinions in Nephrology Hypertension* 23 (1): 46–53.

Main, D.M. and Main, E.K. (1984). *Obstetrics and Gynaecology: A Pocket Reference*. Chicago, IL: Year Book Medical Publishers.

Meltzer, J.S. (2019). Fluid, electrolyte, and hematologic homeostasis. In: *Pharmacology and Physiology for Anasthesia*, 2e (ed. H.C. Hemmings and E.D. Egar). Philadelphia, PA: Elsevier.

Nair, M. and Peate, I. (2021). *Fundamentals of Applied Pathophysiology: An Essential Guide for Nursing Students*, 4e. Oxford: Wiley-Blackwell.

National Institute for Diabetes and Digestive and Kidney Diseases (2010). *Estimating Glomerular Filtration Rate*. Washinton, DC: National Institutes of Health https://www.niddk.nih.gov/health-information/professionals/clinical-tools-patient-management/kidney-disease/laboratory-evaluation/glomerular-filtration-rate/estimating.

National Institute of Health and Care Excellence (2023). Clinical knowledge summary: Urinary tract infection (lower) – women. https://cks.nice.org.uk/topics/urinary-tract-infection-lower-women (accessed 29 June 2023)

Nelson-Piercy, C. (2015). *Handbook of Obstetric Medicine*, 5e. Boca Raton, FL: CRC Press.

Odutayo, A. and Hladunewich, M. (2012). Obstetric nephorlogy: renal hemodynamic and metabolic physiology in Normal pregnancy. *Clinical Journal of American Society of Nephrology* 7 (12): 2073–2080.

Peate, I. and Nair, M. (2016). *Fundamentals of Anatomy and Physiology for Healthcare Professionals*, 2e. Oxford: Wiley-Blackwell.

Tortora, G.J. and Derrickson, B. (2017). *Principles of Anatomy and Physiology*, 15e. Hoboken, NJ: Wiley.

Further Reading

Gao, M., Vilayur, E., Ferreira, D. et al. (2021). Estimating the glomerular filtration rate in pregnancy: the evaluation of the Nanra and CKD-EPI serum creatinine-based equations. *Obstetric Medicine* 14 (1): 31–34.

Peate, I. and Evans, S. (2020). *Fundamentals of Anatomy and Physiology for Healthcare Professionals*, 3e. Oxford: Wiley-Blackwell.

Waugh, A. and Grant, A. (2014). *Ross and Wilson Anatomy and Physiology in Health and Illness*, 12e. Edinburgh: Churchill Livingstone.

Willacy, H. and Tidy, C. (2022). *Physiological Changes in Pregnancy*. Patient UK.

Glossary

Anterior	Front.
Excretion	Elimination of waste products of metabolism.
Filtration	Passive transport system.
Glomerulus	Network of capillaries found in the Bowman's capsule.
Hydronephrosis	Swelling of the renal pelvis and ureter that accommodates increased urine volume.
Hyperfiltration	Increased rate of filtration.
Kidneys	Organs situated in the posterior wall of the abdominal cavity.
Micturition	Urination.
Nephron	Functional unit of the kidneys.
Posterior	Behind.
Renal artery	Blood vessel that takes blood to the kidney.
Renal cortex	Outermost part of the kidney.
Renal medulla	Middle layer of the kidney.
Renal pelvis	Funnel-shaped section of the kidney.
Renal pyramids	Cone-shaped section of the kidney.
Renal vein	Blood vessel that returns filtered blood into the circulation.
Sphincter	Ring-like muscle fibre that can constrict.
Ureter	Membranous tube that drains urine from the kidneys to the bladder.
Urethra	Muscular tube that drains urine from the bladder.

Multiple Choice Questions

1. Which of the following is not a primary function of the organ?
   a. Kidneys filter urine
   b. Ureters transport urine to the bladder
   c. Urinary bladder stores urine
   d. Urethra excretes urine

2. Which of these statements is true about the kidneys?
   a. Increase in size by 30% or 4–5 cm during pregnancy
   b. Take three months to return to their normal size
   c. Increase in size by 30% or 1–1.5 cm during pregnancy
   d. Take 12 months to return to their normal size

3. What is the cause of increased kidney volume?
   a. Increased fluid volume only
   b. Increased number of nephrons only
   c. Increased fluid volume and number of nephrons
   d. Increased fluid volume in the renal pelvis only

4. Urine is formed through which process?
   a. Secretion → selective reabsorption → filtration
   b. Selective absorption → secretion → filtration
   c. Secretion → selective absorption → selective reabsorption
   d. Filtration → selective reabsorption → secretion

5. How do uric acid levels change during pregnancy?
   a. Decreases in GFR result in increased uric acid excretion
   b. Increased GFR results in decreased uric acid excretion
   c. Uric acid as a result of the growing placenta and fetus
   d. Serum and urinary uric acid levels rise

6. How do glucose levels change during pregnancy?
   a. Glucose reabsorption increases during pregnancy
   b. Small amounts of glucose can be lost in the urine
   c. Glucose does not leave the bloodstream and enter the filtrate
   d. An undetectable level of glucose is the same as no glucose

7. How do protein levels change during pregnancy?
   a. Protein levels stay constant during pregnancy
   b. Protein levels increase in the first trimester and then plateau
   c. Protein in the urine is always a sign of pre-eclampsia
   d. Concentration of protein in urine can increase by 50%

8. What composite of urine commonly changes during pregnancy?
   a. Specific gravity
   b. hCG
   c. Urobilinogen
   d. Ketones

9. Electrolyte changes commonly seen in pregnancy include increases in what?
   a. Sodium and potassium storage levels
   b. Sodium and potassium serum levels
   c. Sodium serum and storage levels
   d. Potassium serum and storage levels

10. Which of these statements is true about the urinary bladder?
    a. It is largely unaffected by pregnancy
    b. It relaxes to enable increased urine storage
    c. It is displaced upwards
    d. It is compressed in the first trimester, but this lessens with advancing pregnancy

CHAPTER 13

The Respiratory System

Alison Anderson

AIM

This chapter explores the anatomy and physiology of the respiratory system and the adaptations to their function during pregnancy.

LEARNING OUTCOMES

On completion of this chapter, you will be able to:

- Describe the anatomy of the upper and lower respiratory system.
- Identify the functions of each of the structures found in the respiratory system.
- Describe the respiratory changes which occur in pregnancy.
- Explain the processes of internal and external respiration.

Test Your Prior Knowledge

1. Divide the parts of the respiratory system into the conducting portion and the respiratory portion. In pregnancy, what adaptations must these portions of the respiratory system make?
2. Why is nose breathing preferable to mouth breathing?
3. Describe the processes of inspiration and expiration and the associated volume and pressure changes occurring.
4. Describe the adaptations of the alveoli to its function and how gaseous exchange occurs at the alveoli.

Introduction

The respiratory system ensures that the oxygen needed for cellular respiration is taken from the air we breathe into all the cells of the body where cellular respiration takes place.

Fundamentals of Maternal Anatomy and Physiology, First Edition. Edited by Ian Peate and Claire Leader.
© 2024 John Wiley & Sons Ltd. Published 2024 by John Wiley & Sons Ltd.

Overview of the Respiratory System

The respiratory system provides the exchange of gases needed for cellular respiration (Figure 13.1). Air is inhaled from the atmosphere into the lungs, and oxygen is then transported via the cardiovascular system to the tissues. Carbon dioxide, metabolic waste from respiration, is returned to the lungs and excreted in the air expired. The demand for oxygen and removal of carbon dioxide is greater during pregnancy, labour and the postnatal period due to increased workload. A healthy respiratory system is able to cope with these demands (Wylie 2005).

Structurally, the respiratory system consists of two parts: the *upper respiratory system* (the nose, pharynx, larynx and associated structures) and the *lower respiratory system* (the trachea, bronchi and lungs).

Functionally, the respiratory system can also be separated into two parts: the *conducting* part (consisting of a series of interconnecting cavities and tubes, outside and within the lungs, which filter, warm and moisten air, conducting it into the lungs) and the *respiratory* part (consisting of tissues within the lungs where gas exchange occurs; Tortora and Grabowski 2000).

The Upper Respiratory Tract

The Nose

Air enters the airway through the nose or mouth. The nose is made up of bone and cartilage and houses a large irregular shaped cavity (Figure 13.2). The nasal cavity is divided into two by the nasal septum, with two anterior openings called the nostrils or nares. The septum is made up of part of the ethmoid bone posteriorly and hyaline cartilage anteriorly. Ciliated

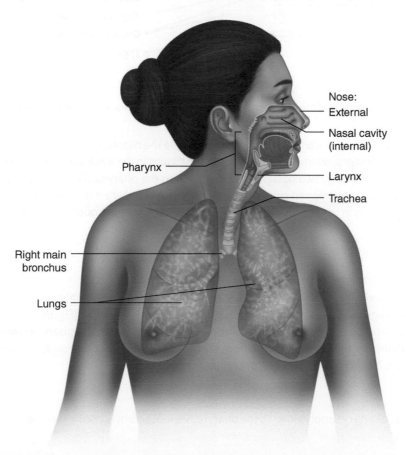

FIGURE 13.1 The respiratory system. Source: Tortora and Derrickson (2021)/John Wiley & Sons.

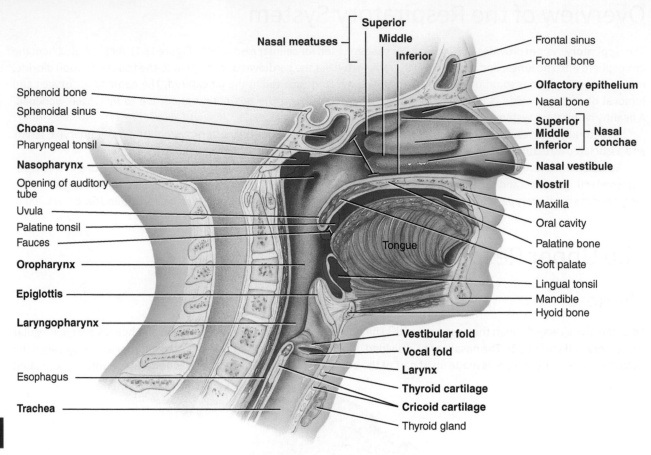

FIGURE 13.2   The anatomical structure of the upper respiratory tract. Source: Tortora and Derrickson (2021)/John Wiley & Sons.

columnar epithelial cells, containing mucus-secreting goblet cells, line the nasal cavity. Air entering via the nasal cavity is filtered by hairs in the nasal passages, warmed by contact with the tissues in the nasal cavity and moistened by cells in the mucous membrane of the nasal cavity. Two posterior nares open into the pharynx. The ciliated cells in the nasal cavity provide a gentle current, moving any trapped mucus towards the pharynx, where it is swallowed, passed to the stomach and digested. Olfactory receptors in the superior mucosa of the nasal cavity detect odours as part of the sense of smell.

The Pharynx

The pharynx is a funnel-shaped tube, beginning at the posterior opening of the two nasal passageways and ending at the larynx, is made up of three regions: the nasopharynx, oropharynx and laryngopharynx (Figure 13.2). Water and food pass through the pharynx in addition to air. As well as transporting air, food and water, the pharynx warms and moistens air further, protects the tympanic membrane or eardrum from changes in atmospheric pressure, acts as a resonance chamber for sound and produces antibodies for infection prevention.

Blood Supply
Several branches of the facial artery supply blood to the pharynx. Venous return is via the facial and internal jugular veins.

Nerve Supply
The pharyngeal plexus contain parasympathetic and sympathetic nerves and supplies the pharynx.

The Nasopharynx

The nasopharynx extends from the nasal cavity to the level of the soft palate of the mouth, and contains the two openings of the auditory or Eustachian tubes that lead to the middle ears. The pharyngeal tonsil or adenoids are also found in the upper region of the nasopharynx. The mucosa of the nasopharynx consists of ciliated columnar epithelium and is continuous with the lining of the nose.

The Oropharynx

The oropharynx extends from the inferior tip of the soft palate to the superior tip of the epiglottis, where the palatine and lingual tonsils are situated. Two folds are formed at the lateral walls on each side of the oropharynx, blending with the soft palate. A collection of lymphoid tissue, called the palatine tonsil, can be found between each pair of folds. The mucosa in the oropharynx changes to tougher stratified squamous epithelium and is continuous with the lining of the mouth and oesophagus. This provides protection from food and other materials passing through during swallowing.

The Laryngopharynx

The laryngopharynx can be found at the inferior aspect of the oropharynx. Air and food pass through the laryngopharynx until the tube divides into two. Anteriorly, the larynx and trachea transport air into the lungs. Posteriorly, the oesophagus transports food and liquid into the stomach. The mucosa in the laryngopharynx also consists of tougher stratified squamous epithelium, continuous with the lining of the mouth and oesophagus.

The Larynx

After the pharynx, the air passes first through the larynx (Figures 13.2 and 13.3), to the trachea, a single tube forming the major airway. Several cartilages are associated with the larynx:

- The *thyroid cartilage*, which consists of hyaline cartilage, is the most prominent cartilage. Its anterior wall projects into the soft tissue of the throat.
- The *cricoid cartilage*, consisting of hyaline cartilage, completely encircles the larynx and lies below the thyroid cartilage.
- Two *arytenoid cartilages*, also made from hyaline cartilage, provide attachment to the vocal cords, thereby affecting the length and tension of the vocal cords.
- The *epiglottis* is made of fibroelastic cartilage, closing off the larynx during swallowing to prevent food or fluids entering the trachea.

    The *vocal cords*, a pair of folds in the mucous membrane, are in the larynx. The vocal cords can vibrate when air passes over them, causing sound waves and allowing speech.

Blood Supply
The superior and inferior laryngeal arteries provide the blood supply of the larynx. Venous return is via the thyroid veins leading to the internal jugular vein.

Nerve Supply
Two branches of the vagus nerve, the superior laryngeal and recurrent laryngeal nerves provide the parasympathetic nerve supply to the larynx. The superior cervical ganglia provide the sympathetic nerve supply.

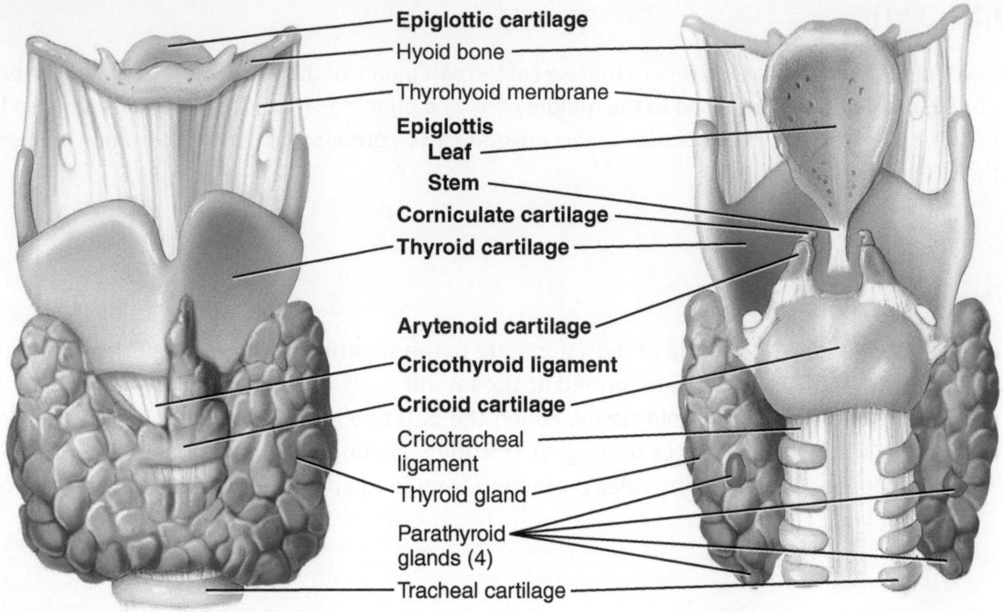

Epiglottic cartilage
Hyoid bone
Thyrohyoid membrane
Epiglottis
    Leaf
    Stem
Corniculate cartilage
Thyroid cartilage

Arytenoid cartilage
Cricothyroid ligament
Cricoid cartilage
Cricotracheal
ligament
Thyroid gland
Parathyroid
glands (4)
Tracheal cartilage

FIGURE 13.3   Anatomy of the larynx. Source: Tortora and Derrickson (2021)/John Wiley & Sons.

The Lower Respiratory Tract

270

After the larynx, air enters the trachea. It then passes through one of two bronchi. The bronchi divide repeatedly into smaller bronchioles before ending in air sacs called alveoli (Figure 13.4):

Trachea → bronchi → bronchioles → terminal bronchioles → respiratory bronchioles → alveoli ducts → alveoli

The Trachea

The trachea lies in front of the oesophagus and is a tube 100–120 mm in length, held open by 16–20 horseshoe-shaped or C-shaped rings of hyaline cartilage (Figure 13.5). The trachea wall has three layers:

- An outer fibrous and elastic tissue layer, enclosing the C-shaped rings of cartilage.
- A middle layer of cartilage, bands of smooth muscle and some areolar tissue, containing blood vessels, lymph vessels and autonomic nerves.
- An inner lining consisting of a mucous membrane containing ciliated epithelium (which beat in a wave-like manner, moving mucus, dust and microorganisms upwards and out of the lungs).

The C-shaped cartilage rings are incomplete on the posterior side, next to the oesophagus. The cartilage rings have two main functions:

- Keeping the trachea patent during pressure changes associated with breathing.
- Allowing for the slight expansion of the oesophagus during swallowing of food or fluid.

Blood Supply

The inferior thyroid and bronchial arteries supply blood to the trachea. Venous return is via the inferior thyroid veins.

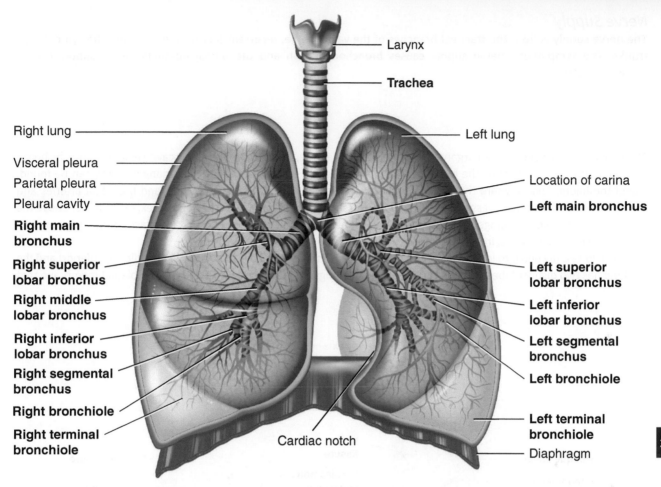

Larynx

Trachea

Right lung

Left lung

Visceral pleura

Parietal pleura

Pleural cavity

Location of carina

Left main bronchus

Right main bronchus

Right superior lobar bronchus

Left superior lobar bronchus

Right middle lobar bronchus

Left inferior lobar bronchus

Right inferior lobar bronchus

Left segmental bronchus

Right segmental bronchus

Left bronchiole

Right bronchiole

Right terminal bronchiole

Cardiac notch

Left terminal bronchiole

Diaphragm

FIGURE 13.4 The anatomical structure of the lower respiratory tract. Source: Tortora and Derrickson (2021)/John Wiley & Sons.

271

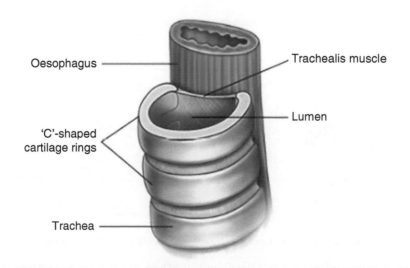

Oesophagus

Trachealis muscle

Lumen

'C'-shaped cartilage rings

Trachea

FIGURE 13.5 The positional relationship of the trachea to the oesophagus. Source: Waugh and Grant (2018)/Elsevier.

Nerve Supply

The nerve supply is from the tracheal branches of the vagus nerve, recurrent laryngeal nerves and the sympathetic trunks. The sympathetic nerve supply causes bronchodilatation and the parasympathetic nerve supply causes bronchoconstriction.

The Lungs

The lungs are large cone-shaped organs with a broad concave base, located in the thoracic cavity (Figure 13.6). The heart, in the mediastinum, separates the two lungs. At the mediastinal surface of the lungs, a triangular area can be found, called the hilum. This is where the bronchus, blood vessels (pulmonary artery and veins, and bronchial arteries and veins), nerves and lymphatic vessels enter the lungs. The superior most part of the lung, the apex, extends just above the clavicles. The base of the lungs is concave and lies just above the diaphragm. The costal surface of the lungs presses against the costal cartilages, intercostal muscles and rib cage.

Each lung is divided into lobes by fissures; the right lung has three distinct lobes (superior, middle and inferior) and the left lung has two distinct lobes (superior and inferior). The lungs are surrounded by a two-layered pleural membrane that

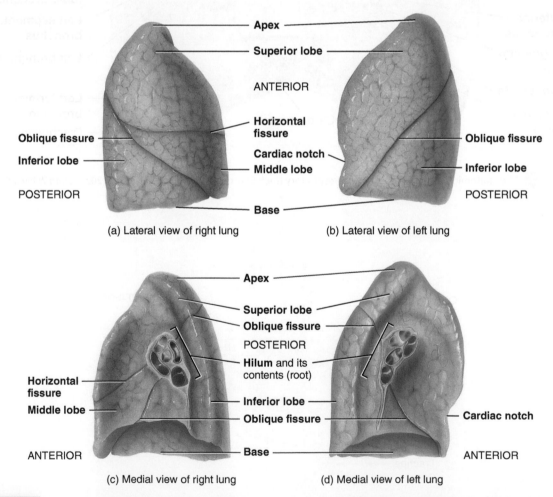

FIGURE 13.6   The external anatomy of the lungs. (a) Lateral view of right lung. (b) Lateral view of left lung. (c) Medical view of right lung. (d) Medical view of left lung. Source: Tortora and Derrickson (2021)/John Wiley & Sons.

secretes pleural fluid from the epithelial cells, which aids the movement of the lungs against the thoracic wall without friction and prevents the pleural layers from separating due to surface tension. The membrane covering the surface of the lungs is the visceral or pulmonary pleura and the part of the membrane covering the thoracic wall and diaphragm is the parietal pleura.

Blood Supply to the Lungs

The lungs function to oxygenate the blood for the other organs and tissues of the body. However, they need their own blood supply. The pulmonary artery delivers deoxygenated blood to the lungs, where it is oxygenated in the pulmonary network of capillaries surrounding the alveoli. The oxygenated blood returns to the left atrium of the heart via the pulmonary veins. The bronchial arteries branch from the aorta and provide the lungs with oxygenated blood for their own cellular respiration. Deoxygenated blood leaves the lungs via the bronchial veins and is deposited in the superior vena cava before entering the right atrium.

The Bronchi

The trachea subdivides into two main branches, the right and left bronchi, which divide repeatedly into smaller and smaller tubes, called bronchi, and then, finally, into bronchioles. The trachea, bronchi and bronchioles contain smooth muscle, which enables them to constrict. The bronchioles lead ultimately to numerous alveoli, where most of the gaseous exchange takes place.

The right bronchus is wider, shorter (approximately 25 mm long) and straighter than the left bronchus (approximately 50 mm long), because of the position of the heart of the left side of the chest. The bronchi enter the lungs at the hilum. The same three layers that exist in the trachea can also be found in the bronchi. The smaller bronchi have smaller cartilage plates, rather than rings, present in their walls, alongside smooth muscle.

Blood Supply

The right and left bronchial arteries supply blood to the walls of the bronchi and bronchioles. Venous return is via the bronchial veins, which lead to the azygous vein on the right side and the superior intercostal vein on the left side.

Nerve Supply

Bronchoconstriction is stimulated by the vagus nerves of the parasympathetic system and bronchodilation is stimulated by the sympathetic nerves.

The Bronchioles

As the bronchi divide into the smaller bronchioles, the rings of cartilage supporting the airways are replaced by smooth muscle. The rings of cartilage reduce in size as the bronchi divide. The lower bronchioles have no cartilage, as it would interfere with the exchange of gases and the expansion of lung tissue. For airflow to be regulated within each lung, the amount of smooth muscle in the bronchioles increases as the cartilage decreases. This smooth muscle increases and decreases the diameter of the airways in response to stimuli, through contraction and relaxation under the control of the autonomic nervous system. The sympathetic nervous system causes bronchodilation, and the parasympathetic nervous system causes bronchoconstriction.

Alveoli

As the bronchi divide, eventually, the smaller passageways are termed terminal bronchioles, then respiratory bronchioles and, finally, alveoli ducts lead to the alveoli or air sacs (Figure 13.7). Alveoli are not part of the conducting region of the respiratory system.

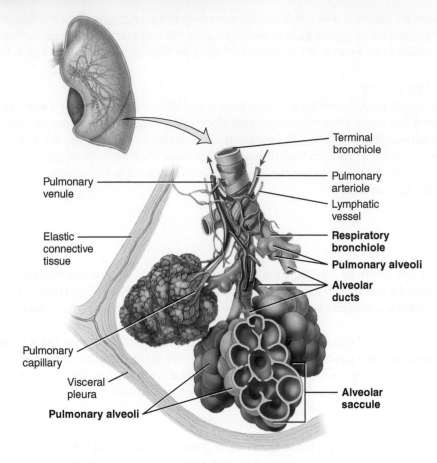

Terminal
bronchiole

Pulmonary
arteriole

Lymphatic
vessel

**Respiratory
bronchiole**

Pulmonary alveoli

**Alveolar
ducts**

**Alveolar
saccule**

Pulmonary
venule

Elastic
connective
tissue

Pulmonary
capillary

Visceral
pleura

Pulmonary alveoli

274

FIGURE 13.7   The structure of a lobule of the lung. Source: Tortora and Derrickson (2021)/John Wiley & Sons.

The lungs form a very efficient gas exchange surface, as they are specially adapted. They provide a large surface area by the presence of an estimated 200–400 million alveoli or air sacs; they have a network of capillaries surrounding each alveolus, and they have a thin exchange surface. There are only two layers of cells, known as the respiratory membrane, between the air in the alveolus and the blood in the capillaries through which oxygen and carbon dioxide diffuse in a process called gaseous exchange (Figure 13.8). These are the alveolar epithelium (squamous epithelial cells) and the cells forming the capillary wall. Alveoli are minute bubble-like air sacs lined with moisture. They are liable to collapse, causing their sides to stick together because of surface tension. Septal cells in the alveolar epithelium secrete surfactant, which greatly reduces the surface tension of the alveoli and keeps them open during expiration, thereby preventing their collapse.

Oxygen and carbon dioxide are exchanged at the respiratory membrane by a process called diffusion, which relies on pressure gradients between the lungs and atmospheric pressure.

The Respiratory Muscles

Diaphragm

Forming the floor of the thoracic cavity, separating it from the abdominal cavity, is the strong dome-shaped muscle of the diaphragm. The diaphragm muscle fibres radiate from a central tendon attaching to the vertebral column, sternum and lower ribs. Contraction of this muscle causes the diaphragm to move downwards and flatten, lifting the rib cage and enlarging the thoracic cavity, causing a decrease in pressure in the thoracic cavity (Figure 13.9). During contraction, the

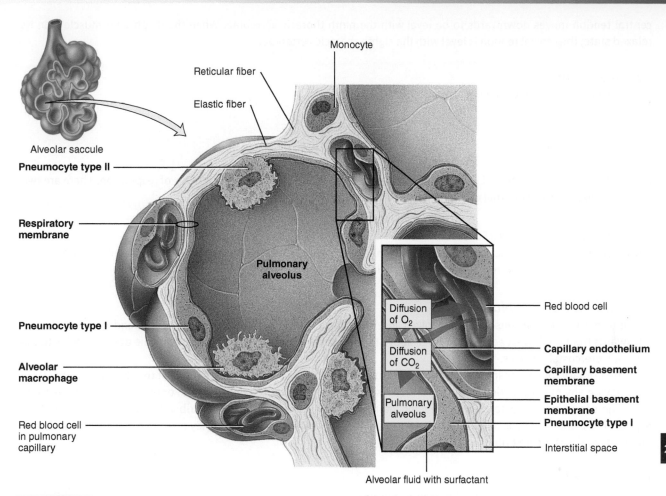

Monocyte

Reticular fiber

Elastic fiber

Alveolar saccule

Pneumocyte type II

Respiratory membrane

Pulmonary alveolus

Pneumocyte type I

Alveolar macrophage

Red blood cell in pulmonary capillary

Diffusion of O_2

Diffusion of CO_2

Pulmonary alveolus

Red blood cell

Capillary endothelium

Capillary basement membrane

Epithelial basement membrane

Pneumocyte type I

Interstitial space

Alveolar fluid with surfactant

FIGURE 13.8 The structure of the alveolus. Source: Tortora and Derrickson (2021)/John Wiley & Sons.

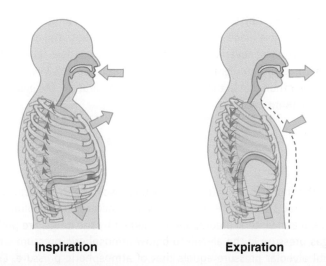

Inspiration

Expiration

FIGURE 13.9 Changes in chest size, intercostal muscles, diaphragm and rib cage positions during inspiration and expiration.

central tendon moves downwards to be level with the ninth thoracic vertebrae. When the diaphragm muscle is in its relaxed state, the central tendon is level with the eighth thoracic vertebrae.

Nerve Supply
The phrenic nerves supply the diaphragm.

Intercostal Muscles

Between the 12 pairs of ribs lie 11 pairs of intercostal muscles, which are accessory muscles of respiration. There are two layers: the external and internal intercostal muscles.

External Intercostal Muscles
The external intercostal muscles are involved in inspiration. They extend downwards and forwards from the lowest edge of the rib above to the uppermost edge of the rib below.

Internal Intercostal Muscles
The internal intercostal muscles are involved in expiration during phases of activity. They extend downwards and backwards from the lowest edge of the ridge above to the uppermost edge of the rib below and lie at right angles to the external intercostal muscles.

    The primary role of the intercostal muscles is to stabilise the ribcage during expansion of the thoracic cavity rather than having any major function in the expansion itself. However, during physical exertion or upper airway obstruction, when there is an increased need for oxygen, the intercostal muscles help to enlarge the ribcage, allowing for further lung expansion. As the first rib is fixed, when the external intercostal muscles contract, they move the ribcage upwards and outwards towards the first rib.

Nerve Supply
The intercostal nerves stimulate the intercostal muscles.

Pulmonary Ventilation (Breathing)

The process of breathing, or pulmonary ventilation, moves air in and out of the lungs. The average adult has a respiratory rate of 12–15 breaths/minute. Breathing is made up of two phases: inspiration and expiration. Inspiration is the movement of air into the lungs and expiration is movement of air out of the lungs. Gases flow from regions of high pressure to regions of low pressure until the pressure gradient is equal, according to Boyle's law. For inspiration to occur, the gas pressure in the alveoli must be lower than that in the atmosphere. For expiration, the gas pressure in the alveoli must be higher than that in the atmosphere (Kent 2000).

Inspiration

Inspiration occurs by enlarging the thoracic cavity (the intercostal muscles contract, drawing the rib cage upwards and outwards, and the diaphragm contracts and moves downwards) and increasing the volume of the lungs. As the ribcage and diaphragm move, the parietal and visceral pleura, and consequently the lungs, are pulled with them, causing lung expansion. This reduces the gas pressure in the alveoli to below atmospheric pressure, creating a pressure gradient, drawing air into the lungs until alveolar pressure equals that of atmospheric pressure. Energy is needed for muscle contraction; inspiration is an active process.

Expiration

During expiration, the respiratory muscles relax, reducing the volume of the thoracic cavity and resulting in an elastic recoil of the lungs and an associated temporary rise in alveolar pressure to above atmospheric pressure occurs. This rise in alveolar pressure causes air to be pushed out of the lungs. Expiration is usually a relatively passive process in resting conditions as energy is not usually required (Kent 2000). The lungs contain a small volume of air after expiration and are prevented from collapse by the pleura.

Factors Affecting Ventilation

Three factors can affect ventilation:

1. *Compliance* or stretchability of the lung tissue and chest wall. In a healthy lung, there should be very little effort needed to inflate the alveoli. In a lung with insufficient surfactant or where the elastic fibres of the lung are damaged, compliance is low and more effort is needed to inflate the lungs.

2. *Elasticity* is in opposition to the compliance of the lungs. Lung elasticity is its ability to return to its resting position and shape after inspiration. Conditions like emphysema can cause a reduction in elasticity.

3. *Airway resistance* is relative to the diameter of the smaller airways in the lungs. During bronchodilation, when the airway diameters are larger, airway resistance is reduced and air moves freely through the bronchioles and alveolar ducts. During bronchoconstriction, when the airway diameters are smaller, resistance increases so more effort is needed to inflate the lungs.

Medications Management: Asthma and Aspirin

Low-dose aspirin is used as a prophylaxis in pregnancy for women at high risk of pre-eclampsia, antiphospholipid syndrome or migraine. Consideration should be given to whether a pregnant woman with asthma has any history of aspirin sensitivity or bronchospasm after having taking aspirin. If a woman has such a history, they should avoid taking low-dose aspirin or non-steroidal anti-inflammatory drugs for pain relief in the postnatal period.

- Dose of prophylactic aspirin: 75–150 mg once a day, at night, until 36 weeks of pregnancy or birth as per local guidance (NICE 2019).

Lung Volumes and Capacities

Lung volumes and capacities are shown in Figure 13.10.

- *Tidal volume* (TV) is the volume of air (usually ~ 500 ml) that passes into and out of the lungs during each cycle of breathing.
- *Inspiratory reserve volume* (IRV) is the volume of air (~ 3100 ml) that can be inhaled forcibly beyond the normal tidal volume.
- *Inspiratory capacity* (IC) is the total amount of air that can be inspired with maximum effort.

$$IC = TV + IRV$$

- *Expiratory reserve volume* (ERV) is the volume of air (~ 1200 ml) that can be exhaled forcibly beyond the normal tidal volume.
- Residual volume (RV) is the volume of air (~ 1200 ml) remaining in the lungs even after forcibly expiring. The residual volume helps to prevent the alveoli from deflating, allowing gaseous exchange to continue between breaths.
- *Vital capacity* (VC) is the maximum amount of air that can be exchanged during inspiration and expiration. This equates to approximately 3100 ml in a healthy young woman.

$$VC = TV + IRV + ERV$$

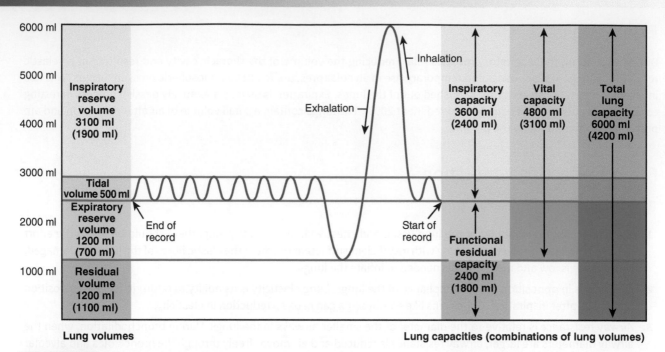

FIGURE 13.10   Lung volumes and capacities. Source: Tortora and Derrickson (2021)/John Wiley & Sons.

- *Total lung capacity* (TLC) is the maximum amount of air the lungs can hold, approximately 6000 ml in an average adult. It cannot be directly measured due to residual volume remaining in the lungs even after forced expiration.

$$TLC = VC + RV$$

- *Alveolar ventilation* is the volume of air that moves in and out of the alveoli per minute. It can be calculated using the following equation:

$$Alveolar\ ventilation = (TV - anatomical\ dead\ space) \times respiratory\ rate$$

$$= (500 - 150) \times 15$$

$$= 5250 ml/min$$

$$= 5.25 l/min$$

A spirometer can be used to measure respiratory capacities as a person breathes. Testing using a spirometer can be useful to determine any respiratory function losses following different respiratory diseases, for example, emphysema or pneumonia.

Reflective Learning Activity

Varicella zoster (chickenpox) pneumonia is a potentially serious condition in pregnancy. It may require admission to hospital and expert advice and treatment. It is important to liaise with the infectious disease consultant at the hospital before planning any care interventions. Approximately 10% of pregnant women with a varicella zoster infection develop pneumonia; severity increases with gestation. There is a 3–14% mortality rate, even with antiviral treatment and optimal intensive care.

- Read the guidance from the UK Health Security Agency (2022a,b) and the Royal College of Obstetricians and Gynaecologists (2015) to write a care plan for a woman presenting with chicken pox.

Gaseous Exchange

Diffusion

Diffusion is the movement of a substance across a semipermeable membrane from an area of high concentration to an area of low concentration to reach equilibrium. Diffusion determines the movement of gases in external and internal respiration. Air is a mixture of gases including oxygen (O_2), nitrogen, carbon dioxide (CO_2) and water vapour. Inspired and expired air contain different percentages of these gases (Table 13.1). The pressure exerted by an individual gas in a mixture is known as its partial pressure (e.g. PO_2 or PCO_2).

Alveolar air is saturated with water vapour and therefore has a reduction in partial pressures of the other gases compared with atmospheric air. It contains decreased oxygen and increased carbon dioxide levels. Gaseous exchange (external respiration) between the alveoli and surrounding blood capillaries is constant.

External Respiration

External respiration is the exchange of gases at the alveolar surface between the alveoli and blood capillaries that surround them (Figure 13.11). Blood arriving at the alveoli in the pulmonary artery from tissue cells of the body have high levels of carbon dioxide (5.8 kPa) and low levels of oxygen (5.3 kPa) compared with alveolar air. Carbon dioxide diffuses down a concentration gradient into the alveoli; oxygen diffuses from the alveoli to the blood in the capillaries. Blood leaving the alveoli has equal carbon dioxide and oxygen concentrations to that of the air in the alveolar space.

Internal Respiration

Internal respiration is the exchange of gases at the level of the cells in the tissues between the systemic capillaries and tissue cells (Figure 13.12). Blood arriving at the cells in the body from the lungs have high levels of oxygen (13.3 kPa) and low levels of carbon dioxide (5.3 kPa). This creates a concentration gradient between the capillaries and tissue cells of the body. Oxygen diffuses down a concentration gradient from the capillaries into the cell; carbon dioxide diffuses from the cells into the blood in the capillaries. Figure 13.13 summarises internal and external respiration processes.

Reflective Learning Activity

The following is a list of different parts of the respiratory system. Research the adaptations that each of these parts has for their function.

- Nose
- Larynx
- Pharynx
- Trachea
- Bronchi
- Bronchioles
- Alveoli
- Capillaries.

Gas	Composition of air (%)		Partial pressure of gases (kPa)		
	Inspired air	Expired air	Alveolar air	Deoxygenated blood	Oxygenated blood
Oxygen	21	16	13.3	5.3	13.3
Carbon dioxide	0.04	4	5.5	5.8	5.3
Nitrogen	78	78	76.4	76.4	76.4
Water vapour	Variable	Variable	6.3	–	–

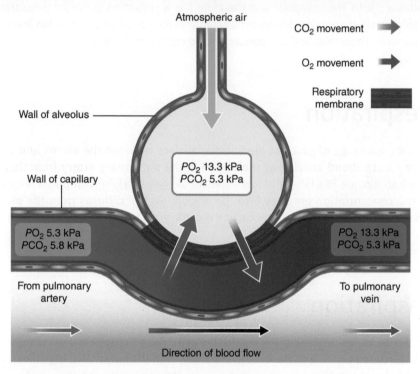

FIGURE 13.11 External respiration. Source: Waugh and Grant (2018)/Elsevier.

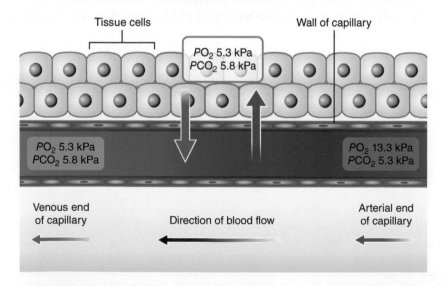

FIGURE 13.12 Internal respiration. Source: Waugh and Grant (2018)/Elsevier.

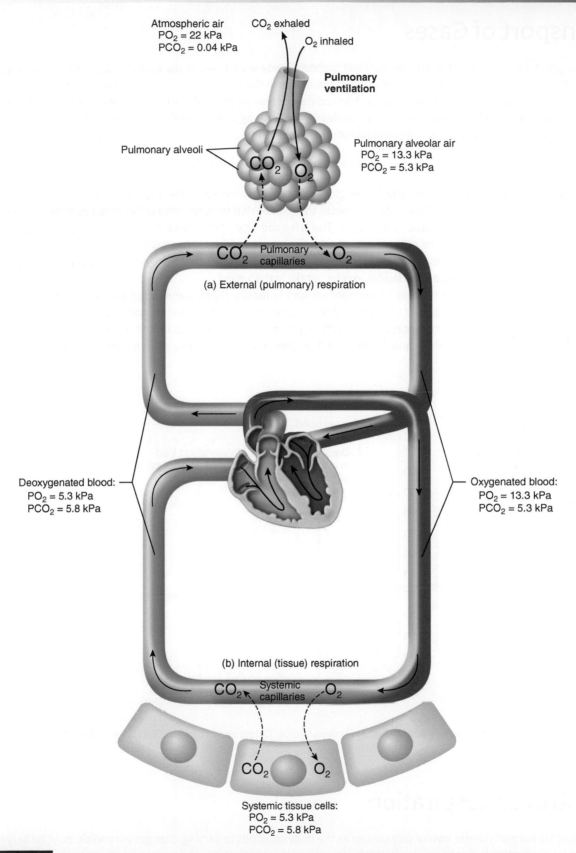

Atmospheric air
PO_2 = 22 kPa
PCO_2 = 0.04 kPa

CO$_2$ exhaled

O$_2$ inhaled

Pulmonary ventilation

Pulmonary alveoli

Pulmonary alveolar air
PO_2 = 13.3 kPa
PCO_2 = 5.3 kPa

CO$_2$ Pulmonary   O$_2$
capillaries

(a) External (pulmonary) respiration

Deoxygenated blood:
PO_2 = 5.3 kPa
PCO_2 = 5.8 kPa

Oxygenated blood:
PO_2 = 13.3 kPa
PCO_2 = 5.3 kPa

(b) Internal (tissue) respiration

CO$_2$ Systemic   O$_2$
capillaries

Systemic tissue cells:
PO_2 = 5.3 kPa
PCO_2 = 5.8 kPa

FIGURE 13.13 Summary of internal and external respiration. Source: Tortora and Derrickson (2021)/John Wiley & Sons.

Transport of Gases

The two gases involved in respiration, oxygen and carbon dioxide are carried in the blood in different ways. Oxygen is mostly (99%) transported attached to haemoglobin molecules in the erythrocytes in the form of oxyhaemoglobin. This reaction is reversible and certain conditions, such as reduced oxygen levels, acidic pH and increased temperatures, cause oxygen to dissociate from haemoglobin and to be released. In this way, oxygen is released to the cells where it is needed most. A small amount of oxygen is also carried dissolved in the plasma.

$$Oxygen + haemoglobin \rightleftharpoons oxyhaemoglobin$$

The equilibrium between oxygen and haemoglobin can be represented by the oxygen–haemoglobin dissociation curve (Figure 13.14). The S-shaped curve demonstrates the relationship between the partial pressure of oxygen and the percentage of haemoglobin saturated with oxygen. The left-hand side of the curve is steep, showing that in low PO_2, haemoglobin releases oxygen to the cells of the body. Small changes in PO_2 at these low levels result in larger changes in haemoglobin saturation. The right-hand side of the curve flattens off, showing that in high PO_2, there are smaller changes in haemoglobin saturation. This demonstrates oxygen uptake in the lungs.

Carbon dioxide is a waste product of metabolism and is mostly (70%) transported in the plasma of blood as bicarbonate ions (HCO_3^-). About 23% of the carbon dioxide is transported in the erythrocytes as carbaminohaemoglobin. It does not affect the oxygen carrying capacity of erythrocytes as carbon dioxide is bound to the globin rather than the haem part of haemoglobin (Stables and Rankin 2010). Approximately 7% of the carbon dioxide is carried in simple solution in plasma.

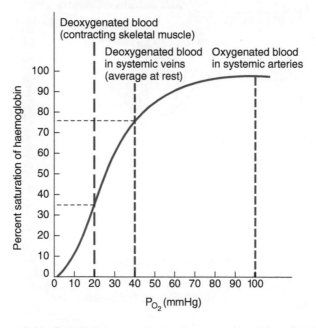

FIGURE 13.14   The oxygen-haemoglobin dissociation curve. Source: Tortora and Derrickson (2021)/John Wiley & Sons.

Control of Respiration

Respiration is normally under involuntary control as the body responds to varying changes in conditions. Voluntary control can be exerted as the need arises; for example, due to speaking. However, involuntary control resumes if carbon dioxide levels in the blood rise (hypercapnia), disrupting homeostasis.

Nervous Control

The respiratory centre is a group of nerves found in the medulla oblongata in the brainstem which control the rate and depth of breathing via inspiratory neurons (Figure 13.15). The pneumotaxic centre (inhibitory, preventing overinflation of the lungs) and the apneustic centre (stimulatory, prolonging inhalation) situated in the pons, higher in the brainstem, adjusts the activity of the respiratory centre (Stables and Rankin 2010; Waugh and Grant 2018).

Chemical Control

Centrally and peripherally located receptors detect changes in arterial PO_2 and PCO_2. Peripheral chemoreceptors can be found in the carotid bodies and in the arch of the aorta. They send impulses to the respiratory centre to alter ventilation when they detect changes to PO_2, PCO_2 and hydrogen ions. The peripheral chemoreceptors are more sensitive to carbon dioxide levels than oxygen levels.

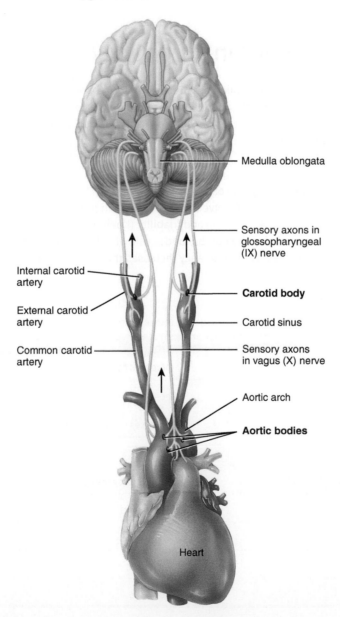

Medulla oblongata

Sensory axons in glossopharyngeal (IX) nerve

Internal carotid artery

Carotid body

External carotid artery

Carotid sinus

Common carotid artery

Sensory axons in vagus (X) nerve

Aortic arch

Aortic bodies

Heart

FIGURE 13.15 Structures involved in the control of respiration. (a) Sagittal section of brainstem. (b) Musculature of thorax.

Central chemoreceptors are found on the surface of the medulla oblongata, primarily responding to hypercapnia (excessive carbon dioxide levels). These central chemoreceptors are bathed in cerebrospinal fluid, so when there is a rise in PCO_2, the carbon dioxide crosses the blood–brain barrier from the cerebral blood vessels to the cerebrospinal fluid where hydrogen ions are released. These hydrogen ions are detected by the central chemoreceptors, which send impulses to the respiratory centre to increase the ventilation rate, thereby decreasing the PCO_2.

Reflective Learning Activity

Home oxygen therapy involves breathing in air that contains more oxygen than normal through a mask or tube connected to a device in the person's home. In instances where a woman may be required to receive oxygen therapy in her own home, what special measures must be taken into account to ensure the safety of all concerned? Take some time to think about and make notes on the safety measures associated with the transportation of oxygen cylinders, the storage of the cylinders, the administration of oxygen and returning used cylinders.

Physiological Changes in Pregnancy

During pregnancy, there are increased metabolic demands on maternal and fetal tissues. To compensate for these demands, there is an increase in metabolic rate and maternal respiratory effort, whereby minute ventilation increases by 15% and approximately 16–20% more oxygen is consumed (Table 13.2). The expanding uterus also affects the respiratory system as it grows. The elevation of the maternal diaphragm in late pregnancy results in functional residual capacity falling by 20% in the third trimester. However, movement of the diaphragm, and therefore vital capacity, remain unchanged.

The upper respiratory tract and airway mucosa are also affected by hormonal changes in pregnancy. Although airway patency and gaseous exchange across the alveoli remain stable in pregnancy, increasing oestrogen levels cause airway mucosal hyperaemia, oedema, hypersecretion and friability (Koehler et al. 2005).

Oestrogen also plays a part in increasing the number and sensitivity of progesterone receptors in the hypothalamus and medulla. Increasing progesterone levels in pregnancy increases the sensitivity of the respiratory centre to carbon

284

TABLE 13.2   **Physiological changes in respiratory function in pregnancy.**

Physiological variable	Change
Oxygen consumption	Increases by approximately 20%
Metabolic rate	Increases by approximately 15%
Minute ventilation	Increases by approximately 15%
Tidal volume	Increases
Functional residual capacity	Decreases by approximately 20% in third trimester
Vital capacity	Unchanged
PO_2	Increases
PCO_2	Decreases
Arterial pH	Increases

dioxide levels. Both hormones also increase the hypoxic sensitivity of peripheral chemoreceptors. A relaxation of the bronchioles can also result from increased levels of progesterone, sometimes leading to dyspnoea.

During labour, an increase in tidal volume and respiratory rate may be caused by pain levels. After delivery, the changes in the respiratory system rapidly return to normal due to delivery of the placenta leading to a fall in progesterone levels.

Snapshot 13.1   Pulmonary Embolism

Background

Suki attends maternity triage at her local hospital with breathlessness and chest pain at 32 weeks of gestation. This is her second pregnancy; her previous child was born two years ago.

Observations

Suki has a body mass index of 32.4 and is a smoker, giving her a venous thromboembolism (VTE) score of 2. Her observations on triage were:
Blood pressure: 124/86 mmHg
Respiratory rate: 28 breaths/minute
Heart rate: 115 beats/minute
Oxygen saturation: 96%
Temperature: 36.6°C
MEWS (maternal early warning score): 4.

Investigations

The midwife called the registrar to review the woman and commenced 15-minute observations while waiting for the review, and continuous fetal monitoring to assess fetal wellbeing. The CTG (cardiotocograph) was normal so was discontinued. After review by the registrar, an ECG (electrocardiogram) was performed showing a sinus tachycardia. After discussion with Suki, a chest x-ray, leg Doppler and ventilation perfusion (VQ) scan were ordered. Until the results of these tests are, low molecular weight heparin is prescribed according to Suki's booking weight.

Reflective Learning Activity

- What were the key elements of good practice highlighted in Snapshot 13.1?
- What considerations need to be discussed with a pregnant woman when considering diagnostic tests for pulmonary embolism of a VQ scan versus computed tomography pulmonary angiogram?
- Using your local VTE scoring chart, what medication and dosage would be prescribed for Suki?
- What are the latest figures from MBRRACE for deaths related to VTE?

Reflective Learning Activity

Women with COVID-19 are more likely to become seriously ill, which can lead to pregnancy problems such as preterm birth or having a baby with a low birth weight. Read the research on COVID-19 in pregnancy and associated outcomes for women and their babies, and produce a timeline of how the disease evolved from March 2020 to March 2021 and its effect and implications on pregnant women and their babies.
Suggested research:

- Pregnancy and COVID-19 (NHS England 2022)
- COVID-19 during pregnancy (Centers for Disease Control and Prevention 2022)
- *SARS-CoV-2* and pregnancy rapid report, March–May 2020 (Knight et al. 2020)
- *SARS-CoV-2* and pregnancy rapid report, June 2020–March 2021 (Knight et al. 2021)

The Respiratory System and the Neonate

In utero, the fetus's lungs are fluid filled and the role of gaseous exchange for the fetus is carried out by the placenta. Respiratory movements can be seen on ultrasound scan in the later stages of pregnancy, drawing small amounts of amniotic fluid into the fetal air passages and causing the development of the lung tissue. The lung fluid begins to be absorbed by the alveolar epithelial cells at the onset of labour, triggered by hormonal changes. The passage of the baby through the vagina during the second stage of labour allows for the remainder of amniotic fluid present in the fetal lungs to be removed. Babies born by elective caesarean section are two to three time more likely to suffer respiratory morbidity as these hormonal and physical changes are not triggered (Hansen et al. 2008; Kamath et al. 2009). Various stimuli at delivery (change in temperature, touch, noise, lights) cause the baby to take their first breath and cry resulting in any remaining fluid to be absorbed by the epithelial cells.

Surfactant

Surfactant is a phospholipid fluid secreted by septal cells in the lungs. Surfactant reduces surface tension in the alveoli, preventing their collapse during expiration. From 35 weeks of gestation, a fetus starts secreting surfactant into the distal air passages and alveoli.

Without surfactant, the lungs cannot function effectively and severe breathing problems can develop. A baby born before 34 weeks of pregnancy may not have accumulated enough surfactant to cope with breathing; they may have immature lungs and can suffer from respiratory distress syndrome. Surfactant can be introduced artificially into the lungs of premature babies to help minimise the effects of respiratory distress syndrome (Jena et al. 2019).

Reflective Learning Activity

The influenza vaccine is seasonally offered to all pregnant women due to the risks for mother and baby if the mother contracts influenza in her pregnancy (UK Health Security Agency 2022c). Research the evidence around influenza in pregnancy and the risks to mother and baby and reflect on how you would share this information with a woman attending for her antenatal clinic appointment.

Snapshot 13.2   Influenza A

Background

Charlene is on the postnatal ward. She reported to the midwife during her daily postnatal check that she had a headache, cough, sore throat, malaise (a feeling of overall weakness), myalgia, arthralgia and rigours. Charlene was three days postnatal after a spontaneous vaginal delivery.

Observations

A set of observations were taken:
Blood pressure 132/83 mmHg
Heart rate 123 beats/minute
Temperature 37.9°C
Respiratory rate 22 breaths/minute
Oxygen saturation levels 98%.

Investigations

A throat swab was sent to the laboratory for testing. Before laboratory confirmation was gained, Charlene was commenced on oseltamivir 75 mg orally twice daily for five days.

Reflective Learning Activity

- What was the MEWS score and associated escalation for Charlene?
- Review the guidelines from Public Health England (PHE) on the use of antiviral agents to treat influenza (PHE 2021). Why do you think treatment is recommended before laboratory confirmation is gained?
- Are you aware of your local policy in managing influenza A in pregnant women?
- What are the implications for the neonate when their mother is diagnosed with influenza A?

Take Home Points

- Respiration is the process where gaseous exchange occurs at the lungs (oxygen is taken from the atmosphere) and the cells of the body (carbon dioxide is returned to the lungs to be expired) to provide the essential reactants for cell metabolism.
- Structurally, the respiratory system consists of two parts: the upper respiratory system and the lower respiratory system.
- Functionally, the respiratory system can also be separated into two parts: the conducting and the respiratory part.
- The parts of the respiratory system have specific adaptations for their function.
- Pregnancy, labour and the postnatal period increases demand on the respiratory system due to increased metabolic demands of the mother and fetus.
- In utero, the functions of the fetal respiratory system are carried out by the placenta; after birth, the respiratory system begins to function in a healthy term neonate.
- There are many diseases affecting the respiratory system; pregnancy is an added risk factor if a woman has any pre-existing respiratory condition or develops a respiratory disease in her pregnancy or the postnatal period.

287

References

Centers for Disease Control and Prevention (2022). *Pregnant and Recently Pregnant People At Increased Risk for Severe Illness from COVID-19*. Washington, DC: National Center for Immunization and Respiratory Diseases (NCIRD), Division of Viral Diseases. https://www.cdc.gov/coronavirus/2019-ncov/need-extra-precautions/pregnant-people.html (accessed 2 November 2023).

Hansen, A.K., Wisborg, K., Uldberg, N., and Henriksen, T.B. (2008). Risk of respiratory morbidity in term infants delivered by elective caesarean section: cohort study. *BMJ* 336: 85–87.

Jena, S.R., Bains, H.S., Pandita, A. et al. (2019). Surfactant therapy in premature babies: SurE or InSurE. *Pediatric Pulmonology* 54 (11): 1747–1752.

Kamath, B.D., Todd, J.K., Glazner, J.E. et al. (2009). Neonatal outcomes after elective caesarean delivery. *Obstetrics and Gynecology* 113: 1231–1238.

Kent, M. (2000). *Advanced Biology*. Oxford: Oxford Publishers.

Knight, M., Bunch, K., Cairns, A. et al. on behalf of MBRRACE-UK (2020). *Saving Lives, Improving Mothers' Care Rapid Report: Learning from SARS-CoV-2-Related and Associated Maternal Deaths in the UK, March–May 2020*. Oxford: National Perinatal Epidemiology Unit, University of Oxford.

Knight, M., Bunch, K., Cairns, A. et al. on behalf of MBRRACE-UK (2021). *Saving Lives, Improving Mothers' Care Rapid Report: Learning from SARS-CoV-2-Related and Associated Maternal Deaths in the UK, June 2020–March 2021*. Oxford: National Perinatal Epidemiology Unit, University of Oxford.

Koehler, K.F., Helguero, L.A., Haldosén, L.A. et al. (2005). Reflections on the discovery and significance of oestrogen receptor beta. *Endocrine Reviews* 26: 465–478.

NHS England (2022). *Pregnancy and COVID-19*. https://www.nhs.uk/conditions/coronavirus-covid-19/people-at-higher-risk/pregnancy-and-coronavirus (accessed 2 November 2023).

NICE (2019). *Hypertension in Pregnancy: Diagnosis and Management*. NICE Guideline NG133. London: National Institute for Health and Care Excellence. www.nice.org.uk/guidance/ng133/chapter/Recommendations (accessed 2 November 2023).

Royal College of Obstetricians and Gynaecologists. (2015). *Chickenpox in Pregnancy*. Green-top Guideline No. 13. London: Royal College of Obstetricians and Gynaecologists. www.rcog.org.uk/guidance/browse-all-guidance/green-top-guidelines/chickenpox-in-pregnancy-green-top-guideline-no-13 (accessed 2 November 2023).

Stables, D. and Rankin, J. (2010). *Physiology in Childbearing*, 3e. London: Elsevier Limited.

Tortora, G.J. and Grabowski, S.R. (2000). *Principles of Anatomy and Physiology*. Hoboken, NJ: Wiley.

Tortora, G. J., and Derrickson, B. H. (2021). *Principles of anatomy and physiology*. 16th Edition. London: Wiley-Blackwell.

UK Health Security Agency. (2021). *Guidance on Use of Antiviral Agents for the Treatment and Prophylaxis of Seasonal Influenza*. Version 11. London: UK Health Security Agency. https://www.gov.uk/government/publications/influenza-treatment-and-prophylaxis-using-anti-viral-agents (accessed 2 November 2023).

UK Health Security Agency. (2022a). *Guidance on the Investigation, Diagnosis and Management of Viral Illness, or Exposure to Viral Rash Illness, in Pregnancy*. London: UK Health Security Agency. https://www.gov.uk/government/publications/viral-rash-in-pregnancy (accessed 2 November 2023).

UK Health Security Agency. (2022b). *Assessment of a Pregnant Woman Reporting Viral Rash Illness, or Exposure to Viral Rash Illness, in Pregnancy: Aide Memoire for Health Professionals*. London: UK Health Security Agency. https://www.gov.uk/government/publications/viral-rash-in-pregnancy (accessed 2 November 2023).

UK Health Security Agency (2022c). *Influenza: The Green Book, Chapter 19*. London: UK Health Security Agency. https://www.gov.uk/government/publications/influenza-the-green-book-chapter-19 (accessed 20 October 2022).

Waugh, A. and Grant, A. (2018). *Anatomy and Physiology in Health and Illness*, 13e. London: Elsevier.

Wylie, L. (2005). *Essential Anatomy and Physiology in Maternity Care*, 2e. London: Elsevier.

288

Further Reading

Bhatia, P. and Bhatia, K. (2000). Pregnancy and the lungs. *Postgraduate Medical Journal* 76: 683–689.

Jensen, D., Webb, K.A., and O'Donnell, D.E. (2007). Chemical and mechanical adaptations of the respiratory system at rest and during exercise in human pregnancy. *Applied Physiology, Nutrition, and Metabolism* 32 (6): 1239–1250.

LoMauro, A., Aliverti, A., Frykholm, P. et al. (2019). Adaptation of lung, chest wall, and respiratory muscles during pregnancy: preparing for birth. *Journal of Applied Physiology* 127 (6): 1640–1650.

Tan, E.K. and Tan, E.L. (2013). Alterations in physiology and anatomy during pregnancy. *Best Practice and Research Clinical Obstetrics and Gynaecology* 27: 791–802.

Conditions Affecting the Respiratory System

Below is a list of conditions that are associated with the respiratory system. Take some time and write notes about each of the conditions. Think about the medications that may be used to treat these conditions and be specific about the pharmacokinetics and pharmacodynamics. Remember to include aspects of patient care. If you are making notes about women, you have offered care and support to you must ensure that you have adhered to the rules of confidentiality.

The condition	Your notes
Asthma	
Tuberculosis	
Pulmonary embolism	
Influenza	
Breathlessness	

Glossary

Alveoli	Tiny air sacs at the end of the alveoli ducts where gaseous exchange occurs.
Chemoreceptors	Sensors that detect changes in the carbon dioxide, oxygen and pH levels in the body; can be central or peripheral.
Cilia	Tiny, threadlike projection from the surface of a cell body.
Diffusion	The movement of a substance from an area of high concentration to an area of low concentration.
Dyspnoea	Difficult or laboured breathing (e.g. breathlessness).
Erythrocytes	A red blood cell, which is biconcave in shape, usually without a nucleus. Erythrocytes contain haemoglobin.
Eustachian tube	Connects the middle ear to the back of your throat. They help equalise air pressure inside your ears and drain fluid.
Hyperaemia	An excess of blood in the vessels supplying an organ or other part of the body.
Hypercapnia	An increase in the partial pressure of carbon dioxide (PCO_2) in the blood.
Intercostal muscles	Accessory muscles to respiration, found in between the 12 ribs.
Mediastinum	The central portion of the thoracic cavity, which contains a group of structures related to the respiratory system including the trachea, nerves and blood vessels.
Medulla oblongata	The lowest part of the brainstem connected to the midbrain by the pons. It plays a critical role in transmitting signals between the spinal cord and the brain in controlling activities such as respiration.
Metabolism	A series of chemical reactions in the body which provide energy for the body's vital processes.
Oestrogen	A sex hormone responsible for the development and regulation of the female reproductive system.
Oxygenated blood	Blood rich in oxygen.
Blood plasma	A straw-coloured liquid component of blood in which blood cells are absent.
Pleural membrane	A serous membrane which folds back on itself to form a two-layered membranous pleural sac around the lungs.
Pons	Part of the brainstem lying inferior to the midbrain and superior to the medulla oblongata. The pons controls unconscious processes such as breathing.
Progesterone	A sex hormone released from the ovary responsible for control of the menstrual cycle and in maintaining the early stages of pregnancy.
Surfactant	A compound of phospholipids and proteins which decreases surface tension in the lungs
Ventilation	The flow of air into and out of the alveoli of the lungs during inspiration and expiration.

Multiple Choice Questions

1. Which part of the respiratory system is a passageway for food and air, as well as playing a role in speech?
    a. Nasal cavity
    b. Pharynx
    c. Larynx
    d. Trachea

2. Which of the following is not a conducting part of the respiratory system?
   a. Trachea
   b. Pharynx
   c. Alveoli
   d. Bronchiole

3. When you inhale, air flows through respiratory structures in which sequence?
   a. Nasal cavity, pharynx, trachea, larynx, bronchus, bronchiole, alveolus
   b. Nasal cavity, pharynx, larynx, trachea, bronchiole, bronchus, alveolus
   c. Nasal cavity, pharynx, larynx, bronchiole, bronchus, trachea, alveolus
   d. Nasal cavity, pharynx, larynx, trachea, bronchus, bronchiole, alveolus

4. When you exhale, the diaphragm does what?
   a. Relaxes moving inferiorly
   b. Relaxes moving superiorly
   c. Contracting moving superiorly
   d. Contracting and moving inferiorly

5. During inspiration, the rib cage moves how?
   a. Upwards and outwards; the diaphragm moves downwards and flattens
   b. Downwards and inwards; the diaphragm moves upwards and becomes dome shaped
   c. Upwards and inwards; the diaphragm moves downwards and becomes dome shaped
   d. Downwards and outwards; the diaphragm moves upwards and flattens

6. Which equation accurately explains the vital capacity of the lungs?
   a. Tidal volume + inspiratory reserve volume + expiratory reserve volume
   b. Tidal volume + residual volume
   c. Residual volume + inspiratory reserve volume + expiratory reserve volume
   d. Tidal volume × respiratory rate

7. Which of the following has the smallest diameter?
   a. Bronchus
   b. Trachea
   c. Terminal bronchioles
   d. Respiratory bronchioles

8. What percentage increase is there in oxygen consumption in pregnancy?
   a. 10%
   b. 15%
   c. 20%
   d. 25%

9. What type of cellular transport moves oxygen and carbon dioxide between the alveoli and the blood capillaries surrounding the alveoli?
   a. Diffusion
   b. Osmosis
   c. Active transport
   d. Deflation

10. Where can the central chemoreceptors responsible for the control of respiration be found?
    a. Carotid bodies
    b. Medulla oblongata
    c. Pons
    d. Aortic arch

CHAPTER **14**

The Nervous System

Claire Ford

AIM

This chapter aims to support midwifery students' practice by providing information about the anatomy and physiology of the nervous system. It also uses case study examples and highlights red flag alerts to assist students with the integration of the theory into practice.

LEARNING OUTCOMES

On completion of this chapter, you will be able to:

- Describe how the nervous system interacts with other bodily systems.
- Understand the structure and function of the nervous system and how these adapt and change during the perinatal journey.
- Demonstrate an awareness of some of the red flag alerts associated with the central and peripheral nervous system to provide safe and effective care to women.
- Appreciate the role of the midwife in relation to managing and treating some conditions affecting the nervous system.

Test Your Prior Knowledge
1. Can you name five pairs of cranial nerves?
2. How many lobes are found in the cerebrum if the brain?
3. What organs are part of the central nervous system?
4. Can you articulate difference between the autonomic and somatic nervous systems?
5. Can you name the three layers of the meninges?

Introduction

The nervous system is composed of two major systems: the central nervous system, largely consisting of the brain and spinal cord, and the peripheral nervous system, which is separated into autonomic and somatic responses (Figure 14.1). These systems, in collaboration with the endocrine system, maintain the balance of the body and control several rapid

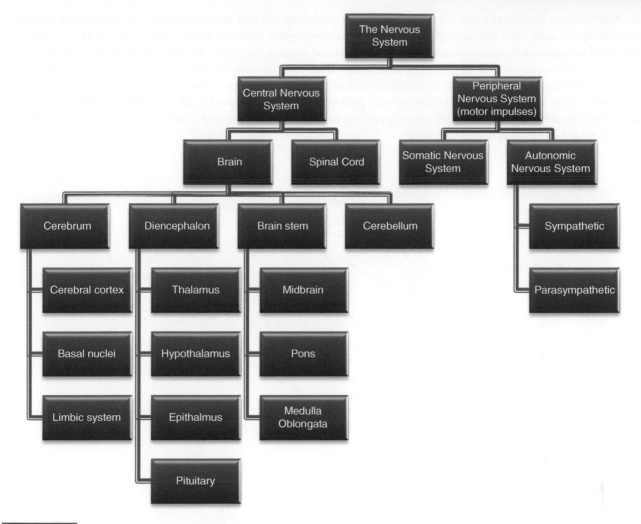

FIGURE 14.1 The organisation of the nervous system.

and more sustained essential bodily functions, such as motor function, breathing and thermoregulation (McErlean and Migliozzi 2017). Throughout this chapter, the nervous system is explored in greater depth and reference is made to the specific knowledge needed by midwives and midwifery students to provide safe and effective care to women during their perinatal journey. We start with the two main cells that are the functional building blocks of the central nervous system: neurons and neuroglia.

Neurons

There are estimated to be over 100 billion neurons within the body. These cells are different from other body cells as they can both initiate and conduct nerve impulses, thus, generating an action potential for sending and receiving information (Boore et al. 2021). There are three types of neurons: *sensory neurons* carry signals from the body to the spinal cord and brain and are therefore afferent neurons; *motor neurons* are efferent pathways that relay impulses from the brain and spinal cord to either muscle or epithelial tissue, and *interneurons* are connecting neurons that carry impulses from sensory to motor neurons.

Neurons also have three parts: the *cell body*, which is considered the core and main part of the neuron, *axons*, which transfer signals away from the cell body, and *dendrites*, which forward impulses towards the cell body. The axon is the stalk and is wrapped in myelin, a white fatty protective coat that plays an essential role in the conductivity of the impulses and covers sections of the axon length, separated by the nodes of Ranvier. Dendrites are branched projections that surround the cell body and are shaped in a way which increases the surface area, enhancing the effectiveness and speed of the signal (Figure 14.2). Neurons communicate with each other by sending nerve impulses, known as action potentials, along the axon and then to another cell across a gap (synaptic cleft) separating two neurons, by a chemical or electrical synaptic relay facilitated by neurotransmitters.

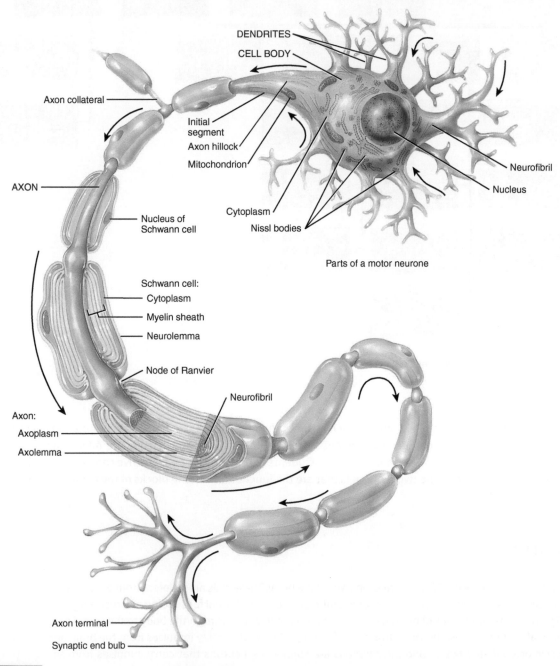

Parts of a motor neurone

FIGURE 14.2 A neuron. Source: Peate and Evans (2016)/John Wiley & Sons.

Snapshot 14.1   Multiple Sclerosis

Background

Louise Gent is 23-year-old woman expecting her first child. Within her second trimester, she contacted her midwife as she was experiencing some pain in the soles of her feet and was worried as she had been losing weight throughout the pregnancy and always seemed tired.

The midwife gained consent to obtain a more thorough history of her presenting symptoms, such as what made the pain in her feet worse, whether she could describe the pain and provide an intensity score, and asked her other questions about her diet and any other digestive symptoms.

Observations

She also carried out vital observations, an abdominal examination and fetal assessment. Louise's vital observations were within normal parameters; the fetal heart sounds were normal, but the fundal height was lower than it should be for the gestation. The pain in Louise's feet was also concerning at it was having a debilitating impact on her mobility and was severe, even at rest. The weight loss was also not explained by any major changes to her nutritional intake and Louise was not experiencing any nausea or vomiting.

Investigations and Diagnosis

The midwife was unsure of the cause and needed further advice. She made a referral to the pregnancy assessment unit, where further investigations could be made, including blood tests, ultrasounds scans and an examination by the medical team.

After further investigations by the obstetric consultant, referral to a neurologist and MRI (magnetic resonance imaging), Louise was diagnosed with multiple sclerosis (MS) and was offered support from the wider multidisciplinary team, such as occupational therapists, physiotherapist. She was advised that during extreme periods of relapse, a short course of steroids could be prescribed.

While it is not a complication of pregnancy, some women can display MS symptoms for the first time during pregnancy. The reason for this presentation is unknown, but most people develop MS between the ages of 20–40 years and women are twice as likely to experience the condition than men (Waugh and Grant 2018); it is thus often discovered when women of childbearing age interact with healthcare professionals. For individuals affected by MS, areas of demyelinated white matter (plaques) replace myelin and grey matter in the spinal cord and brain.

While MS does not prevent women from becoming pregnant, it can sometimes result in babies with smaller birth weight and can also make delivery more difficult, due to symptoms of reduced sensation and feeling; there is therefore an increased need for forceps or vacuum assistance during delivery (Dobson et al. 2019; NICE 2022).

Medications Management: Corticosteroids

Corticosteroids (also known as steroids) may be used to treat relapses or acute exacerbations of MS, as they can reduce inflammation in the central nervous system. Methylprednisolone is the steroid most often prescribed; it is considered safe to administer during pregnancy. However, it should only to be prescribed for short periods of time due to its adverse effects and the associated complications of long-term use.

Dose: 500 mg once daily for five days.

For further information, see:

- British National Formulary. Methylprednisolone: https://bnf.nice.org.uk/drugs/methylprednisolone
- National Institute for Health and Care Excellence. Multiple sclerosis: https://www.nice.org.uk/guidance/conditions-and-diseases/neurological-conditions/multiple-sclerosis

Neuroglia

There are around one trillion neuroglial cells within the central nervous system. They play a huge supporting role, protecting the neurons, holding neurons together and regulating neuronal functions. As with the overall structure of the nervous system, there are central and peripheral divisions, which vary in size and shape (Figure 14.3 and Table 14.1). Microglia, as

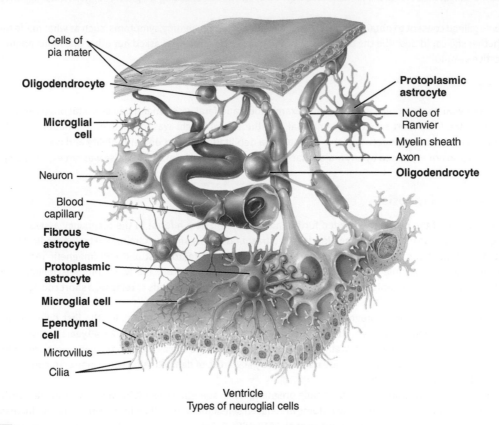

Cells of pia mater
Oligodendrocyte
Protoplasmic astrocyte
Node of Ranvier
Myelin sheath
Axon
Oligodendrocyte
Microglial cell
Neuron
Blood capillary
Fibrous astrocyte
Protoplasmic astrocyte
Microglial cell
Ependymal cell
Microvillus
Cilia
Ventricle
Types of neuroglial cells

FIGURE 14.3   A neuroglia. Source: Tortora and Derrickson (2017)/John Wiley & Sons.

TABLE 14.1   **Types of neuroglia.**

Name	Location	Function
Astrocytes	Central nervous system	Form blood–brain barrier, secure neurons to the blood supply and regulate external chemical environment
Microglia	Central nervous system	Protect neurons from pathogens as they are capable of phagocytosis
Oligodendrocytes	Central nervous system	Produce myelin which coats the axons of neurons and increases the speed of action potential
Ependymal	Central nervous system	Create, secrete, circulate and reabsorb cerebrospinal fluid
Schwann	Peripheral nervous system	Produce myelin, which coats the axons of neurons and increases the speed of action potential. Also protects as removes debris and is capable of phagocytosis
Satellites	Peripheral nervous system	Regulate external chemical environment and play a role in inflammation process during injury

Source: Adapted from Boore et al. (2021).

the name suggests, are smaller and play a large role in the inflammatory process and oligodendrocytes are longer and produce the myelin sheath that coats the neuron axon and due to its consistency also holds some nerve fibres together.

The Brain

The brain is considered the personal computer of the body. It receives information and undertakes the complex process of interpreting the data and then advising the body on how to react, either immediately or at a much later date. It is such an important organ that is it housed in its own protective shell (the cranium, which consists of several irregular bones), protective membranes (known collectively as the meninges) and protective fluid (cerebrospinal fluid). It also receives 15% of the entire cardiac output and has a unique blood delivery system, constructed in such a way that it enables equal oxygenated blood distribution, even in the event of damage to arteries supplying the brain (McErlean and Migliozzi 2017).

The brain is a fascinating and complex organ, weighing approximately 1400–1600 g. It is constructed from grey matter: nerve cell bodies that undertake higher brain functions, and white matter: nerve cell axons that relay messages and act as brain connectors. Tto understand its complexity, textbooks have described the brain in various ways; however, for the purpose of this chapter, we have separated these structures from the exterior to interior and superior to inferior, rather than the traditional description of the forebrain, midbrain and hindbrain (Figure 14.1 for the organisation of the brain flowchart and Figure 14.4 for a drawing of the brain with the associated structures).

Cerebrum

This is the largest part of the brain and is divided into two hemispheres (right and left) by the longitudinal fissure and separated from the cerebellum by the transverse fissure (Waugh and Grant 2018). What can sometimes be confusing when assessing neurological functioning is that the brain is contralateral, which means that the left hemisphere controls the functions associated with the right side of the body and the right hemisphere with those aligned to the left side.

297

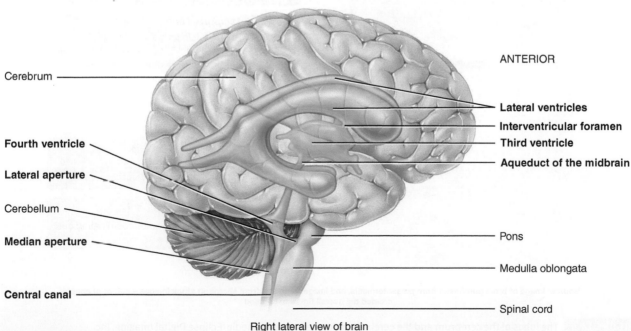

Right lateral view of brain

FIGURE 14.4 The brain and associated structures. Source: Tortora and Derrickson (2017)/John Wiley & Sons.

These hemispheres communicate with each other via nerve axons found in a large collection of white matter deep inside the brain, called the corpus callosum. Conversely, grey matter is found in the outer sections of the brain (the cerebral cortex), with some islands of grey matter surrounded by white matter (nuclei), responsible for unconscious bodily functions, also found in other inner regions of the brain (Boore et al. 2021).

To aid the description of the external structure of the brain, the right and left hemispheres are further divided into four lobes, which are named after the cranial bones directly protecting the underlying section of the cerebrum, with the exception of the fifth lobe (insular lobe) folded deep within the lateral sulcus and thus hidden (Figure 14.5).

Cerebral Cortex

The brain has an extremely large surface area, created by hundreds of concave and convex folds of matter, tightly packed together, the grooves (sulci) are known as fissures and the ridges (gyri) are referred to as convolutions. This provides two main benefits: it enables the amount of grey matter to be increased within the cortex area and ensures that its overall shape and dimensional size are small enough, so it can fit into the protective skull.

The cerebral cortex is associated with higher-order function, sensory perception and voluntary movement. All the main functional areas have been mapped (Figure 14.6), with the anterior sections of both hemispheres being aligned with motor function and the sections found posteriorly to the central sulcus with sensory functions. However, it is important to state that while these functions have been associated with special locations within the cerebral cortex, they are not always exclusive and individual variations have been noted.

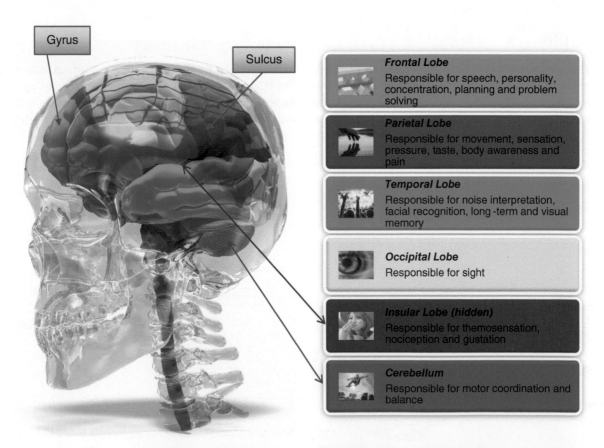

Gyrus

Sulcus

Frontal Lobe
Responsible for speech, personality, concentration, planning and problem solving

Parietal Lobe
Responsible for movement, sensation, pressure, taste, body awareness and pain

Temporal Lobe
Responsible for noise interpretation, facial recognition, long-term and visual memory

Occipital Lobe
Responsible for sight

Insular Lobe (hidden)
Responsible for themosensation, nociception and gustation

Cerebellum
Responsible for motor coordination and balance

Source: Image of brain purchased from presentermedia, and images with text from Microsoft stock images – author of chapter created the overall figure to be used

FIGURE 14.5   The lobes of the cerebrum and the cerebellum.Source: presentermedia/Eclipse Digital Imaging, Inc.

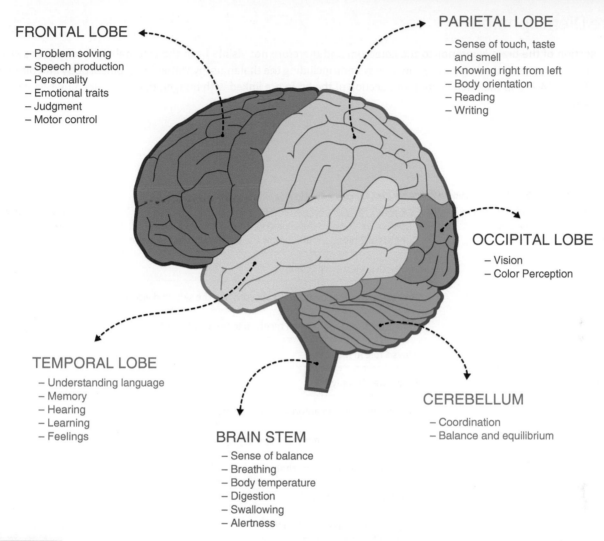

FRONTAL LOBE
- Problem solving
- Speech production
- Personality
- Emotional traits
- Judgment
- Motor control

PARIETAL LOBE
- Sense of touch, taste and smell
- Knowing right from left
- Body orientation
- Reading
- Writing

OCCIPITAL LOBE
- Vision
- Color Perception

TEMPORAL LOBE
- Understanding language
- Memory
- Hearing
- Learning
- Feelings

CEREBELLUM
- Coordination
- Balance and equilibrium

BRAIN STEM
- Sense of balance
- Breathing
- Body temperature
- Digestion
- Swallowing
- Alertness

FIGURE 14.6 Functions associated with the cerebral cortex. fatmasniper/Adobe Stock Photos

Basal Nuclei (Ganglia)

The basal ganglia (nuclei) is a group of five pairs of nuclei: the caudate nucleus, putamen, globus pallidus, subthalamic nucleus and substantia nigra, which are subcortical structures found deep within the white matter. These structures fine tune voluntary movements (Boore et al. 2021). They work in conjunction with the limbic systems to achieve this.

Limbic System

The limbic system is the part of the brain involved in emotional and behavioural responses, the interpretation of facial expressions and the formation of episodic memories. It is located deep within the brain, inferior to the cerebral cortex and superior to the brainstem and two of the major structures are the hippocampus, responsible for short-term and long-term memory and the amygdala, which regulates emotional learning and stores emotional experiences as memories.

The Diencephalon

This section of the brain is inferior to the cerebrum and therefore not visible from the external view. It houses several important structures linked with the endocrine system, including the thalamus, hypothalamus, pineal body and pituitary gland (Table 14.2) and the nuclei within this section of the brain are linked with hunger, thirst and sleeping (Waugh and Grant 2018).

TABLE 14.2   Functions associated with the cerebral cortex.

Structure	Description and functions
Thalmus	Consists of 2 masses found below the corpus callosum on either side of the third ventricle
	Has both grey and white matter
	Processes information from the receptors in the skin and viscera
	Relays the basic information received to the cerebral cortex
	Plays a role in memory
Hypothalamus	Small; weighs only 7 g
	Situated inferior and anterior to the thalmus
	Secretes antidiuretic hormone and oxytocin
	Regulates hormone levels that are released from the pituitary gland
	Regulates temperature
	Regulates water balance and thirst
	Regulates appetite
	Associated with emotional reactions and circadian rhythms
Pineal body/gland	Secretes melatonin responsible for sleep–wake cycles
Pituitary gland	Secretes hormones such as:
	• Luteinising hormone
	• Adrenocorticotrophic hormone
	• Thyroid-stimulating hormone
	• Prolactin
	• Follicle-stimulating hormone
	• Growth hormone
	• Melanocyte-stimulating hormone

Brainstem

The brainstem is a stalk-like structure below and partially covered by the cerebellum. It consists of three sections: the pons, midbrain and medulla oblongata.

Midbrain

The midbrain is situated between the cerebellum (anterior) and the pons (inferior) and relays motor and sensory information, specifically in relation to the visual and auditory impulses. It is able to carry out these functions because it consists of many nuclei and nerve fibres connecting the cerebrum with the lower parts of the brain and spinal cord.

Pons

The pons is situated anterior to the cerebellum, inferior to the midbrain and superior to the medulla oblongata. It also relays sensory and motor visual and auditory impulses but also works with the medulla oblongata to control the rate and depth of breathing.

Medulla Oblongata

The medulla oblongata is the most inferior part of the brainstem. It is about 2.5 cm long and is continuous with the spinal cord. Unlike the cerebrum, the outer matter is white and the central matter is grey. There are also many nuclei, which are associated with autonomic reflexes, so this part of the brainstem is often referred to as housing the cardiovascular, respiratory and reflex centres for most involuntary responses, such as the rate of cardiac, diaphragm and intercostal muscle contractions, coughing and sneezing, vomiting and swallowing.

Cerebellum

The cerebellum is also a convoluted structure, oval in shape and situated posteriorly to the pons and inferior to the posterior section of the cerebrum. This structure, like the cerebrum, has two hemispheres and a white matter centre, known as the arbour vitae (tree of life), and a grey matter cortex. There are also nuclei providing essential roles in the balance of the body, posture and voluntary muscle activity; consequently, damage to the cerebellum results in an altered gait and uncoordinated movements, which can limit an individual's ability to undertake precise movements (Waugh and Grant 2018).

Reflective Learning Activity

As the brainstem is central to vital bodily functions, it is possible to receive a traumatic head injury and survive, as long as the brainstem is protected and remains intact. Often, individuals are nutritionally maintained and remain in a coma until they can recover. However, once the brainstem is severely compromised, brain death is usually declared.

Meninges

As previously mentioned, the brain has many protective mechanisms, one of which is the meninges, which lie between the skull and the brain and are continuous with the spinal cord (discussed later in the chapter). The meninges are constructed from three main layers: the pia mater, dura mater and arachnoid mater, with space between them, referred to as the subdural and subarachnoid space (Figure 14.7).

Dura Mater

The dura mater is constructed from two dense layers of tough fibrous connective tissue, one of which is closest to the inner surface of the skull wall (periosteal layer) and one protecting the outer side of the brain (meningeal layer). The space

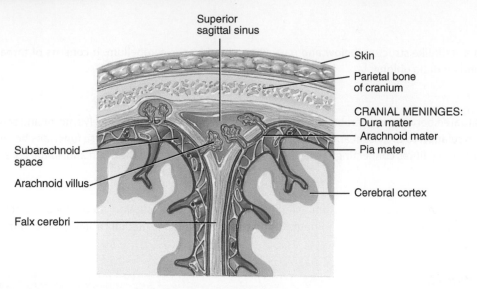

Superior
sagittal sinus

Skin

Parietal bone
of cranium

CRANIAL MENINGES:
Dura mater
Arachnoid mater
Pia mater

Subarachnoid
space

Arachnoid villus

Cerebral cortex

Falx cerebri

FIGURE 14.7   Meninges. Source: Peate and Evans (2016)/John Wiley & Sons.

between these two layers is extremely thin, except in three specific locations of the brain, where natural sinuses occur, owing to the more prominent ridges of the cerebral cortex, which act as dividing groves between the left and right cerebral hemispheres (falx cerebri), the two cerebellar hemispheres (falx cerebelli) and the cerebrum and cerebellum (tentorium cerebelli).

Arachnoid Mater

The arachnoid mater is a fibrous layer that is separated from the dura mater by the smaller subdural space, where a small amount of serous fluid is found, and from the pia mater by the larger subarachnoid space, which contains cerebrospinal fluid (CSF) and also some large blood vessels.

Pia Mater

The pia mater layer consists of delicate connective tissue, with a rich blood supply. It adheres directly to the brain, tightly following the folds and ridges of the surface area.

Reflective Learning Activity

The meninges in the brain and spinal cord are usually well protected; however, they can become infected (via head injuries, the bloodstream or medical procedures) by bacteria, viruses, protozoa and fungi. Bacterial infection in the meninges is known as meningitis and is a life-threatening condition, most commonly found in babies and children. The annual incidence of bacterial meningitis in the UK is 1 : 100 000. With swift diagnosis and treatment, the outcomes are very favourable (NICE 2020). Symptoms of meningitis include:

- Headache
- Neck stiffness
- Photophobia
- Pyrexia
- Petechial rash.

Cerebrospinal Fluid and Ventricles

Interspersed throughout the brain are cerebrospinal fluid-filled cavities known as ventricles, which secrete CSF via the choroid plexus at a rate of 0.5 ml/minute. This protective fluid (approximately 150 ml) is then circulated via the subarachnoid space, around the brain and spinal cord, through the action of pulsating blood vessels, changes in posture and respiration (Waugh and Grant 2018). Lateral ventricles 1 and 2 are in the cerebrum, ventricle 3 is located in the diencephalon and ventricle 4 can be found between the cerebellum and the medulla oblongata (Figure 14.8).

CSF is a clear, slightly alkaline fluid that is mostly water containing plasma proteins, mineral salts, glucose and small amounts of urea and creatinine. It supports and protects the brain by acting as a shock absorber between the hard skull and the soft delicate tissue of the brain and also maintains a moist environment, which enables the transfer of nutrients and waste (McErlean and Migliozzi 2017).

Intracranial Pressure

The pressure within the cranium must be closely regulated and maintained to around 10 cm H_2O when lying and 30 cm H_2O when standing, as the brain, the cerebral blood vessels and the CSF are housed within the cavity, which is fixed and rigid (Waugh and Grant 2018). The total force exerted by the contents of the cranium (brain tissue 78%, blood 12% and CSF 10%) is referred to as intracranial pressure (ICP). If one of the components increases in volume, the others must decrease to keep the pressure inside the skull steady. For example, if a patient has a brain tumour, there will be extra brain tissue volume, thus, blood and CSF must decrease in volume to keep the pressure from rising. Conversely, if a patient has excess CSF (hydrocephalus) then blood and tissue must decrease in volume to prevent the ICP from rising. The process of altering the changes in volume to limit overall rises in pressure is known as compensation, or autoregulation, which is a function controlled by the autonomic nervous system. However, in some circumstances, there comes a point when increased ICP exceeds the limits of compensation and autoregulation fails. If ICP continues to rise and is not recognised and treated, it can eventually lead to death; thus, raised or rising intracranial pressure is an emergency situation.

303

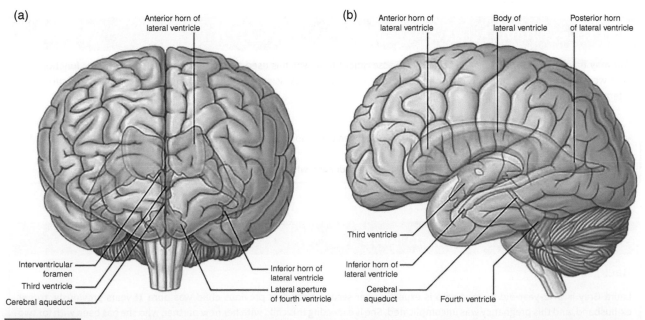

(a)

Anterior horn of lateral ventricle

Interventricular foramen

Third ventricle

Cerebral aqueduct

Inferior horn of lateral ventricle

Lateral aperture of fourth ventricle

(b)

Anterior horn of lateral ventricle

Body of lateral ventricle

Posterior horn of lateral ventricle

Third ventricle

Inferior horn of lateral ventricle

Cerebral aqueduct

Fourth ventricle

FIGURE 14.8 Anterior and lateral view of the ventricles. Source: Grays Anatomy The Anatomical Basis of Clinical Practice / Elsevier.

Red Flag Alert: Raised Intracranial Pressure

There are certain aspects of life that can temporarily increase ICP. These include activities such as drinking alcohol, being constipated, stressed, and during labour and delivery. It is therefore important that midwives and midwifery students closely observe women in labour for signs of raised ICP, especially if they already have hypertension, when some form of neurological assessment should be undertaken.

Signs of raised ICP include:

- Headaches
- Vomiting
- Papilloedema
- Photophobia
- Bradycardia
- Hypertension
- Erratic respirations.

Key Areas of Neurological Assessment

- The *Glasgow Coma Scale* – this scale reflects diffuse brain function. Where a patient has raised ICP, consciousness levels will be impaired. Consciousness is controlled by nerve impulses continually bombarding the cerebral cortex from an area of the brain called the reticular activating system (RAS). Increased cranial pressure disrupts the blood and oxygen supply to the cerebral cortex or RAS; therefore, subtle changes in conscious level can alert the midwife to potential neurological deterioration.
- *Vital signs* – ischaemia and pressure on the vasomotor centre causes vasoconstriction, which raises the blood pressure. It also leads to changes in the respiratory centres and changes to cardiac function; these signs are known as Cushing's triad.
- *Focal signs* – motor fibres are located at the back of the frontal lobe. Motor fibres descend through the brainstem to the spinal cord and out to the extremities. Any pressure on the cerebral cortex will decrease strength and movement of the limb on the opposite side because the fibres cross over or decussate. The oculomotor nerve rises in the midbrain near the base of the cerebrum and causes the pupils of the eye to constrict. The oculomotor nerve becomes compressed against this hard surface as pressure within the skull rises. Compression interrupts the nerve impulses to the muscles of the iris and the pupil becomes dilated. They may react sluggishly to light at first and then fail to react at all. This is a very late sign and will not occur unless the pressure is extreme.

Reflective Learning Activity

You may have heard of the Glasgow Coma Scale assessment tool, which is used to assess verbal response, motor function and limb weaknesses. However, this is only one part of the neurological assessment and it is also often subject to various subjective interpretation.

- What do you already know about this assessment tool?
- Do you think this is something you would need to use when caring for women during pregnancy?
- Would you feel confident using this tool in practice?
- If you suspected neurological changes in the women in your care, what would you do?

Snapshot 14.2   Pre-eclampsia in Pregnancy

Background

Laura Gray is a 42-year-old woman who is expecting her second baby. Her previous child was born 15 years previously, to her ex-husband, and this pregnancy was uncomplicated. She is expecting this child with her new partner, who she has been with for two years. Laura has been experiencing severe headaches, flashing lights and her hands and feet are swollen.

Observations

The midwife undertakes some vital observations, urinalysis, abdominal examination and fetal assessment. Laura's blood pressure is high, at 156/106 mm/Hg, and the urinalysis test confirms proteinuria.

Interventions

The midwife refers Laura to a specialist in hypertensive disorders of pregnancy, to discuss the risks and benefits of treatment. She also provides lifestyle advice, such as weight management, exercise, healthy eating and lowering the amount of salt in her diet and discusses the need to increase prenatal visits to monitor her hypertension, proteinuria and fetal health more closely.

Clinical Notes

In pre-eclampsia, the placenta's blood supply is compromised, disrupting the blood flow between mother and baby and damaging the placenta. The subsequent substances released affect the mother's blood vessels, causing hypertension and proteinuria (NICE 2023a).

Medications Management: Eclampsia

Eclampsia describes a type of convulsion that pregnant women can experience, usually from 20 weeks of pregnancy. It presents as involuntarily, repetitive, jerky movements of the arms and legs, and the neck and jaw will twitch. The convulsion usually lasts less than 60 seconds. Most women make a full recovery; however, if the seizures are severe, there is a small risk of permanent disability or brain damage. Magnesium sulphate has been shown to halve the risk of eclampsia and is now widely used to treat women who have or may be at risk of developing eclampsia, as it can trigger cerebral vasodilation and reduce cerebral vasospasm and ischaemia.

Dose: Initially 4 g by intravenous injection over 5–15 minutes, then continue intravenous infusion of 1 g/hour for 24 hours. If further seizures occur, an additional dose of 2–4 g by intravenous injection over 5–15 minutes can be given.

For further information, see:

- British National Formulary. Magnesium sulfate: https://bnf.nice.org.uk/drugs/magnesium-sulfate.
- NICE (2023a).

305

Blood Supply

The brain is supplied by four main arteries, the right and left common carotid arteries, and the right and left vertebral arteries They all contribute to the circulus arteriosus (circle of Willis; Figure 14.9), which lies in the subarachnoid space on the underside of the brain (Waugh and Grant 2018). This network ensures that the brain receives an adequate blood supply, even when one of the arteries is damaged or occluded due to extreme movements of the head.

Cranial Nerves

While the brain can be referred to as the computer, the cranial nerves, which are paired, are the wired cables, transmitting signals from and/or to the brain to the head and neck, as each paired nerve is constructed from either sensory or motor nerves, or both (Figure 14.10 and Table 14.3). There are 12 pairs of nerves, each one categorised due to their unique function and these mainly originate from the nuclei in the brainstem. They are always described chronologically, in the order in which they connect to the brain.

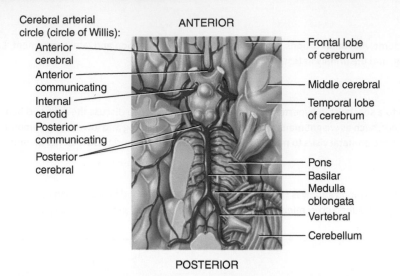

FIGURE 14.9   Circle of Willis. Source: Peate and Evans (2016)/John Wiley & Sons.

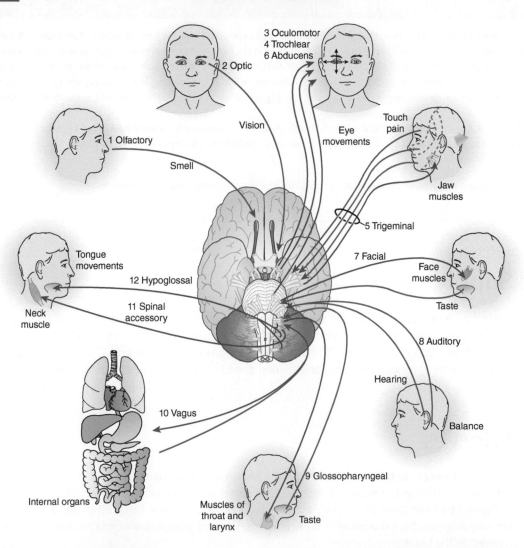

FIGURE 14.10   Function and organisation of the cranial nerves. Source: Peate and Evans (2016)/John Wiley & Sons.

TABLE 14.3 Cranial nerves and primary function.

Number	Name	Sensory/ motor	Function
I	Olfactory	Sensory	Relays signals from the nasal cavity to temporal lobe
II	Optic	Sensory	Relays signals from the retinae of the eyes to the occipital lobe
III	Oculomotor	Motor	Arise from nuclei near the cerebral aqueduct and supply information to the six extrinsic muscles that move the eyeball. The intraocular muscles shape the lens, focus the retina and constrict the pupil and the levitator palpebrae muscles raise the upper eyelids
IV	Trochlear	Motor	Arise from nuclei near the cerebral aqueduct and relay instructions to the superior oblique muscles and extrinsic muscles of the eyes
V	Trigeminal	Both	Sensory impulses transmit signals from pain, temperature and touch from the face and head, oral and nasal cavity and teeth and motor fibres stimulate muscles for mastication
VI	Abducent	Motor	Arise from nuclei under the fourth ventricle and relay instructions to the lateral rectus muscles and intrinsic muscles of the eyeballs that cause abduction
VII	Facial	Both	Fibres arise from the nuclei in the pons, motor fibres signal facial muscles and sensory fibres convey impulses from the taste buds to the cerebral cortex
VIII	Vestibulocochlear	Sensory	Connect the semicircular canals of the inner ear to the cerebellum and the cochlear nerves connect the coati of the inner ear to the auditory cortex in the temporal lobe
IX	Glossopharyngeal	Both	Motor fibres arise from the nuclei on the medulla oblongata and stimulate tongue muscles and cells of the salary glands. The sensory fibres rely upon impulses from the cerebral cortex to the posterior area of the tongue tonsils, and pharynx to activate swallowing and gag reflexes
X	Vagus	Both	These are the longest nerves reaching down into the thorax and abdomen. They relay information to smooth muscles and secretary glands and from the nuclei in the medulla to the pharynx, larynx, trachea and other organs and blood vessels in the thoracic and abdominal cavity
XI	Accessory	Motor	Arise from the nuclei of the medulla oblongata and in the spinal cord, supplying the sternocleidomastoid and trapezius muscle and other associated muscles in the neck
XII	Hypoglossal	Motor	Arise from nuclei in the medulla oblongata and supply muscles of the tongue and the hyoid bone responsible for swallowing and speech

Source: Adapted from Waugh and Grant (2018).

Spinal Cord

The spinal cord, which is continuous with the medulla oblongata, is cylindrical, and is suspended in the vertebral canal. It extends from the first cervical vertebra to the end of the first lumbar vertebra. There are three groups of neurons in the spinal cord: the ascending carry signals upwards to the brain, the descending carry instructions away from the brain and down the spinal cord and interneurons act as connectors between the ascending and descending neurons. The spinal

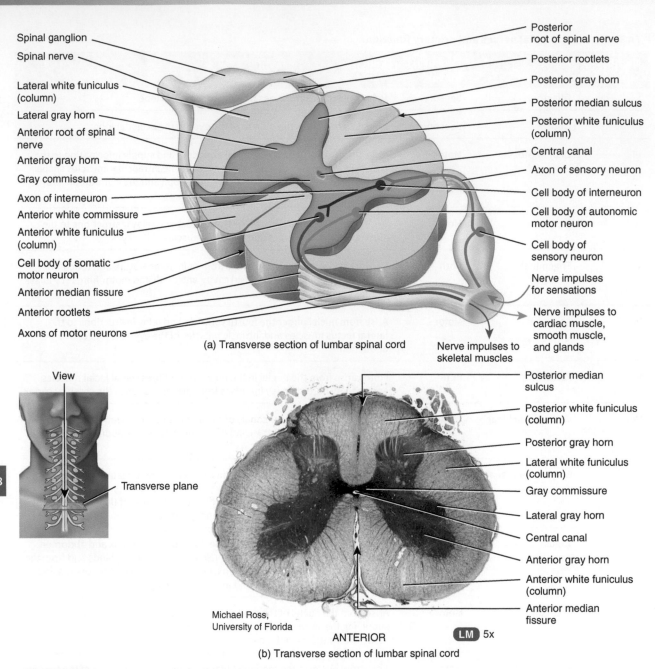

(a) Transverse section of lumbar spinal cord

Spinal ganglion
Spinal nerve
Lateral white funiculus (column)
Lateral gray horn
Anterior root of spinal nerve
Anterior gray horn
Gray commissure
Axon of interneuron
Anterior white commissure
Anterior white funiculus (column)
Cell body of somatic motor neuron
Anterior median fissure
Anterior rootlets
Axons of motor neurons

Posterior root of spinal nerve
Posterior rootlets
Posterior gray horn
Posterior median sulcus
Posterior white funiculus (column)
Central canal
Axon of sensory neuron
Cell body of interneuron
Cell body of autonomic motor neuron
Cell body of sensory neuron
Nerve impulses for sensations
Nerve impulses to cardiac muscle, smooth muscle, and glands

Nerve impulses to skeletal muscles

View

Transverse plane

Posterior median sulcus
Posterior white funiculus (column)
Posterior gray horn
Lateral white funiculus (column)
Gray commissure
Lateral gray horn
Central canal
Anterior gray horn
Anterior white funiculus (column)
Anterior median fissure

Michael Ross, University of Florida

ANTERIOR   LM 5x

(b) Transverse section of lumbar spinal cord

FIGURE 14.11   Spinal cord. Source: Tortora and Derrickson (2017)/John Wiley & Sons.

cord is approximately 42–45 cm long and, like the brain, it is surrounded by the meninges and CSF. However, unlike the brain, its grey matter is central, set out in an H shape (Figure 14.11) and divided into horns. The anterior (ventral) horn contains cell bodies found along the entire length of the spinal cord and stimulates the skeletal muscle. The posterior (dorsal) horn contains sensory neurons and also runs the length of the spinal cord and the lateral horns contain cells that stimulate smooth muscles (Boore et al. 2021).

White matter surrounds the grey matter and also has three columns, the posterior and lateral columns, which are then divided into tracts. The ascending tract, as the name suggests, transmits signals to the brain and the descending away from the brain. Three main pathways on either side of the spinal cord, for sensory information, are the dorsal column tract (fine touch and vibration to the cerebral cortex), the spinothalamic tract (temperature, pain to the cerebral cortex) and the spinocerebellar tract (posture and position from all parts of the body).

Spinal Nerves

There are 31 pairs of spinal nerves attached to the subdivisions of the spinal column, so they are often categorised in numerical order and identified by the first letter of the associated section of the spine. Thus, in the cervical sections of the spine, you will find eight pairs (C1–C8), within the thoracic segments two pairs (T1–T12), and five pairs in the lumbar region (L1–L5), with another five in the sacral area (S1–S5). The last pair is attached to the coccygeal division (Figure 14.12). Once these spinal nerves leave the spinal cord, they break off to form the network of nerves in the body and limbs, some of which combine and entwine to form braided branches – plexuses. These nerves serve as the highway by which impulses are sent to and from all other areas of the body (that the cranial nerves do not control and respond to), via the sophisticated pathway referred the peripheral nervous system, which contains both sensory and motor fibres. These nerves, therefore, make possible movement and sensation; thus, if they are injured or impaired, it can result in a loss of movement or feeling in specific parts of the body. A detailed map of this network is therefore important for healthcare professionals to confirm injury or reduced sensation via testing of the body dermatomes (Figure 14.13).

Red Flag Alert: Epidural Anaesthesia/Analgesia

An epidural is a procedure that involves injecting a medication into the space around the spinal nerves known as the epidural space, to provide pain relief (analgesia) or a total block (anaesthesia). However, while it is considered a safe procedure and is used routinely during labour, there are some complications and risks that midwives and midwifery students need to be cognisant of, as delays in recognition and treatment could result in neurological damage. Because of these risks, and the additional levels of skill needed to insert the needle, epidurals are normally only offered in obstetric units. Blood pressure and fetal heart rate need to be closely monitored. Complications include:

- Hypotension
- Incontinence
- Nausea and vomiting
- Headache
- Bradypnoea
- Temporary or permanent nerve damage
- Infection.

For further information, see NICE (2023b), Roderick et al. (2017) and Yentis et al. (2020).

Reflective Learning Activity

Roderick et al. (2017) conducted a national survey to examine the monitoring of recovery after neuraxial anaesthesia. They found that. within the UK, practice varied widely and only 56% of obstetric units had a policy in place to monitor this treatment. Reflect on what you have witnessed in practice.

- Have you undertaken checks especially related to the assessment of neuraxial anaesthesia?
- Are there specific documents and tools that are used in practice to assist midwives in assessing the level and effectiveness of the types of anaesthesia and analgesia?
- Would you feel confident using these in practice?
- If you suspected neurological changes in the women in your care, what would you do?

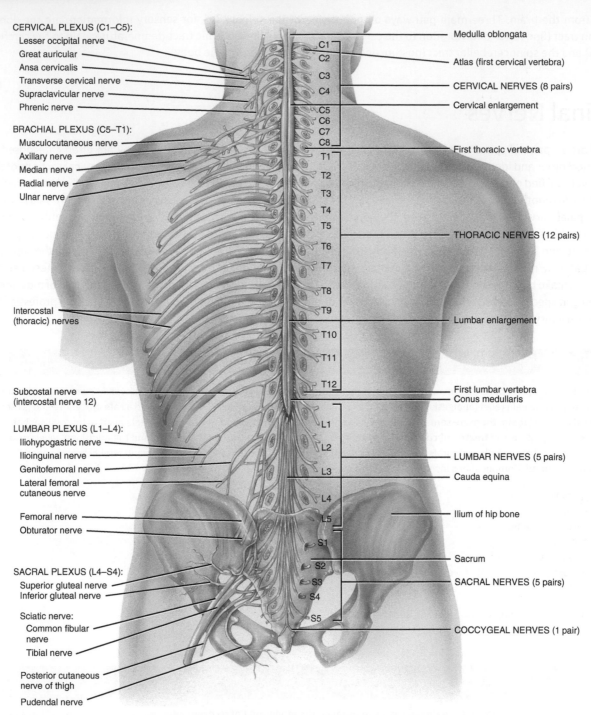

CERVICAL PLEXUS (C1–C5):
  Lesser occipital nerve
  Great auricular
  Ansa cervicalis
  Transverse cervical nerve
  Supraclavicular nerve
  Phrenic nerve

BRACHIAL PLEXUS (C5–T1):
  Musculocutaneous nerve
  Axillary nerve
  Median nerve
  Radial nerve
  Ulnar nerve

Intercostal
(thoracic) nerves

Subcostal nerve
(intercostal nerve 12)

LUMBAR PLEXUS (L1–L4):
  Iliohypogastric nerve
  Ilioinguinal nerve
  Genitofemoral nerve
  Lateral femoral
  cutaneous nerve

  Femoral nerve
  Obturator nerve

SACRAL PLEXUS (L4–S4):
  Superior gluteal nerve
  Inferior gluteal nerve

  Sciatic nerve:
    Common fibular
    nerve
    Tibial nerve

  Posterior cutaneous
  nerve of thigh
  Pudendal nerve

Medulla oblongata

Atlas (first cervical vertebra)

CERVICAL NERVES (8 pairs)

Cervical enlargement

First thoracic vertebra

THORACIC NERVES (12 pairs)

Lumbar enlargement

First lumbar vertebra
Conus medullaris

LUMBAR NERVES (5 pairs)

Cauda equina

Ilium of hip bone

Sacrum

SACRAL NERVES (5 pairs)

COCCYGEAL NERVES (1 pair)

C1
C2
C3
C4
C5
C6
C7
C8
T1
T2
T3
T4
T5
T6
T7
T8
T9
T10
T11
T12
L1
L2
L3
L4
L5
S1
S2
S3
S4
S5

Posterior view of entire spinal cord and portions of spinal nerves

FIGURE 14.12   The spinal nerves. Source: Peate and Evans (2020)/John Wiley & Sons.

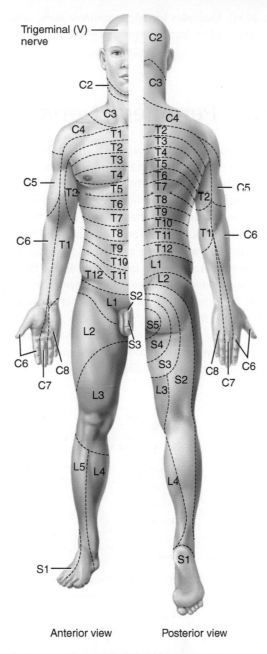

Anterior view   Posterior view

FIGURE 14.13   Dermatomes. Source: Tortora and Derrickson (2017)/John Wiley & Sons.

Sensory Division of the Peripheral Nervous System

As we have seen from the red flag alert on epidural anaesthesia/analgesia, the brain must receive sensory information from visceral and somatic sensations, internal and external structures, for the maintenance of homeostasis and to detect tissue damage. This information is forwarded to the brain through afferent neurons connecting either directly to the cranial nerves or via the ascending tract of the spinal cord. However, before a signal can be transmitted a primary signal needs to be initiated via the activation of sensory receptors. These are organs converting energy from light, pressure and heat into an action potential and these receptors vary depending on their location, the level of sensitivity and the speed of the action required (Boore et al. 2021). Examples include enteroreceptors, which are associated with the internal environment, exteroceptors, with the external environment located in the skin, and proprioceptors, which are related to the position of parts of the body.

Motor Division of the Peripheral Nervous System

The motor division of the peripheral nervous system is associated with the transfer of information away from the brain and spinal cord. It consists of two major pathways, the somatic and autonomic nervous systems. The somatic nervous system voluntarily controls skeletal muscles. It begins in the ventral horn of the spinal cord where it connects to the spinal nerves terminating at striated muscles. The autonomic nervous system involuntarily controls smooth muscles in blood vessels, cardiac muscles, airways and glandular epithelial tissue and is thus associated with bodily functions not under conscious control, such as heart rate, blood pressure and perspiration. These nerves are found in the lateral horn and are not connected directly to muscles, but rather make a synapse in the ganglia of the central nervous system that acts as a junction, connecting preganglionic fibres with the lateral horn and to the muscle via postganglionic fibres.

There are also two branches of the autonomic nervous system, the sympathetic (fight or flight) and parasympathetic (rest and digest) branches (Figure 14.14). The sympathetic nervous system is also referred to as the thoracolumbar division as it includes nerve fibres originating from the thoracic and lumber sections of the spine. Its main role is to control body functions when stressors are present, enabling muscles to react quickly and adrenaline to be released. Conversely, the parasympathetic nervous system is largely active when the body is at rest and is referred to as the craniosacral division due to the fact that it is associated with the spinal nerves emanating from the lower end of the spine.

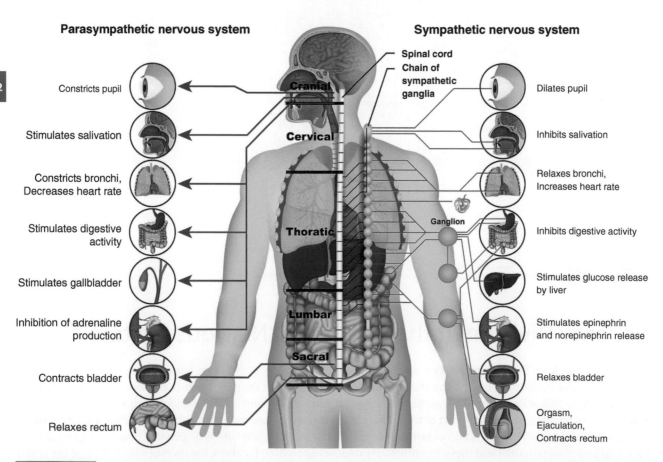

FIGURE 14.14   Sympathetic and parasympathetic branches of the autonomic nervous system. bilderzwerg/Adobe Stock Photos.

> ## Take Home Points
>
> - When caring for any woman, it is important to have a sound understanding of the anatomy and physiology of the nervous system.
> - This knowledge enables midwives to carry out procedures safely but also to recognise disease and neurological disorders that may impact the perinatal journey.
> - It is also essential to include women and their partners in their care and not to make a decision for women, but with women.
> - Any decisions made must be tailored to the individual needs of the woman and need to take into consideration their holistic picture.

Summary

The central nervous system plays an essential role in bodily functions, responses and maintaining homeostasis. Additionally, stressors placed upon the body during pregnancy and labour will initiate changes and adaptations to the central nervous system which impact how women function physically and emotionally during the perinatal journey. Midwives and midwifery students must understand anatomy and physiology and appreciate how the nervous system connects mind and body to be able to practise safely and effectively and to ensure that their care is woman centred, individualised and holistic.

References

Boore, J., Cook, N., and Shepherd, A. (2021). *Essentials of Anatomy and Physiology for Nursing Practice*, 2e. London: Sage.

Dobson, R., Dassan, P., Roberts, M. et al. (2019). UK consensus on pregnancy in multiple sclerosis: 'Association of British Neurologists' guidelines. *Practical Neurology* 19: 106–114.

McErlean, L. and Migliozzi, J.G. (2017). The nervous system. In: *Fundamentals of Anatomy and Physiology for Nursing and Healthcare Students*, 2e (ed. I. Peate and M. Nair), 403–438. Chichester: Wiley.

NICE (2020). *Meningitis: Bacterial Meningitis and Meningococcal Disease*. Clinical Knowledge Summaries. London: National Institute for Health and Care Excellence https://cks.nice.org.uk/topics/meningitis-bacterial-meningitis-meningococcal-disease.

NICE (2022). *Multiple Sclerosis in Adults: Management*. NICE Guideline NG220. London: National Institute for Health and Care Excellence https://www.nice.org.uk/guidance/ng220.

NICE (2023a). *Hypertension in Pregnancy: Diagnosis and Management*. NICE Guideline NG133. London: National Institute for Health and Care Excellence https://www.nice.org.uk/guidance/ng133.

NICE (2023b). *Intrapartum Care*. NICE Guideline NG235. London: National Institute for Health and Care Excellence https://www.nice.org.uk/guidance/ng235.

Peate, I. and Evans, S. (2020). *Fundamentals of Anatomy and Physiology*, 3e. Oxford: Wiley-Blackwell.

Roderick, E., Hoyle, J., and Yentis, S.M. (2017). A national survey of neurological monitoring practice after obstetric regional anaesthesia in the UK. *Anaesthesia* 72: 755–759.

Tortora, G.J. and Derrickson, B.H. (2017). *Tortora's Principles of Anatomy and Physiology*, 15e. Chichester: Wiley.

Waugh, A. and Grant, A. (2018). *Ross and Wilson Anatomy and Physiology in Health and Illness*, 13e. London: Elsevier.

Yentis, S.M., Lucas, D.N., Brigante, L. et al. (2020). Safety guidelines: neurological monitoring associated with the obstetric neuraxial block. *Anaesthesia* 75: 913 919.

313

Online Resources

Multiple Sclerosis Society. Pregnancy, birth, breastfeeding and MS: www.mssociety.org.uk/about-ms/what-is-ms/women-and-ms/pregnancy-and-birth

Multiple Sclerosis Trust. Pregnancy and MS: https://mstrust.org.uk/a-z/pregnancy

Meningitis Research Foundation: https://www.meningitis.org

Glossary

Action potential	A rapid sequence of changes in the voltage across a membrane.
Adrenaline	A hormone released from the adrenal glands to prepare the body for 'fight or flight' responses.
Afferent	Inwards or towards.
Anterior	Near the front.
Autonomic	Involuntary or unconscious.
Concave	A surface that curves inwards.
Contralateral	Relating to the opposite side of the body to which a particular structure or condition occurs.
Convex	A surface that curves inwards.
Convoluted	Intricately folded.
Efferent	Outwards or away.
Endocrine system	A messenger system comprising a collection of ductless glands that produce hormones and secrete them into the circulatory system.
Epidural	On or around the dura mater.
Epithelial tissue	A type of body tissue that forms the covering on all internal and external surfaces of the body.
Ganglion	A neuronal body found in the peripheral nervous system.
Gestation	The period related to the development of the fetus inside the womb between conception and birth.
Gyri	A ridge or fold between two clefts on the cerebral surface in the brain.
Hemispheres	One half of a sphere.
Homeostasis	A self-regulating process where biological systems maintain the stability of internal, physical and chemical conditions.
Inferior	Situated lower down.
Lateral	Of or relating to the side.
Lobe	A roundish and flattish projecting divided by a fissure.
Perinatal	Time immediately before, during and after birth.
Periosteal	Situated around or produced external to bone.
Posterior	Situated behind.
Receptor	An organ or cell able to respond to light, heat or other external stimulus and transmit a signal to a sensory nerve.
Reticula formation	A network of nuclei responsible for consciousness.
Second trimester	Weeks 13 through 27 of pregnancy.
Somatic	Relating to, supplying, or involving skeletal muscle.
Subcortical	Below the cortex.
Sulci	A groove in the cerebral cortex.
Superior	Situated higher up.
Synapse	A gap between two nerve cells, where impulses cross by diffusion of a neurotransmitter.
Thermoregulation	A process that allows the body to maintain its core internal temperature within certain tight parameters.
Viscera	Internal organs in the main cavities of the body, especially those in the abdomen.

Multiple Choice Questions

1. What does the abbreviation CSF stand for?
    a. Cerebrospinal fluid
    b. Cerebellum sebaceous fluid
    c. Cerebrum sebaceous fluid
    d. Central spinal fluid

2. Where is CSF made?
    a. Hypothalamus
    b. Pons
    c. Medulla
    d. Ventricles

3. How many pairs of cranial nerves are there in the brain?
    a. 10
    b. 11
    c. 12
    d. 13

4. How many lobes are in the cerebrum?
    a. 3
    b. 4
    c. 5
    d. 6

5. Which cranial nerve is responsible for the movement of the upper eyelid?
    a. Oculomotor
    b. Trochlear
    c. Abducent
    d. Trigeminal

6. Which lobe of the cerebrum is associated with taste?
    a. Temporal
    b. Parietal
    c. Frontal
    d. Occipital

7. What is the most inferior layer of the meninges?
    a. Dura mater
    b. Pia mater
    c. Arachnoid mater
    d. Subdural mater

8. What part of the diencephalon is associated with melatonin?
    a. Hypothalamus
    b. Thalamus
    c. Pineal body
    d. Pituitary

9. What does ICP mean?
    a. Intercranial pressure
    b. Intracranial pressure
    c. Intercerebrial pressure
    d. Intracerebral pressure

10. Where is the cardiac centre of the brain located?
    a. Pons
    b. Midbrain
    c. Cerebellum
    d. Medulla Oblongata

CHAPTER 15

The Endocrine System

Rosalind Haddrill

AIM

This chapter provides an overview of the endocrine system and the role of hormones in the body, particularly in relation to conception, pregnancy, birth and the postnatal period.

LEARNING OUTCOMES

By the end of the chapter, you will be able to:

- Explain the function of the endocrine system and its relationship to the nervous system.
- Identify parts of the body responsible for the production of hormones and the principal hormones related to reproduction.
- Explain the function of these hormones in relation to maternal health and wellbeing, from conception, through pregnancy, labour and birth, to the puerperium.
- Discuss the impact of hormones on the development of the embryo and fetus and the care of the neonate, particularly in relation to infant feeding.

Test Your Prior Knowledge

1. List as many glands and hormone-producing locations in the pregnant female body as you can. Can you name the hormones they produce?
2. What are the roles of prolactin and oxytocin in human lactation (breastfeeding)? What is the impact of reducing the number or length of breastfeeds on prolactin and oxytocin production?
3. Identify the principal thyroid hormones. What are their functions and how do they change during pregnancy? What impact might this have on the woman, fetus and neonate?
4. Consider the body's response to stress and the 'fight or flight' mechanism? Which hormones are involved, what do they do and why?

Fundamentals of Maternal Anatomy and Physiology, First Edition. Edited by Ian Peate and Claire Leader.
© 2024 John Wiley & Sons Ltd. Published 2024 by John Wiley & Sons Ltd.

Introduction

This chapter considers the anatomy and physiology of the endocrine system, the changes that occur during normal pregnancy and birth and their impact, considering each of the important hormone-producing structures in the body in turn.

Body systems influence and respond to each other. The endocrine system was previously considered to be a discrete system; however, it is now recognised as working with the nervous and immune systems, coordinating and regulating the body's physiology in response to changes inside and outside the body. Many endocrine responses are initiated by neural triggers and the hormones (chemical messengers) produced often also act as neurotransmitters. However, whereas the nervous system responds rapidly, endocrine responses can range from seconds to days, providing slower but more precise adjustments to body functions. A comparison can be seen in Table 15.1.

Hormones produced by the endocrine system are responsible for maintaining homeostasis, a stable internal environment within the body. This includes regulating tissues, organs and the composition of body fluids, sustaining body functions such as the menstrual cycle, triggering survival mechanisms in response to changes in external environment and activating or inhibiting the immune system. The endocrine system is intrinsic to metabolism and growth, but also behaviour and sexual differentiation and development. It plays a key role in all aspects of female reproduction, from the release of the mature ovum, successful implantation and the maintenance of the embryo in early pregnancy, through the development of the fetus, placenta and uterus, to the physiology of labour and birth, lactation and early relationships.

The human endocrine system involves the production of around 50 hormones from a number of glands and cells throughout the body (Figure 15.1). *Endocrine* means secreted into the bloodstream, in contrast to *exocrine*, which means secreted into a duct or opening (e.g. sweat, tears or saliva). Glands consist of groups of secretory cells, which synthesise the hormones, surrounded by a network of diffusion cells, which facilitate transfer of the hormones around the body. Endocrine glands are very vascular, making it easy for hormones to diffuse into the bloodstream. They are distinct structures, such as the pituitary, thyroid or adrenal glands. However, hormones are also produced in endocrine cells within organs and tissues, such as the gastrointestinal tract, pancreas or ovaries. Some hormones are produced in several places. For example, melatonin, a hormone associated with sleep and biorhythms, is produced in the pineal gland but also in a wide range of organs and tissues in the body.

Changes During Pregnancy

During pregnancy, production of many hormone increases. Temporary structures like the placenta and decidua (the modified endometrium, or lining, of the uterus) are responsible for significant hormone production; the fetus can also produce some hormones. Many endocrine changes in pregnancy are the result of hormonal signals from the fetal–placental unit, critical in directing the initiation, maintenance and adaptations of pregnancy, fetal development and the birth process. The fetal endocrine system is largely functional by the end of pregnancy, although some hormones are not produced until puberty. Immediately after birth and expulsion of the placenta, many hormone levels drop or change to facilitate lactation. The endocrine system gradually returns to its prepregnancy state, although levels of some hormones may take up to 12 weeks to do so. Table 15.2 summarises the major hormones relevant to human reproduction.

TABLE 15.1   The nervous system compared with the endocrine system.

	Nervous system	Endocrine system
Speed of action	Seconds	Minutes to hours (or days)
Duration of action	Seconds to minutes	Minutes to days
Method of transmitting messages	Electrical	Chemical
Transport method	Neurones	Hormones

HORMONES

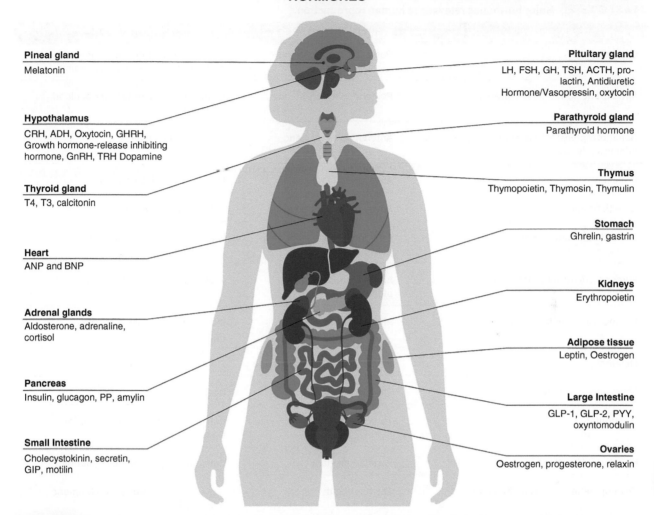

Pineal gland
Melatonin

Hypothalamus
CRH, ADH, Oxytocin, GHRH,
Growth hormone-release inhibiting
hormone, GnRH, TRH Dopamine

Thyroid gland
T4, T3, calcitonin

Heart
ANP and BNP

Adrenal glands
Aldosterone, adrenaline,
cortisol

Pancreas
Insulin, glucagon, PP, amylin

Small Intestine
Cholecystokinin, secretin,
GIP, motilin

Pituitary gland
LH, FSH, GH, TSH, ACTH, pro-
lactin, Antidiuretic
Hormone/Vasopressin, oxytocin

Parathyroid gland
Parathyroid hormone

Thymus
Thymopoietin, Thymosin, Thymulin

Stomach
Ghrelin, gastrin

Kidneys
Erythropoietin

Adipose tissue
Leptin, Oestrogen

Large Intestine
GLP-1, GLP-2, PYY,
oxyntomodulin

Ovaries
Oestrogen, progesterone, relaxin

319

FIGURE 15.1 The endocrine system in women. LH: Luteinising hormone; FSH: Follicle stimulating hormone; GH: Growth hormone; TSH: thyroid-stimulating hormone; ACTH: adrenocorticotrophic hormone; CRH: corticotrophin-releasing hormone; ADH: anti-diuretic hormone (vasopressin); GHRH: Growth hormone releasing hormone; GHRIH: Growth hormone-release inhibiting hormone (somatostatin); GnRH: gonadotrophin-releasing hormone; TRH: Thyrotrophin-releasing hormone; PTH: Parathyroid hormone; T3: Triiodothyronine; T4: Thyroxine; ANP: Atrial Natriuretic Peptide; BNP: Brain natriuretic peptide; PP: Pancreatic polypeptide; GLP-1, GLP-2: Glucagon-like peptides 1 and 2; PYY: Peptide YY; GIP: Glucose-dependent insulinotropic peptide. pikovit/Adobe Stock Photos

Secretion, Transportation and Action of Hormones

Hormones are transported round the body in the blood, either in the plasma (water-soluble hormones) or bound to transport proteins (fat-soluble hormones). Some act locally on adjacent cells, known as paracrine signalling. Hormones bind to target cells, altering the function of these cells. Some act on specific target cells (i.e. those with specific receptors in their cell membranes). Others affect a wide range cells in the body (e.g. thyroxine, which is produced by the thyroid gland).

The action of hormones depends on how they are secreted and the response of their target cells, the number of receptors on the target cells or how quickly the hormone is dissipated or broken down in the bloodstream. For example, the increased number of oxytocin receptors on the uterus by the end of pregnancy increases its sensitivity to this hormone, which is essential for labour and birth. Secretion and regulation is influenced by many factors: by the nervous

TABLE 15.2   Major hormones relevant to human reproduction.

Name	Primarily secreted from	Action
Oxytocin	Posterior pituitary gland	Uterine contraction, lactation – milk ejection, social behaviour, bonding
Antidiuretic hormone/vasopressin	Posterior pituitary gland	Fluid balance, maintenance of blood pressure
Gonadotrophins: follicle-stimulating hormone, luteinising hormone	Anterior pituitary gland	Ovulation (in females)
Prolactin	Anterior pituitary gland	Lactation – milk production
Growth hormone	Anterior pituitary gland	Cell growth, energy for fetus
Thyroid-stimulating hormone	Anterior pituitary gland and placenta	Production of thyroid hormones
Adrenocorticotrophic hormone	Anterior pituitary gland, placenta	Production of cortisol
Melanocyte-stimulating hormone	Anterior pituitary gland	Increased melanin: affects skin pigmentation
Melatonin	Pineal gland, various organs	Regulates sleep and biorhythms
Thyroxine, triiodothyronine	Thyroid gland	Regulates metabolism
Calcitonin	Thyroid gland	Calcium and phosphate regulation, transfer to fetus
Parathyroid hormone	Parathyroid gland	Calcium and phosphate regulation
Thymopoietin, thymosin, thymulin	Thymus gland	Stimulate T-cell production (immune response)
Glucocorticoids: cortisol, corticosterone	Adrenal gland cortex, placenta and uterus	Response to stress, glucose regulation, fluid balance, BP maintenance
Mineralocorticoids (e.g. aldosterone)	Adrenal gland cortex	Fluid/electrolyte balance
Gonadocorticoids (sex hormones): oestrogens (e.g. oestriol), androgens (e.g. testosterone), progesterone	Adrenal gland cortex, ovaries, placenta and fetus	Fertility, male/female characteristics, libido
		Oestrogen: stimulates uterine growth and activity, blood supply, preparation of breasts for lactation
		Progesterone: acts on smooth muscle, inhibits uterine activity in pregnancy
Catecholamines (stress hormones): adrenaline, noradrenaline, dopamine	Adrenal medullae; dopamine also produced by hypothalamus	Response to stress, muscular contraction, cardiovascular and respiratory function; inhibit oxytocin
Glucagon	Pancreas	Converts glycogen into glucose

TABLE 15.2 *(Continued)*

Name	Primarily secreted from	Action
Insulin	Pancreas	Converts glucose into glycogen, encourages glucose uptake, fat storage
Relaxin	Ovaries and decidua (endometrium of uterus)	Stimulates uterine and cardiovascular changes, relaxes pelvic ligaments
Human chorionic gonadotrophin	Trophoblast cells and placenta	Stimulates thyroid, maintains corpus luteum, linked to nausea and vomiting
Human placental lactogen	Trophoblast cells and placenta	Metabolic modification to supply energy to fetus
Serotonin	Central nervous system, intestine, placenta	Mood, cognition, gastrointestinal function, fetal brain development

system (neural stimulation), the availability of binding proteins, chemicals or nutrients in the blood (humoral), environmental changes, or through the influence of other releasing or inhibiting hormones (hormonal). For example, insulin is released from the pancreas in response to rising blood glucose levels following the consumption of carbohydrate; light inhibits the release of melatonin from the pineal gland. Some hormones show temporal patterns of release (e.g. prolactin release is higher at night) whereas others are released in pulses to optimise their effect (e.g. oxytocin, as part of the milk ejection reflex in breastfeeding).

Regulation

Hormone release and levels are regulated through the processes of positive and negative feedback. Positive feedback speeds up processes. For example, the production of prolactin from the anterior pituitary gland during lactation. Prolactin directs lactocyte cells within the breast to produce milk. Suckling by the infant stimulates the production of prolactin and thus milk production increases. However, if this suckling decreases or stops then prolactin production will be reduced and subsequently the amount of milk produced declines. This positive feedback is optimised through early and regular responsive breastfeeding.

Negative feedback slows down processes and maintains homeostasis. For example, the production of thyroid-stimulating hormone (TSH) by the anterior pituitary gland stimulates the thyroid gland to produce thyroid hormones such as thyroxine (T_4). As the levels of T_4 rise, this inhibits the further production of TSH, thus slowing production and maintaining the optimal level in the blood. The hormone insulin lowers blood glucose levels, whereas glucagon converts glycogen stored in the liver and muscles into glucose, to raise blood glucose levels; they work together to maintain normal blood glucose levels (normoglycaemia).

Excretion

Hormones can be excreted via the kidneys in the urine. Some hormones have a short life; oxytocin, for example, has a half-life of a few minutes, whereas others are longer lasting, such as steroid hormones like the oestrogens and cortisol.

The Hypothalamus

The hypothalamus is a small but complex region at the base of the brain, which acts as the 'control centre', linking the nervous and endocrine systems. It receives information from the brain and organs, monitoring levels of chemicals in the body and responding if levels are low or high, controlling hormone release from the endocrine glands. The hypothalamus produces both releasing and inhibiting hormones, which act on the pituitary gland (Figure 15.2, Table 15.3), affecting pituitary hormone production. It also produces hormones such as oxytocin and antidiuretic hormone (ADH), which are transported to the posterior pituitary gland for release, also dopamine, which affects prolactin secretion and gonadotrophin-releasing hormone (GnRH).

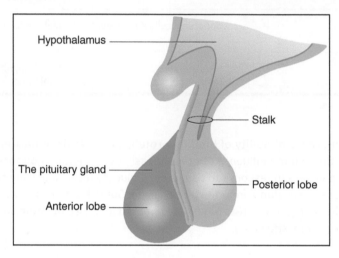

FIGURE 15.2   The hypothalamus and pituitary gland.

TABLE 15.3   **Hypothalamus hormones and their impact on the anterior pituitary gland.**

Hypothalamus hormone	Anterior pituitary gland hormone released/inhibited	Target organ or tissues	Action
Growth hormone-releasing hormone	Growth hormone	Many (including bones, muscles, organs)	Stimulates growth of body cells, facilitates energy to the foetus
Growth hormone-release inhibiting hormone	Inhibits release of growth hormone, thyroid-stimulating hormone, prolactin	Many	Inhibits hormone production in many parts of the body
Thyrotrophin-releasing hormone	Thyroid-stimulating hormone and prolactin	Thyroid gland	Stimulates thyroid hormone release
Corticotrophin-releasing hormone	Adrenocorticotropic hormone	Adrenal cortex	Stimulates corticosteroid release
Prolactin-releasing hormone (theoretical)	Prolactin	Milk producing cells in the breasts	Stimulates milk production
Prolactin-inhibiting hormone (dopamine)	Inhibits release of prolactin	Milk producing cells in the breasts	Inhibits milk production
Gonadotrophin-releasing hormone	Follicle-stimulating hormone, luteinising hormone	Gonads – ovaries	Stimulates ovulation

The Pituitary Gland

The pituitary gland, situated at the base of brain below the hypothalamus, plays a vital role in homeostasis. It has anterior and posterior lobes and a rich blood supply, and is physically connected to the hypothalamus by nerve fibres in the pituitary stalk (Figure 15.2). The posterior lobe of pituitary is composed of specialised secretory cells and nerve fibres from the hypothalamus and brain. It secretes two hormones, oxytocin and ADH, which are both produced in the hypothalamus but stored in and released from the posterior lobe; the posterior lobe does not manufacture hormones itself. The anterior pituitary, sometimes called the 'master endocrine gland', secretes six key hormones in response to hormones released from the hypothalamus (Table 15.3). The anterior pituitary increases in size in pregnancy by approximately 30–50%, mainly due to an increase in lactotrophs (prolactin-releasing cells). It is susceptible to blood loss, particularly in pregnancy, as it is vulnerable to vasospasm following a sudden decrease in arterial blood supply (e.g. as a result of haemorrhage), which can lead to the endocrine disorder Sheehan syndrome (hypopituitarism).

Anterior Pituitary Hormones

The gonadotrophins consist of follicle-stimulating hormone (FSH) and luteinising hormone (LH). FSH stimulates the ovary to produce a Graafian follicle containing a mature ovum in females and stimulates sperm production in males. LH triggers ovulation and maintains the corpus luteum, which develops from an ovarian follicle. The corpus luteum secretes progesterone and relaxin and is essential for establishing and maintaining a pregnancy. In males, LH stimulates production of testosterone in the testes. Both FSH and LH are inhibited during pregnancy, as a result of the influence of the fetoplacental hormones and elevated levels of prolactin.

Production of prolactin is stimulated by a number of hormones produced in the hypothalamus, such as ADH and GnRH; no specific prolactin-releasing hormone has been identified. Prolactin is inhibited by the stress hormone dopamine, also produced by the hypothalamus. Prolactin receptors are found in the breasts and ovaries but also in many other tissues and organs in the body. In non-pregnant females, prolactin leads to breast tenderness and swelling before menstruation. Levels of prolactin rise from early pregnancy, stimulating the development of structures in the breast essential for lactation. However, prolactin's influence on milk production is inhibited by high levels of oestrogen and progesterone antenatally. These levels drop abruptly after delivery of the placenta and increased levels of prolactin directs lactocytes in the breast to produce milk, thus initiating breastmilk production. Figure 15.3 illustrates how hormone levels change during pregnancy and postnatally.

323

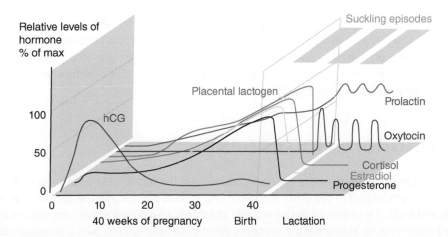

FIGURE 15.3 Different hormone levels during pregnancy and during breastfeeding. Source: Grattan and Ladyman (2020).

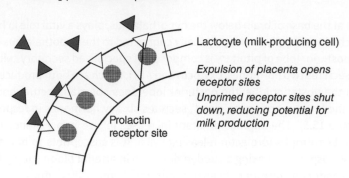

Surges of prolactin when
feeding prime the receptor sites

Lactocyte (milk-producing cell)

*Expulsion of placenta opens
receptor sites*

*Unprimed receptor sites shut
down, reducing potential for
milk production*

Prolactin
receptor site

FIGURE 15.4   The prolactin receptor theory.

The prolactin receptor theory (Figure 15.4) suggests that early breastfeeding, soon after birth, increases the number of prolactin receptors in breast tissue, which optimises milk production (Wambach and Watson 2021). Regular stimulation of the nipple by the infant suckling and removal of milk from the breast results in further release of prolactin and maintains milk production. Levels of prolactin are highest at night. Raised levels of prolactin delay ovulation by inhibiting the ovarian response to FSH, contributing to the contraceptive effect of breastfeeding. If a woman does not breastfeed, prolactin levels drop rapidly and reach non-pregnant levels by around seven days postpartum.

Growth hormone stimulates cells to grow and divide, determining the growth of bone, tissues such as muscles, and organs, including the kidneys and liver. It stimulates protein synthesis and the use of fats for fuel, also glucose conservation. In pregnancy, this helps to facilitate the energy supply to the fetus. Growth hormone stimulates the production of insulin-like growth factors in the liver and regulates other metabolic hormones, including thyroid hormones. The secretion of growth hormone follows a diurnal cycle, being highest during sleep, demonstrating the importance of sleep for recovery from illness and injury. Hyper- or hyposecretion of growth hormone in childhood can lead to excess or diminished growth.

Thyroid-stimulating hormone (TSH) is produced by the anterior pituitary gland but is also synthesised by the placenta during pregnancy. Its release affects the production of hormones by the thyroid gland (see below).

Adrenocorticotrophic hormone (ACTH) is also produced by the anterior pituitary gland, in response to the release of corticotropin-releasing hormone (CRH) from the hypothalamus and is also synthesised by the placenta during pregnancy. ACTH stimulates blood flow to the adrenal glands and the production of glucocorticoids such as cortisol in response to stress, as part of the hypothalamic–pituitary–adrenal (HPA) axis (see below).

Melanocyte-stimulating hormone (MSH) affects skin pigmentation. Melanocytes are responsible for the production of melanin, a group of pigments that affect hair, eye and skin colour. Melanoctyes are primarily found in the outer layer of the skin and the epidermis. Production of melanin is initiated in response to exposure to ultraviolet radiation. A temporary increase in MSH and melanin production during pregnancy, stimulated by oestrogen and progesterone, leads to hyperpigmentation in the majority of women, especially those with darker skin. This condition is called melasma. It manifests itself as dark patches on the skin, usually the face. Pregnant women are also more sensitive to sunburn. Hyperpigmentation also results in the linea nigra, a thin dark line on the skin that runs from the fundus or naval to the pubic area. Hyperpigmentation fades gradually after birth.

Posterior Pituitary Hormones

Oxytocin is a small neuropeptide, or signalling molecule, produced in the hypothalamus but released from the posterior pituitary gland. It is also synthesised in the ovaries, adrenal and thymus glands, and the pancreas, and has widespread effects on the brain and body. It is produced during sex and childbirth, also during social interactions and in response to stress. Oxytocin reduces stress by activating the parasympathetic nervous system, which promotes calm, healing and growth. It also reduces activity in the sympathetic nervous system, which reduces fear and stress, and the production of catecholamines (stress hormones), and increases sociability (Buckley 2015).

Levels increase gradually during pregnancy, and during the first and second stages of labour, with increasing size and frequency of pulses, with a surge around the time of birth itself, stimulating the 'fetal ejection reflex' (Uvnäs-Moberg et al. 2019). Oxytocin levels are particularly elevated in multiparous women during pregnancy. This suggests that oxytocin may mediate some of the physiological changes that are required to give birth for the first time, and these changes may leave the body permanently sensitised to oxytocin (Prevost et al. 2014).

Oxytocin is involved in uterine muscle contraction in labour and also postnatally, helping to minimise blood loss. Peptides cannot enter cells, so bind to receptors located on the surface of the cell. The concentration of uterine oxytocin receptors increases during pregnancy, especially in the upper part of the myometrium, the muscle layer of the uterus, reaching up to 200-fold by the end of pregnancy (Walter et al. 2021). Oxytocin is released in labour due to the stretching of the cervix by the presenting part of the fetus, a neurohormonal feedback mechanism known as Ferguson's reflex (Figure 15.5), which results in an increase in uterine activity. This can be effectively blocked by medical interventions such as epidural analgesia, affecting the progress of labour (Uvnäs-Moberg et al. 2019). Oxytocin release can also be inhibited by stress hormones such as adrenaline, which underpins the use of alternative therapies and coping strategies to promote calm and relaxation during labour and birth.

The use of synthetic oxytocin in labour and postnatally is widespread to augment and induce labour and control postnatal bleeding. However, oxytocin is similar in structure to ADH; it is an ADH agonist, binding to the same receptor sites in the kidneys and eliciting the same response (i.e. water retention). Excessive and sustained use of synthetic oxytocin, for example during labour, can therefore lead to oedema (swelling). Synthetic oxytocin must be used with caution, especially in women with impaired kidney function; for example, as seen in pre-eclampsia, a pathological condition of pregnancy associated with hypertension and proteinuria.

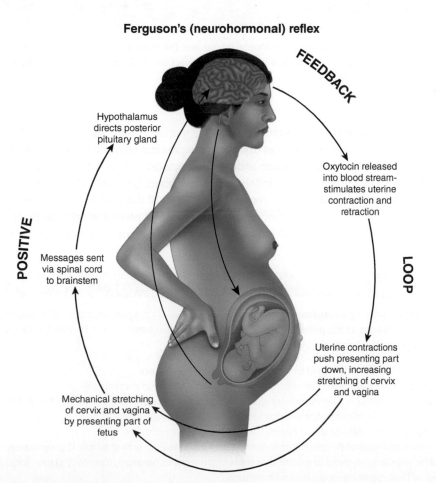

Ferguson's (neurohormonal) reflex

FEEDBACK

Hypothalamus directs posterior pituitary gland

Oxytocin released into blood stream- stimulates uterine contraction and retraction

POSITIVE

LOOP

Messages sent via spinal cord to brainstem

Uterine contractions push presenting part down, increasing stretching of cervix and vagina

Mechanical stretching of cervix and vagina by presenting part of fetus

FIGURE 15.5 Diagram of Ferguson's reflex.

Snapshot 15.1   Induction of Labour

Farida is being induced at 41 weeks of gestation for prolonged pregnancy and is being given an intravenous infusion of synthetic oxytocin to stimulate contractions. Prolonged exposure to high concentrations of oxytocin in labour leads to a reduction in the number of oxytocin receptors on the uterus (known as downregulation), requiring increasing amounts to maintain effective contractions. Overstimulation of the uterus during labour can have a negative impact on the fetus, as blood flow through the cord and subsequently fetal oxygen levels are reduced during each contraction, necessitating close monitoring of the fetal heartrate.

Continuous electronic fetal monitoring is used during Farida's labour. This type of monitoring would be indicated during labour to assess the wellbeing of the fetus and monitor uterine contractions. It involves the use of cardiotocography (CTG) to monitor the baby's heart rate and the mother's uterine contractions in real time.

The dose of synthetic oxytocin given to Farida is monitored and adjusted regularly throughout labour, to balance stimulation of the uterus and effective contractions with fetal wellbeing. Farida is also given intramuscular oxytocin following the birth of her baby, to help to deliver the placenta and reduce her risk of haemorrhage.

Oxytocin has a wide range of neuroendocrine effects, influencing behaviours such as social interaction, communication and aggression, but also parent–infant attachment. Production of oxytocin and ADH by the neonate affects infant brain development and is itself affected by parental oxytocin production. Disruption to this process may have long-term consequences for the development of the 'social brain', impacting on mental wellbeing and adult social behaviour, for example (Hammock 2015).

Reflective Learning Activity

Consider the use of synthetic oxytocin to augment or induce labour and the mechanism for its administration. How is oxytocin administered to optimise uterine contractions, while minimising the impact on the fetus during labour? How do we ensure that a woman is not given too much oxytocin?

Synthetic oxytocin given as an infusion does not cross into the mother's brain because of the blood–brain barrier and does not influence brain function in the same way as oxytocin during normal labour (Uvnäs-Moberg et al. 2019). However, studies suggest that synthetic oxytocin may influence endogenous oxytocin release, via a feedback inhibitory mechanism (Moberg and Prime 2013). The quantity of oxytocin administered during labour is directly related to maternal plasma oxytocin levels at two months postpartum, suggesting a possible long-term effect of this routine intervention (Prevost et al. 2014). Given its neuroendocrine effect, while the use of synthetic oxytocin has clear physiological benefits, the psychological and neurological benefits or harms of elevated oxytocin exposure for mother and infant remain unclear (Hammock 2015).

Red Flag Alert: Fetal Distress

Key concerns in relation to monitoring throughout the administration of oxytocin are the potential risks associated with hyperstimulation of the uterus. This is defined as the presence of more than five uterine contractions in 10 minutes, lasting up to 60 seconds with accompanying abnormal fetal heart rate. Monitoring should include:

- Continuous fetal monitoring should be used to observe for signs of fetal distress.
- Uterine contractions should be palpated and recorded and the infusion titrated accordingly.
- The infusion should be increased in 30-minute intervals until contractions are stabilised at four to five in 10 minutes.
- If contractions exceed five in 10 minutes, the infusion should be reduced or stopped.
- If contractions do not establish despite the optimum dose, request obstetric review.
- Four-hourly abdominal and vaginal examinations should be performed to ensure that labour is progressing.
- Vital signs should be regular monitored to ensure that the woman remains haemodynamically stable, including fluid balance, because of the risk of fluid retention associated with oxytocin.

Oxytocin infusion should be stopped immediately and a medical review requested if any of the following occur:

- Pathological CTG trace
- Antepartum haemorrhage (APH)
- Suspected uterine rupture
- Signs of obstructed labour
- Cord prolapse
- Abnormal fetal presentation (e.g. breech, arm)
- Contractions of more than five in 10 minutes with fetal compromise.

Oxytocin also acts on the myoepithelial cells in the alveoli of the breasts in response to the infant suckling. This results in contraction of these cells, which releases milk from the lactocytes they surround into branching ducts that flow to the nipple (Figure 15.6). The pulsatility of oxytocin release is a critical aspect of the action of oxytocin in such milk ejection. This 'let-down reflex' can also occur in the mother following sensory stimulation, such as the sight, sound or smell of her infant, and becomes a conditioned response (Moberg and Prime 2013; Figure 15.7).

Reflective Learning Activity

Reflect on your experience of supporting a woman who is breastfeeding.

- How can you support 'responsive feeding'?
- What is the physiology behind this process?

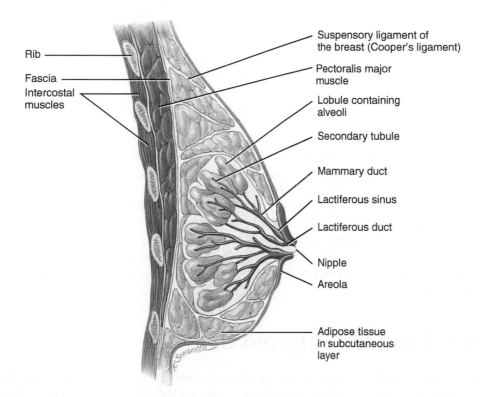

Rib

Fascia

Intercostal muscles

Suspensory ligament of the breast (Cooper's ligament)

Pectoralis major muscle

Lobule containing alveoli

Secondary tubule

Mammary duct

Lactiferous sinus

Lactiferous duct

Nipple

Areola

Adipose tissue in subcutaneous layer

Sagittal section

FIGURE 15.6 Breastfeeding – the structure of the breast.

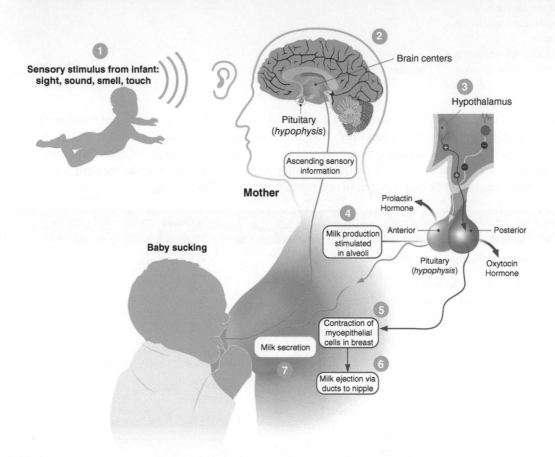

The pituitary gland control milk secretion

1 Sensory stimulus from infant: sight, sound, smell, touch

2 Brain centers

3 Hypothalamus

Pituitary (*hypophysis*)

Ascending sensory information

Mother

Prolactin Hormone

4 Milk production stimulated in alveoli

Anterior

Posterior

Pituitary (*hypophysis*)

Oxytocin Hormone

Baby sucking

5 Contraction of myoepithelial cells in breast

Milk secretion

7

6 Milk ejection via ducts to nipple

FIGURE 15.7   Breastfeeding – the role of oxytocin and prolactin. Source: Alden (n.d.). PATTARAWIT/Adobe Stock Photos

ADH acts on the nephrons in the kidneys to reabsorb water and reduce urine production, in response to a decrease in blood fluid volume or blood pressure, monitored by receptors in the hypothalamus. These receptors are reset in pregnancy to accommodate the increased circulating blood volume. ADH also acts as a vasoconstrictor to help maintain blood pressure, for example during haemorrhage. ADH release is stimulated by pain and drugs such as nicotine and morphine, whereas alcohol and excess water consumption inhibit ADH release, resulting in diuresis: increased or excessive production of urine. ADH is sometimes called vasopressin and, like oxytocin, is also involved in human social behaviour and bonding (Hammock 2015).

The Thyroid and Parathyroid Glands

The thyroid and parathyroid glands are situated in the neck, in front of the trachea and behind the larynx. The parathyroid gland is found on the posterior surface of the thyroid gland. The thyroid is the largest endocrine gland and is extremely vascular. It is supplied with blood through thyroid arteries branching from the carotid and subclavian arteries. The glands secrete thyroxine (T_4), triiodothyronine (T_3) and calcitonin from follicular and parafollicular cells. Iodine in the diet is required for the production of thyroid hormones.

Thyroxine (T_4) and triiodothyronine (T_3) are produced by the thyroid in response to TSH being released from the anterior pituitary gland. These hormones are essential for metabolic processes, physical and mental growth, regulating metabolic rate, the metabolism of carbohydrates (via the pancreas), fats and proteins, also the functioning of cardiac, nervous and reproductive systems, so have an impact on most cells of the body. The release of T_4 and T_3 is highest at night, with a negative feedback system controlling levels (high levels of TSH result in low secretion of T_4 and T_3, and vice versa).

Overall, thyroid function remains normal during most pregnancies, balanced by changes in the metabolism of iodine, requirements for which double in pregnancy. During early pregnancy, the maternal thyroid gland provides the fetus with thyroxine, stimulated by an increase in several hormones, including human chorionic gonadotrophin (hCG) and oestrogen. As a result, the size and activity of the thyroid glands increase. Increased T_4 and hCG are linked to nausea and vomiting during this period. Increased T_4 and T_3 production leads to an increase in metabolic rate, which optimises glucose provision to the fetus. From around 12 weeks of gestation, both maternal and fetal glands produce T_4. In the neonate, thyroid hormones contribute to metabolism, including the metabolism of brown fat to help with temperature regulation, and surfactant production, which affects lung function. After birth, maternal thyroid hormones take approximately 6–12 weeks to return to their prepregnancy levels.

Hyperthyroidism is caused by an overactive thyroid gland, hypothyroidism underactive. Both affect fertility. The treatment of women with either condition can be affected by pregnancy: careful monitoring is needed, as drug requirements may change due to altered metabolic demands. Thyroid hormones are essential for maturation of the fetal brain and fetal growth. Low levels during pregnancy can result in congenital hypothyroidism in the newborn, which requires treatment in the neonatal period to prevent permanent neurological damage. Congenital hypothyroidism is screened for on day 5, as part of the UK Newborn Screening Programme (Public Health England 2018).

Calcitonin is secreted in response to high levels of calcium and phosphate in the blood. It regulates the levels of these minerals, for example by reducing the amount of calcium released from bone and promoting uptake and increasing the amount secreted by the renal system. Calcitonin levels increase in pregnancy and during breastfeeding, facilitating the transfer of maternal calcium to the fetus/infant while protecting the maternal skeleton from bone loss (Canul-Medina and Fernandez-Mejia 2019).

Parathyroid hormone (PTH) is secreted by the parathyroid gland. PTH maintains calcium homeostasis. It works as an antagonist to calcitonin to regulate calcium and phosphate, via the bones and kidneys. It also promotes formation of calcitriol (the active form of vitamin D) in the kidneys, which is involved in absorption of calcium and other minerals in the intestine and may affect the function of the placenta (Wagner and Hollis 2022). Levels of calcitriol increase in pregnancy.

329

The Adrenal Glands

The adrenal gland is situated above each kidney. The gland consists of an inner medulla (part of the sympathetic nervous system) and an outer cortex. The cortex is responsible for the secretion of a range of steroid (cholesterol-based, fat-soluble) hormones: corticosteroids (glucocorticoids and mineralocorticoids) and gonadocorticoids (sex hormones).

Adrenal Cortex Hormones

Glucocorticoids include cortisol and corticosterone, which have a wide range of effects throughout the body, in all cells and organs. They maintain homeostasis and regulate metabolism, particularly the metabolism of carbohydrates, to maintain a steady level of plasma glucose. Cortisol can also increase vasoconstriction to maintain blood pressure and fluid balance, and increase circulatory efficiency; they also control sodium and water absorption in the kidneys. Cortisol acts as an anti-inflammatory and can suppress or regulate the immune system. The increase in steroid levels during pregnancy may also lead to an improvement in certain conditions such as rheumatoid arthritis and eczema.

Glucocorticoids are also produced as part of the body's response to stress. Stress in this context is any challenge that has the potential to disrupt homeostasis, including physical stressors like infection or injury, exposure to adverse

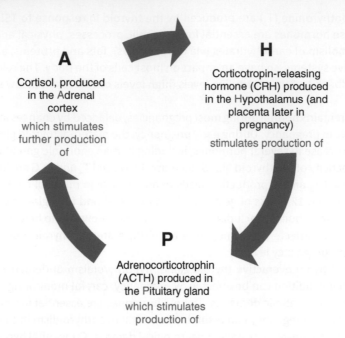

A
Cortisol, produced
in the Adrenal
cortex
which stimulates
further production
of

H
Corticotropin-releasing
hormone (CRH) produced
in the Hypothalamus (and
placenta later in
pregnancy)
stimulates production of

P
Adrenocorticotrophin
(ACTH) produced in
the Pituitary gland
which stimulates
production of

FIGURE 15.8   The hypothalamic–pituitary–adrenal axis.

environments and psychological stress such as fear or anxiety. This systemic stress response combines both the suppressive and stimulating actions of glucocorticoids, to provide energy for a 'flight or fight' response (see also catecholamines).

The production of glucocorticoids is stimulated by the release of ACTH from the anterior pituitary in response to the release of CRH from the hypothalamus and following a circadian pattern, increasing after sleep. This is called the hypothalamic–pituitary–adrenal (HPA) axis (Figure 15.8).

During pregnancy, the HPA axis is stimulated and levels of glucocorticoids rise, in response to oestrogen and progesterone, resulting in increased metabolic activity and cardiac output. This enables body systems to adapt to the requirements of pregnancy. In the second half of pregnancy, the fetal adrenal glands begin to produce cortisol, which promotes maturation of fetal organs, such as the lungs, in preparation for extrauterine life. Synthetic steroids can be used to help to mature the lungs and reduce the chance of respiratory distress in the neonate if born prematurely. The fetus, decidua and placenta also stimulate the maternal HPA axis in late pregnancy; increased cortisol contributes to the onset of labour, increasing the production of prostaglandins and oestrogens, which enhance uterine contractility. However, studies suggest that fetal exposure to excess maternal cortisol, for example as a result of chronic stress, may impact on birth outcomes and result in impaired brain development and increased risk of chronic illness in later life (Duthie and Reynolds 2013).

Mineralocorticoids include aldosterone, which is involved in the reabsorption of sodium in kidneys, sweat and saliva, and the removal of hydrogen ions in urine, to maintain the water–electrolyte balance. Aldosterone is part of the renin-angiotensin mechanism, which controls blood volume and pressure and the amount of water and electrolytes in extracellular fluid by affecting sodium and potassium concentrations. In pregnancy, levels are increased as a result of the actions of oestrogen and progesterone.

Gonadocorticoids comprise a group of structurally related sex hormones, including oestrogens, androgens and progesterone. All are produced by both men and women, but in different amounts. They are involved in changes at puberty, being produced by the gonads (the primary reproductive organs): the testes in the male and the ovaries in the female. Androgens such as testosterone facilitate the maintenance of male characteristics and fertility, also libido in both men and women; oestrogens such as oestradiol facilitate the maintenance of female characteristics and fertility.

In pregnancy, levels of oestrogens and progesterone rise significantly, being produced initially by the corpus luteum, then the placenta and fetus. For example, the primary oestrogen is oestriol, which increases by 1000 times during pregnancy. This rise ensures the continuation of pregnancy, for example by facilitating uterine growth, activity and enhanced blood supply, also preparation of the breasts for lactation. Oestrogen stimulates the formation of oxytocin receptors on uterine muscle (myometrium), to prepare the uterus for labour and birth, and acts on the thyroid gland to increase production too.

Progesterone increases threefold by end of pregnancy. It has many functions, including relaxing smooth muscle, for example blood vessels and in the gastrointestinal and renal systems. The increased level of progesterone delays gastric emptying, which may be linked to nausea and vomiting in early pregnancy. It acts as an immunosuppressant and stimulates the formation of the decidua (the maternal part of placenta) from the endometrium and also inhibits uterine action until the end of pregnancy.

Snapshot 15.2   Haemorrhoids and Varicose Veins

Amie is visiting her community midwife Jo for an antenatal appointment at 34 weeks of gestation in her first pregnancy. She asks Jo about the haemorrhoids and varicose veins in her legs that she is experiencing, also about constipation. Jo explains that increased progesterone levels relax blood vessels and may result in varicose veins during pregnancy. Many women experience this.

The increasing size of the uterus in late pregnancy also affects venous return in the legs. Resting and elevating her legs, and performing gentle leg exercises, will help. Haemorrhoids are a type of varicose vein too. Jo explains about the impact of progesterone on the digestive system, which slows the passage of food through the intestine, increasing water absorption. She advises Amie to increase the amount of fruit and vegetables in her diet, also the amount of water she drinks each day, as these will help reduce the constipation and pressure on the haemorrhoids. Jo advises that varicose veins diminish in size after birth but may return in future pregnancies.

Adrenal Medulla Hormones

The adrenal medulla is part of the sympathetic nervous system. It produces the catecholamines (stress hormones) adrenaline and noradrenaline, together with dopamine (which can be modified to form adrenaline). Dopamine is also produced by the hypothalamus and suppresses the secretion of prolactin from the pituitary gland.

This is part of the body's acute stress response – a physiological state of hyperarousal in response to short-term stress that threatens homeostasis. This triggers a response in the hypothalamus, resulting in the release of hormones from the pituitary and adrenal glands, including ACTH, adrenaline and cortisol. These hormones increase muscular contraction, cardiovascular and respiratory function, and decrease digestion. Catecholamines stimulate the liver to produce glucose and prepare the body for action: 'flight or fight'. The heart increases its rate and strength, peripheral blood supply is reduced to prioritise essential organs such as the heart, brain and muscles, resulting in paleness. Dilation of pupils occurs, tear production and salivation are inhibited, release of blood clotting factors is increased, to protect the body from possible injury.

Neuroendocrine evidence from animal and human studies suggests that oxytocin, in conjunction with female reproductive hormones, such as oestrogen and endogenous opioids, may be responsible for downregulating this stress response, activating the parasympathetic nervous system and reducing activity in the sympathetic nervous system. However, oxytocin release itself can be inhibited by catecholamines, impacting the progress of labour and birth.

Reflective Learning Activity

Reflect on your experience of caring for a woman during spontaneous/physiological labour and birth.

- How do midwives support the woman and her partner and manage the birth environment?
- How might this help to optimise oxytocin production and minimise production of stress hormones such as cortisol and adrenaline? Why does this matter?

The Thymus Gland

Situated in between lungs, the thymus gland secretes hormones such as thymopoietin, thymosin and thymulin to stimulate production of T cells (T lymphocytes) in the bone marrow, as part of an immune response. Increased levels of some T cells help to balance the body's immune response to pregnancy, protecting the fetus (Hellberg et al. 2019)

The Pineal Gland

Melatonin is produced in the pineal gland in the brain but also in a wide range of organs and tissues in the body, including the uterus, placenta and immune system cells. It is secreted in a circadian manner, with highest levels at night: its secretion is stimulated by darkness and inhibited by light. It has an impact on biorhythms, for example daily variations in temperature, sleep and appetite, and a critical role in homeostasis. Melatonin has antioxidant and anti-inflammatory properties and impaired levels have been linked to diseases that develop in adult life, through the concept of fetal programming (Kvetnoy et al. 2022). It regulates the production of prolactin, FSH and LH. Melatonin appears to be linked to successful pregnancy outcomes in animal and human studies, with reduced levels associated with reproductive dysfunction and pregnancy complications such as pre-eclampsia and intrauterine growth restriction, linked to placental function. Melatonin levels increase during pregnancy, particularly in the third trimester, and are neuroprotective to the fetus through the regulation of fetal sleep patterns. Melatonin is provided to the infant through breastmilk; production in the infant is not fully functioning until weeks or months after birth (Voiculescu et al. 2014)

Endocrine Cells in the Body

Endocrine cells exist in the many organs and tissues in the body, including the ovaries, testes, placenta, pancreas and digestive system. Individual cells can produce hormones too but the function of these is not always clear.

The pancreas is made up of both exocrine and endocrine cells. In the islets of Langerhans, different cells have different functions. This includes alpha cells, which secrete glucagon when blood glucose levels are low. Glucagon converts glycogen, stored in the liver and muscles, into glucose. Beta cells secrete insulin when blood glucose levels are high. Insulin converts glucose into glycogen for storage, increases the uptake of glucose by cells, especially muscle cells, and the storage of fats in adipose tissue. Other cells in the pancreas secrete hormones which regulate the secretion of glucagon, insulin and digestive enzymes.

Placental hormones result in a state of progressive insulin resistance during pregnancy. Diabetes with onset during pregnancy (gestational diabetes) results from reduced capacity to compensate for this resistance, resulting in maternal hyperglycaemia (high blood glucose) and an increase in plasma glucose availability to the fetus. Strict carbohydrate restriction or insulin therapy may be required to minimise risks to the fetus, for example from excessive fetal growth (macrosomia), as a result of this.

Reflective Learning Activity

How is fetal growth monitored during pregnancy? What is a normal weight for a newborn? What actions should be taken antenatally if growth is restricted or excessive?

Relaxin

Relaxin is released initially by the corpus luteum and later produced by the placenta and the decidua. Levels are highest at the end of the first trimester of pregnancy. Relaxin stimulates endometrial decidualisation – changes to the cells of the endometrium in preparation for, and during, pregnancy – and other changes to facilitate successful implantation of the embryo and development of the placenta. It facilitates many of the cardiovascular and renal adaptations of pregnancy and inhibits uterine contractions, having vasodilation and antifibrotic properties (Sarwar et al. 2017). Relaxin affects the cervix to facilitate softening and ripening. Similar in structure to insulin, elevated concentrations of maternal relaxin during pregnancy are associated with preterm birth and low levels associated with increased insulin resistance (Goldsmith and Weiss 2009).

Relaxin relaxes pelvic ligaments and is thought to soften the symphysis pubis, to allow the growth of the uterus into the abdomen. Some studies have suggested a relationship between higher relaxin levels in pregnant women with pelvic joint instability and pelvic girdle pain, but other studies have not (Aldabe et al. 2012). Pelvic girdle pain is common, affecting about 20% of pregnant women, especially those with a previous history of low back pain. Women have reduced mobility and struggle to function during pregnancy and are at increased risk of postnatal depressive symptoms (Fishburn and Cooper 2015).

Human Chorionic Gonadotrophin

Human chorionic gonadotrophin (hCG) is initially produced by embryonic trophoblast cells and then the placenta. This hormone stimulates the thyroid gland, affects appetite, thirst and fluid balance, through ADH release. It also stimulates ovulation, also progesterone production, for example in the corpus luteum in early pregnancy, until the placenta takes over. Increased levels of hCG are an early positive sign of pregnancy: the presence of hCG can be detected in urine two weeks after conception, which is used in some pregnancy tests. Low levels are associated with early pregnancy failure. hCG peaks around the end of the first trimester, at 12–14 weeks, mirroring the incidence of nausea and vomiting in pregnancy, suggesting an association, alongside the rise in T_4.

Human Placental Lactogen

Human placental lactogen (hPL) is also produced by trophoblast cells and the placenta. It is only present during pregnancy. Similar to growth hormone, hPL modifies the metabolic state of the mother to facilitate the energy supply to the fetus. It is antagonistic to insulin, and has a diabetogenic effect, increasing maternal metabolism and the use of fat for energy and reducing the uptake of glucose by cells, so blood glucose levels remain higher for fetal use. hPL increases as hCG falls, in parallel with the size of the placenta. Low levels are associated with pregnancy failure. hPL mimics prolactin and competes with it for receptors on the breast. It is unclear what role hPL plays in human lactation, but a fall in hPL after birth of the placenta is associated with a rise in prolactin.

Prostaglandins

Prostaglandins are an example of 'eicosanoids' or local hormones, present and synthesised in most tissues, including the myometrium of the uterus, the cervix, ovaries, placenta and fetal membranes. They act on the tissue that secretes them (autocrine) or adjacent tissues (paracrine). Their functions are wide ranging; prostaglandins are short-lived vasodilators, inhibit blood clotting, influence muscle contraction and the body's inflammatory response. They also stimulate uterine contractions. Synthetic prostaglandins have been used to induce labour since the 1960s.

333

Reflective Learning Activity

Consider the use of synthetic prostaglandins in maternity care.

- How are synthetic prostaglandins used to induce labour?
- How are they administered and what risks are associated with their use?

Serotonin

Serotonin is produced in the brainstem and the intestine and has a wide range of functions, including regulation of mood, appetite, digestion and sleep. Serotonin also has some cognitive functions, influencing memory and learning. Drugs that alter serotonin levels are used in treating depression and anxiety. Levels rise in pregnancy: the placenta provides serotonin to the fetal brain, which may be important for normal brain development (Bonnin and Levitt 2011).

Take Home Points

- The endocrine system works with the nervous and immune systems, coordinating and regulating the body's physiology in response to internal and external changes.
- Around 50 hormones (chemical messengers) are produced in glands and cells throughout the body. These play a key role in body functions, including all aspects of female reproduction.
- During pregnancy, production of many hormones increases; the placenta, uterus and fetus also produce hormones, which direct the adaptations necessary for pregnancy, promote fetal development, facilitate the birth process and breastfeeding.
- Midwifery care aims to monitor maternal adaptations and optimise the physiology of birth, lactation and early relationships between mother and infant.

Summary

This chapter has provided readers with detail regarding intricate interplay between the endocrine system and maternal health, exploring the hormonal changes that occur throughout pregnancy, labour and postpartum. Understanding the endocrine adaptations is crucial for midwives and other health and care professionals involved in maternal care, as these changes bring together the physiological transformations necessary to support a healthy pregnancy and successful childbirth. The chapter bridges theoretical knowledge with practical applications, fostering a holistic understanding of the endocrine system's role in maternity care ensure that the woman is at the centre of all that is done.

References

Aldabe, D., Ribeiro, D.C., Milosavljevic, S., and Dawn Bussey, M. (2012). Pregnancy-related pelvic girdle pain and its relationship with relaxin levels during pregnancy: a systematic review. *European Spine Journal* 21 (9): 1769–1776.

Alden, K. R. (n.d.). Newborn nutrition and feeding, Chapter 18. *Nursekey* https://nursekey.com/newborn-nutrition-and-feeding-2 (accessed 4 November 2023).

Bonnin, A. and Levitt, P. (2011). Fetal, maternal, and placental sources of serotonin and new implications for developmental programming of the brain. *Neuroscience* 197: 1–7. https://doi.org/10.1016/j.neuroscience.2011.10.005.

Buckley, S.J. (2015). Executive summary of hormonal physiology of childbearing: evidence and implications for women, babies, and maternity care. *Journal of Perinatal Education* 24 (3): 145–153. https://doi.org/10.1891/1058-1243.24.3.145.

Canul-Medina, G. and Fernandez-Mejia, C. (2019). Morphological, hormonal, and molecular changes in different maternal tissues during lactation and post-lactation. *Journal of Physiological Sciences* 69 (6): 825–835. https://doi.org/10.1007/s12576-019-00714-4.

Duthie, L. and Reynolds, R.M. (2013). Changes in the maternal hypothalamic-pituitary-adrenal axis in pregnancy and postpartum: influences on maternal and fetal outcomes. *Neuroendocrinology* 98 (2): 106–115. https://doi.org/10.1159/000354702.

Fishburn, S. and Cooper, T. (2015). Pelvic girdle pain: are we missing opportunities to make this a problem of the past? *British Journal of Midwifery* 23 (11): 774–778. https://doi.org/10.12968/bjom.2015.23.11.774.

Goldsmith, L.T. and Weiss, G. (2009). Relaxin in human pregnancy. *Annals of the New York Academy of Sciences* 1160: 130–135. https://doi.org/10.1111/j.1749-6632.2008.03800.x.

Grattan, D.R. and Ladyman, S.R. (2020). Neurophysiological and cognitive changes in pregnancy. *Handbook of Clinical Neurology* 171: 25–55.

Hammock, E.A. (2015). Developmental perspectives on oxytocin and vasopressin. *Neuropsychopharmacology* 40 (1): 24–42.

Hellberg, S., Mehta, R.B., Forsberg, A. et al. (2019). Maintained thymic output of conventional and regulatory T cells during human pregnancy. *Journal of Allergy and Clinical Immunology* 143 (2): 771–775.e777. https://doi.org/10.1016/j.jaci.2018.09.023.

Kvetnoy, I., Ivanov, D., Mironova, E. et al. (2022). Melatonin as the cornerstone of neuroimmunoendocrinology. *International Journal of Molecular Sciences* 23 (3): 1835.

Moberg, K.U. and Prime, D.K. (2013). Oxytocin effects in mothers and infants during breastfeeding. *Infantry* 9 (6): 201–206.

Prevost, M., Zelkowitz, P., Tulandi, T. et al. (2014). Oxytocin in pregnancy and the postpartum: relations to labor and its management. *Frontiers in Public Health* 2: https://doi.org/10.3389/fpubh.2014.00001.

Public Health England. (2018). Newborn blood spot screening: programme overview. https://www.gov.uk/guidance/newborn-blood-spot-screening-programme-overview (accessed 4 November 2023).

Sarwar, M., Du, X.J., Dschietzig, T.B., and Summers, R.J. (2017). The actions of relaxin on the human cardiovascular system. *British Journal of Pharmacology* 174 (10): 933–949. https://doi.org/10.1111/bph.13523.

Uvnäs-Moberg, K., Ekström-Bergström, A., Berg, M. et al. (2019). Maternal plasma levels of oxytocin during physiological childbirth – a systematic review with implications for uterine contractions and central actions of oxytocin. *BMC Pregnancy and Childbirth* 19 (1): 285. https://doi.org/10.1186/s12884-019-2365-9.

Voiculescu, S., Zygouropoulos, N., Zahiu, C., and Zagrean, A. (2014). Role of melatonin in embryo fetal development. *Journal of Medicine and Life* 7 (4): 488.

Wagner, C.L. and Hollis, B.W. (2022). The extraordinary metabolism of vitamin D. *eLife* 11: e77539. https://doi.org/10.7554/eLife.77539.

Walter, M.H., Abele, H., and Plappert, C.F. (2021). The role of oxytocin and the effect of stress during childbirth: neurobiological basics and implications for mother and child. *Frontiers in Endocrinology* 12: 1409.

Wambach, K. and Spencer, B. (2021). Anatomy and physiology of lactation. In: Breastfeeding and Human Lactation, 6e, (ed. K. Wambach and B. Spencer), 49–84. Burlington, MA: Jones and Bartlett Learning.

335

Online Resources

British Thyroid Foundation: https://www.btf-thyroid.org
The Pituitary Foundation. What are hormones? www.pituitary.org.uk/information/hormones
The Society for Endocrinology. You and your hormones: https://www.yourhormones.info

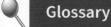

Glossary

Agonist	A chemical that binds to and activates cell receptors to produce a biological response.
Antagonist	A chemical that interferes with or inhibits the physiological action of another.
Autocrine	Where a hormone acts on the cells/tissues where it is produced.
Catecholamines	Hormones such as adrenaline and noradrenaline produced by the adrenal gland in response to stress.
Circadian rhthym	Physical, mental and behavioural changes in the body that follow a 24-hour cycle.

Corpus luteum	A structure in the ovary that secretes hormones essential for establishing and maintaining a pregnancy.
Downregulation	A decrease in the number of receptors on the surface of target cells, making them less sensitive to a hormone.
Endocrine	Secreted into the bloodstream.
Endogenous	Developing or originating within the body.
Endometrium	The lining of the uterus; it is shed during menstruation and modified in pregnancy to become the decidua, the maternal part of the placenta.
Exocrine	Secreted into a duct or opening (e.g. sweat, tears or saliva).
First trimester	The first 12 weeks of pregnancy.
Homeostasis	The state of balanced internal physical and chemical conditions maintained by the body.
Myometrium	The muscle layer of the uterus. Contracts and retracts during labour under the influence of oxytocin, to facilitate the birth of the fetus.
Neurotransmitters	Chemical messengers in the nervous system that transmit messages between neurons or from neurons to muscles.
Neuropeptide	Chemical messenger made up of small chains of amino acids (proteins), such as oxytocin, which affects the nervous system and other cells.
Osmoreceptor	Receptor in the central nervous system that responds to changes in the osmotic pressure of the blood.
Paracrine	Where a hormone acts on nearby cells close to where it is produced.
Steroid	A fat-soluble organic compound with a specific molecular configuration. Includes all the hormones produced by the adrenal cortex, such as the sex hormones.
Third trimester	The final part of pregnancy, from 28 weeks onwards.

Multiple Choice Questions

1. Which term means 'secreted into the bloodstream'?
   a. Exocrine
   b. Paracrine
   c. Endogenous
   d. Endocrine

2. Which hormone is responsible for the production of milk by lactocytes in the breast?
   a. Oxytocin
   b. Prostaglandin
   c. Prolactin
   d. Human placental lactogen

3. Steroid hormones, produced in the adrenal gland, are cholesterol-based and fat-soluble. Which of these is an example of a steroid hormone?
   a. Oxytocin
   b. Cortisol
   c. Calcitonin
   d. Antidiuretic hormone

4. Which hormone is important in labour, acting on the myometrium (muscle layer) of the uterus to produce contractions?
   a. Oxytocin
   b. Oestrogen
   c. Adrenalin
   d. Relaxin

5. Which hormone/hormones are involved in the 'fight or flight' response to stress?
   a. Adrenaline
   b. Cortisol
   c. Noradrenaline
   d. All of the above

6. What are the two key hormones produced by the pancreas that are responsible for regulating glucose levels in the blood?
   a. Insulin and glycogen
   b. Insulin and glucagon
   c. Glycogen and glucose
   d. Glucagon and glucose

7. Which hormone is responsible for the relaxation of smooth muscle during pregnancy, for example in the gastrointestinal system, which may result in nausea and vomiting?
   a. Progesterone
   b. Relaxin
   c. Prolactin
   d. Prostaglandin

8. Where is the hormone oxytocin produced?
   a. Adrenal gland
   b. Hypothalamus
   c. Posterior pituitary gland
   d. Anterior pituitary gland

9. Hormones produced by the endocrine system are responsible for maintaining a stable internal environment within the body. What is this process known as?
   a. Haemostasis
   b. Hypothermia
   c. Homeostasis
   d. Normoglycaemia

10. Triiodothyronine (T_3) is an important hormone affecting metabolism. Where does it come from?
    a. Thymus gland
    b. Thyroid gland
    c. Parathyroid gland
    d. Placenta

CHAPTER **16**

The Immune System

Angela Frankland

AIM

The aim of this chapter is to explain the role of the immune system, together with adaptations in pregnancy and implications for clinical practice.

LEARNING OUTCOMES

By the end of this chapter, you will be able to:

- Understand how the body responds to infection.
- Explain the difference in the innate and adaptive immune systems.
- Discuss the inflammatory response.
- Describe adaptations to the immune system during pregnancy.

Test Your Prior Knowledge

1. List the organs of the immune system.
2. What is the role of a macrophage?
3. What is cell-mediated immunity?
4. What type of immunity is passed from mother to fetus?

Introduction

Throughout a human's life, the body is under constant attack from many sources including bacteria, viruses, parasites, fungi, cancer, foreign cells and tissues. To prevent the body from becoming overwhelmed and destroyed by these invaders, it has its own in-built defence mechanism (innate or non-specific immunity) and can adapt its immunity (adaptive or specific immunity) to protect itself against future threats. During pregnancy, some immunity responses are reduced and the body enters an immunocompromised state to prevent rejection of fetal tissue, which is seen as 'foreign' or 'non-host'.

Fundamentals of Maternal Anatomy and Physiology, First Edition. Edited by Ian Peate and Claire Leader.
© 2024 John Wiley & Sons Ltd. Published 2024 by John Wiley & Sons Ltd.

Although this adaptation prevents rejection, it does leave the body with an increased susceptibility to viral, bacterial and fungal infections. The effects of pregnancy on the immune system are discussed in more detail later. First, we describe the anatomy and physiology of the non-pregnant immune system.

Non-specific or Innate Immunity

Innate immunity is the body's pre-existing defence system with which a person is born. It recognises and responds to pathogens but it does not give long-lasting immunity. The innate immune system:

- Is a first line of defence, acting as a physical and chemical barrier to harmful microbes.
- Identifies and removes foreign substances by specialised white blood cells.
- Activates the complement cascade.
- Recruits immune cells to infection sites by producing chemical factors, including cytokines.
- Activates the adaptive immune system through antigen presentation.

Non-specific or innate defence mechanisms are the natural barriers that protect the body from daily threats (Table 16.1).

Physical Barriers

The epithelium is a type of body tissue that forms the covering on all internal and external surfaces of the body. It lines body cavities and hollow organs and is the major tissue in glands. The skin forms the largest organ in the human body, with a surface area of approximately 1.5–2 m^2 in adults (Figure 16.1).

The epidermis is the outer layer of the skin. It provides a physical and biological barrier to the external environment, preventing penetration by microorganisms, mechanical and chemical trauma, maintains internal homeostasis and prevents the loss of water. The epidermis contains dendritic cells.

The thicker inner layer of the skin, the dermis, sustains and supports the epidermis. Scattered within this layer are several specialised cells, including mast cells, and structures such as blood vessels, lymphatic vessels, sweat glands and nerves.

The skin carries a diverse community of commensal bacteria. These bacteria play a vital role in defence by acting on the host's immune system to induce protective responses that prevent colonisation and invasion by pathogens, so few bacteria can establish themselves on healthy skin. Antibacterial and antifungal substances are also present in sebum and sweat on the skin, which provide further protection.

Epithelial membranes line the body cavities and hollow passageways that are open to the external environment; these include the digestive, respiratory, excretory and reproductive tracts. Although these membranes are more delicate

339

TABLE 16.1   Non-specific or innate defence mechanisms.

Defence mechanism	Location	Barrier type
First line	Surface membrane	Physical barriers (skin and mucous membranes)
Second line	Cellular and chemical	Natural antimicrobial substances
		Phagocytosis
		Inflammatory response
		Complement
		Pyrexia

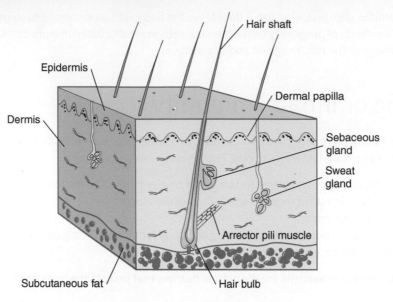

Epidermis

Dermis

Hair shaft

Dermal papilla

Sebaceous gland

Sweat gland

Arrector pili muscle

Subcutaneous fat

Hair bulb

FIGURE 16.1   Layers of the skin. Source: Peate and Evans (2020)/John Wiley & Sons.

than the epidermis, they provide effective defences. The epithelia produce antibacterial secretions, which are often acidic and contain enzymes and antibodies that can trap irritants such as dust, smoke or microbes.

Hairs in the nose act as a coarse filter, and the sweeping action of the cilia in the respiratory system moves mucus and inhaled foreign material towards the throat, where it can be swallowed or expelled through coughing.

The risk of ascending infections in the bladder and uterus is minimised by the one-way flow of urine and the presence of acidic secretions in the vagina that discourage microbial growth.

Natural Antimicrobial Substances

Antimicrobial substances protecting from invading microbes include:

- *Lysozyme* – a naturally occurring enzyme found in bodily secretions such as tears and saliva. Lysozyme functions as an antimicrobial agent, breaking down excess or wornout cell parts and destroying invading microbes.
- *Saliva* – secreted by the salivary glands in the mouth, saliva contains water, mucus antibodies, lysozyme and buffers that neutralise bacterial acid in the mouth and wash away food debris which may otherwise encourage bacterial growth.
- *Stomach secretions* – made up of hydrochloric acid, enzymes and a mucus coating that protects the lining of the stomach. Hydrochloric acid not only helps in the breakdown of food but it also kills the majority of ingested microbes.
- *Interferons* – proteins secreted from virally infected T lymphocyte and macrophage cells that inhibit virus replication and therefore reduce the spread of infection around the body.

Phagocytosis

Phagocytosis is the mechanism used to remove any unwanted pathogens and dead and dying cells from the body by engulfing and destroying them (Figure 16.2). Many cells are capable of phagocytosis, but some cells perform it as part of their main function (e.g. neutrophils and macrophages, the body's first line of cellular defence).

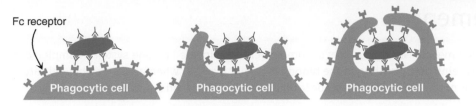

FIGURE 16.2 Phagocytosis. Source: Coico (2021)/John Wiley & Sons.

The Inflammatory Response

The inflammatory response is a physiological response to damaged cells or invasion of the physical barriers by harmful stimuli, such as pathogens, damaged tissues or cells and toxins. With the body's defences broken, it mobilises the inflammatory response, rapidly producing localised swelling, redness, heat, pus formation (suppuration) and pain at the site of damage or infection. Although the symptoms of the immune response may seem detrimental, they are beneficial as they stop the spread of infection and damage to surrounding tissues, removing dead, damaged and harmful cells, alerting the adaptive immune system and starting the healing process (Table 16.2).

Pyrexia

As a result of invasion by microorganisms, the body releases chemicals called pyrogens that act on the hypothalamus, which is the body's thermostat, to raise the temperature above the normal level, increasing the metabolic rate of cells in the tissue, which in turn speeds up the repair process aiding recovery.

TABLE 16.2 Symptoms of the inflammatory response.

Sign	Clinical response
Localised swelling	Increased capillary permeability, fluid leaves the blood vessel and enters the interstitial space
	An increase in protein-rich fluids into the tissue spaces sweeps foreign material for processing in the lymph nodes via the lymphatic vessel
	Transports complement and clotting factors to the site of damage/infection
Localised heat and redness	Caused by an increase in blood flow to the site
Pus formation	White or yellow exudate at a wound
	Formed from a collection of dead cells, microbes and phagocytes as well as fibrin and inflammation exudate at the site
Pain	Localised swelling compressing the sensory nerves causing pain

Complement

A complement is a mechanism that assists or complements the innate immune system. Complements are a group of more than 30 proteins that circulate in the blood when inactive, but when activated they initiate the complement cascade. The steps of the complement cascade facilitate the search for and removal of antigens by:

- Binding to the blood vessels to increase permeability.
- Tagging pathogens for elimination by phagocytes (opsonisation).
- Attacking the pathogens cell membrane creating holes and causing its degeneration.
- Promoting inflammation.

Organs of the Immune System

The organs of the immune system are all lymphoid organs and are part of the lymphatic system, which is a specialised system made up of vessels, nodes and organs. Their main functions are:

- The production of platelets and red and white blood cells.
- Removing damaged red blood cells.
- Maturation of immune cells.
- Trapping foreign material.

The components of the lymphatic system are outlined in Figure 16.3.

Lymphatic Vessels

The lymphatic vessels make up a one-way transport system for fluid called lymph, a clear watery fluid similar to plasma. Interstitial fluid continually leaks out of the blood stream and into the interstitial tissues and the lymphatic vessels collect and return it to the blood circulatory system. It also serves as a major transport route for immune cells. There are two main types of lymphoid organs:

- Primary lymphoid organs (primary as this is where most of the immune cells originate from):
  - Bone marrow
  - Thymus.
- Secondary lymphoid organs:
  - Spleen
  - Lymph nodes.

Bone Marrow

Bone marrow is a spongy substance found in the central cavity of long bones such as the femur, tibia and humerus, and flat bones such as the pelvis, ribs and sternum. Bone marrow produces stem cells, which rapidly multiply to make billions of blood cells each day; this process is known as haematopoiesis (Figure 16.4). Embryological haematopoiesis occurs at the following times in the fetus during pregnancy:

- Day 7: blood cells are made in the yolk sac.
- Weeks 13–24: the spleen, lymph nodes and liver take over production.
- Weeks 20–24: bone marrow takes over most haematopoietic functions so that, at birth, the whole skeleton is filled with red bone marrow.

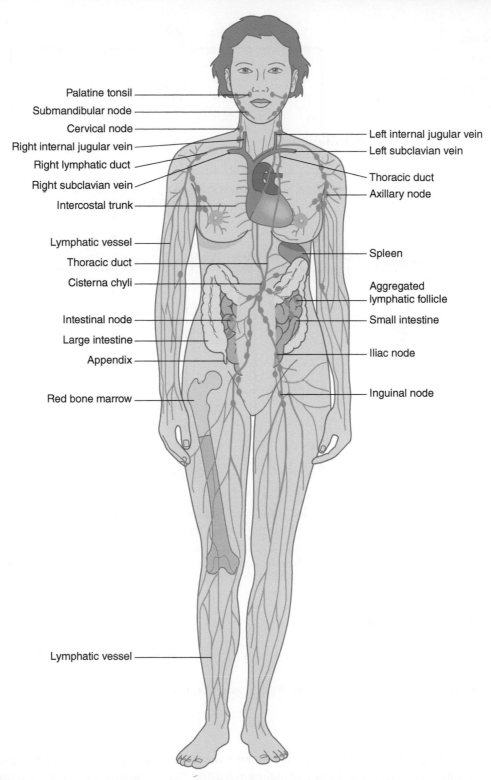

Palatine tonsil

Submandibular node

Cervical node

Right internal jugular vein

Right lymphatic duct

Right subclavian vein

Intercostal trunk

Lymphatic vessel

Thoracic duct

Cisterna chyli

Intestinal node

Large intestine

Appendix

Red bone marrow

Left internal jugular vein

Left subclavian vein

Thoracic duct

Axillary node

Spleen

Aggregated lymphatic follicle

Small intestine

Iliac node

Inguinal node

Lymphatic vessel

343

FIGURE 16.3 Components of the lymphatic system. Source: Peate and Mitchell (2022)/John Wiley & Sons.

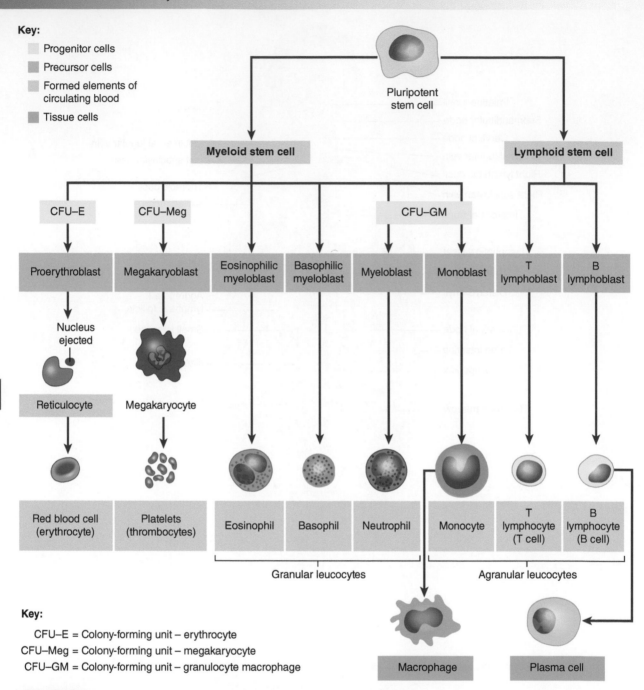

Key:

- ■ Progenitor cells
- ■ Precursor cells
- ■ Formed elements of circulating blood
- ■ Tissue cells

Pluripotent stem cell

Myeloid stem cell

Lymphoid stem cell

CFU–E

CFU–Meg

CFU–GM

Proerythroblast

Megakaryoblast

Eosinophilic myeloblast

Basophilic myeloblast

Myeloblast

Monoblast

T lymphoblast

B lymphoblast

Nucleus ejected

Reticulocyte

Megakaryocyte

Red blood cell (erythrocyte)

Platelets (thrombocytes)

Eosinophil

Basophil

Neutrophil

Monocyte

T lymphocyte (T cell)

B lymphocyte (B cell)

Granular leucocytes

Agranular leucocytes

Macrophage

Plasma cell

Key:

CFU–E = Colony-forming unit – erythrocyte
CFU–Meg = Colony-forming unit – megakaryocyte
CFU–GM = Colony-forming unit – granulocyte macrophage

FIGURE 16.4   Haematopoiesis. Source: Peate and Mitchell (2022)/John Wiley & Sons.

Thymus

The thymus is a bilobed organ found just the below the sternum above the heart (Figure 16.5). T cells originate from the bone marrow, and some will travel to the thymus, to mature into active T cells. A proportion of these mature T cells continually migrate from the thymus into the blood, spleen and lymph nodes, where they play a major role in the body's adaptive immune response.

The size of the thymus reduces with age, changing into fatty tissue post adolescence, when most of the body's T cells have matured.

344

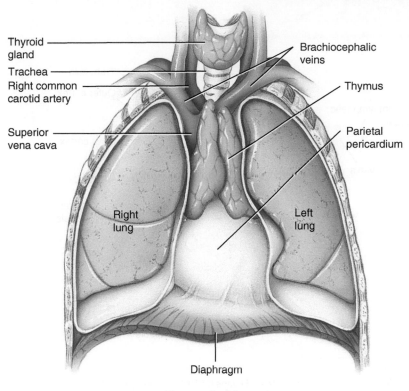

Thyroid gland

Trachea

Right common carotid artery

Superior vena cava

Right lung

Brachiocephalic veins

Thymus

Parietal pericardium

Left lung

Diaphragm

Thymus of adolescent

FIGURE 16.5 Position of the thymus gland (adolescent). Source: Peate and Evans (2020)/John Wiley & Sons.

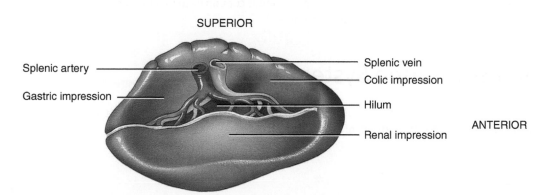

SUPERIOR

Splenic artery

Gastric impression

Splenic vein

Colic impression

Hilum

Renal impression

ANTERIOR

FIGURE 16.6 The spleen. Source: Tortora and Dickenson (2017)/John Wiley & Sons.

The Spleen

The spleen is an oval-shaped, highly vascular organ situated in the upper left side of the abdomen, behind the ribs and next to the stomach (Figure 16.6). The primary function of the spleen is to act as a filter for the blood, bringing it into close contact with scavenging phagocytes and lymphocytes to remove unwanted pathogens.

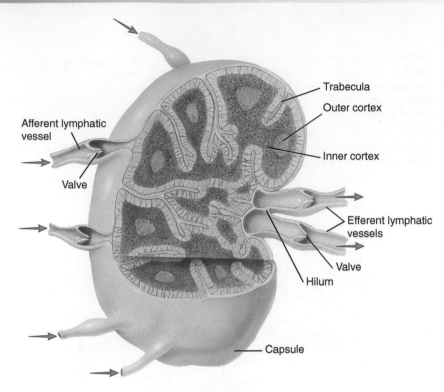

FIGURE 16.7   Structure a lymph node. Source: Peate and Evans (2020)/John Wiley & Sons.

Lymph Nodes

Found in clusters around the body, lymph nodes vary in size and shape, but are typically small, bean-shaped structures (Figure 16.7). Antigens entering the body are swept along the lymphatic vessels and enter the lymph nodes, together with any bacteria, dead or wornout cells and inhaled particles, the nodes contain fixed macrophages, which detect and destroy pathogens and have a role in the adaptive immune system.

Cells of the Immune System

As well as organs, the immune system also includes a complex network of cells, each with their own unique role to play in protecting the body again the constant threat of harm (Figure 16.8).

Macrophages

Macrophages are specialised white blood cells involved in the detection and destruction of bacteria and other harmful organisms. In addition, they can present antigens to T cells and initiate inflammation by releasing cytokines (Figure 16.9).

Dendritic Cells

Named for their probing 'tree-like' shape, dendritic cells are a type of fixed macrophage cell found in the epidermis and dermis (Figure 16.10).

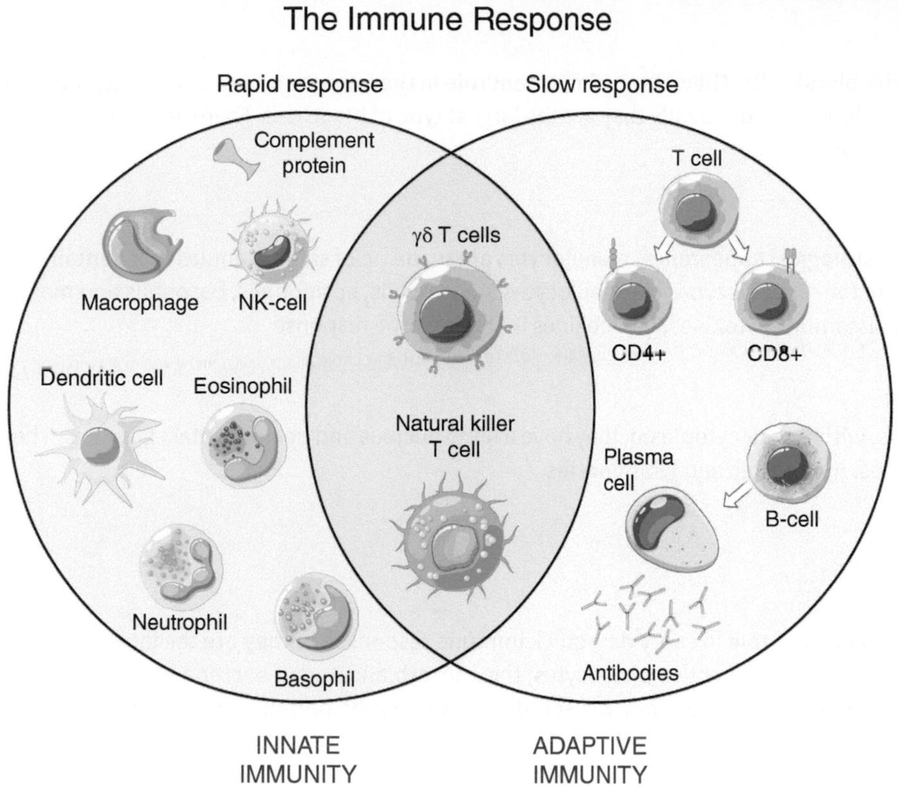
The Immune Response
Rapid response
Slow response
Complement protein
Macrophage
NK-cell
γδ T cells
T cell
CD4+
CD8+
Dendritic cell
Eosinophil
Natural killer T cell
Plasma cell
B-cell
Neutrophil
Basophil
Antibodies
INNATE IMMUNITY
ADAPTIVE IMMUNITY

FIGURE 16.8 Innate and adaptive immune cells. designua/Adobe Stock Photos

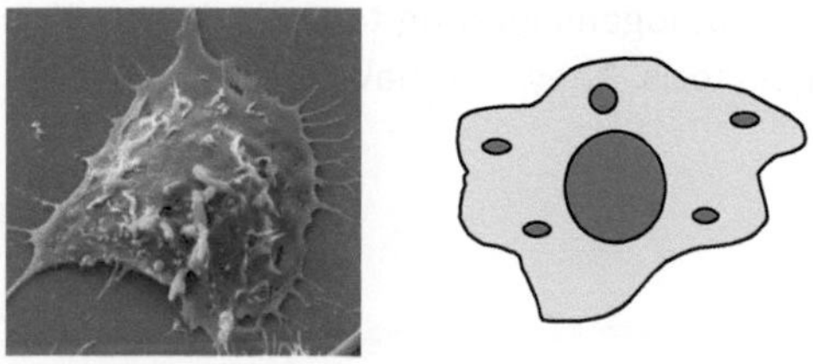

FIGURE 16.9 Macrophages. Source: Delves et al. (2017)/John Wiley & Sons.

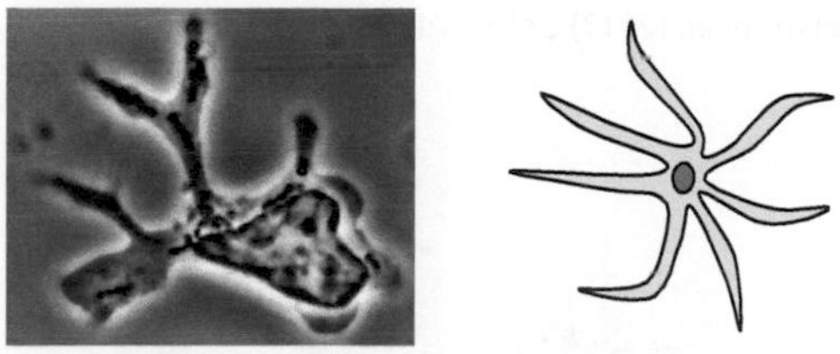

FIGURE 16.10 Dendritic cells. Source: Delves et al. (2017)/John Wiley & Sons.

Leucocytes

Leucocytes are white blood cells. They play an important role in the immune system. They only make up about 1% of the total blood volume, although individually they are the largest type of blood cell. There are two types of leucocytes: granulocytes and agranulocytes.

Granulocytes

Named after their histological appearance, granulocytes are made up of small granules that contain proteins within their cytoplasm. There are four specific types of granulocytes: neutrophils, eosinophils, basophils and mast cells. They release molecules such as histamine, cytokines, chemokines in the immune response

Agranulocytes

Unlike granulocytes, within their cytoplasm, they have a large nucleus and do not contain granules. There are two specific types of granulocytes: monocytes and lymphocytes.

Neutrophils

Neutrophils play a significant role in every day, quick immune responses as they are the largest group of innate immune cells in the body. They are very effective phagocytes; they absorb and engulf bacteria but if they become overwhelmed and are surrounded by the pathogens, they will self-destruct releasing harmful enzymes all over the bacteria around it (Figure 16.11).

Eosinophils

Eosinophils are also phagocytes, although they are not as active as neutrophils. They also contain enzymes in their granules, which are toxic to invading pathogens leading to their destruction. Eosinophils are effective against parasites that are too large for phagocytosis. They also have a role in allergic inflammation such as asthma and hayfever (Figure 16.12).

FIGURE 16.11   A neutrophil. Source: Delves et al. (2017)/John Wiley & Sons.

FIGURE 16.12   Eosinophil. Source: Delves et al. (2017)/John Wiley & Sons.

Basophils

Basophils are the largest of the granulocytes. During an immune response, it is the basophils that are responsible for inflammatory reactions. This causes the release of histamine, a vasodilator, which promotes blood flow to tissues, and heparin, an anticoagulant, which prevents blood from clotting too quickly to maintain blood flow to the tissues (Figure 16.13).

Mast Cells

Similar to basophils in an immune response, mast cells release histamine and heparin to promote and maintain blood flow (Figure 16.14).

Monocytes

The largest of the white blood cells, monocytes circulate in the blood and when needed can be phagocytic or can they migrate from blood into tissues and develop into macrophages (Figure 16.15).

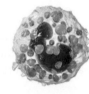

FIGURE 16.13 Basophil. Source: Delves et al. (2017)/John Wiley & Sons.

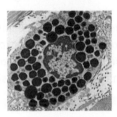
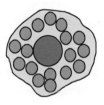

FIGURE 16.14 Mast cells. Source: Delves et al. (2017)/John Wiley & Sons.

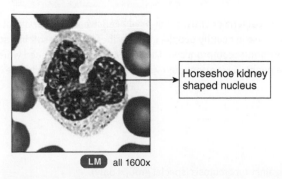

Horseshoe kidney shaped nucleus

LM all 1600x

FIGURE 16.15 Monocyte. Source: Peate and Nair (2016)/John Wiley & Sons.

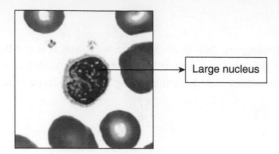

FIGURE 16.16   Lymphocyte. Source: Peate and Nair (2016)/John Wiley & Sons.

Lymphocytes

Lymphocytes are mostly found in lymphatic tissue. They are smaller than monocytes but, unlike monocytes, they are not phagocytic. Each lymphocyte recognises only one specific antigen (Figure 16.16):

- *B lymphocyte cells* originate in the bone marrow; B cells produce antibodies.
- *T lymphocyte cells* derive their name from the thymus, where they mature after originating in the bone marrow.
- *Natural killer (NK) cells* are lymphocytes that patrol the body in search of abnormal cells or harmful cells. Once found, they respond quickly to destroying it.

The organs and the cells of the immune system work together to protect the body, from both immediate and future threats. To do this, there are inbuilt defence mechanisms and adaptations that the body can make to protect itself. Specialised NK cells are also found in the placenta and may play an important role in pregnancy.

Specific or Adaptive Immunity

Specific or adaptive immunity is also known as acquired immunity. Unlike innate immunity, it is not pre-existing in the body. When the body is exposed to an antigen to which it has not previously been exposed, it adapts its immune system for future attacks by memorising the antigen. A healthy immune system can memorise millions of different antigens, producing both short- or long-term protection. Acquired immunity can be either passive or active and naturally or artificially acquired (Table 16.3).

Medications Management: Live Attenuated Vaccines

Live attenuated vaccines contain whole bacteria or viruses that have been 'weakened' or attenuated. They generate a protective immune response but do not cause disease in healthy people. Live vaccines usually result in a strong and lasting immunity. They may not be suitable for those who are immunocompromised. This is because the weakened viruses or bacteria could multiply too much and may cause disease in these people. Live attenuated vaccines used in the UK schedule include:

- Rotavirus
- measles, mumps and rubella
- Nasal flu
- Shingles
- Chickenpox (special groups only)
- BCG (bacillus Calmette– Guérin) against tuberculosis (special groups only).

TABLE 16.3 Acquired immunity.

Mode	Natural	Artificial
Active	Having a disease or infection stimulates the body to make antibodies	Short- or long-term immunity in response to having a dead or live vaccine
Passive	Short term immunity acquired from the mother via the placenta or breastmilk	Immunity from ready-made antibodies in donor human or animal serum

If the first-line barriers or second-line defence mechanisms of the innate immune system are invaded, the adaptive immune system is activated.

Key points of the adaptive immune system include:

- For subsequent exposures to an antigen, the body recognises the antigen and mounts a faster and stronger response.
- It recognises specific antigens to enable a targeted response.
- Following the initial infection, the antigen is recognised throughout the body, not just the initial infection site.
- Healthy cells display 'self' markers (proteins) on their membrane, which are ignored by patrolling immune cells to prevent destruction of the body's normal host cells.

Adaptive immune responses fall into two categories:

1. Antibody-mediated immunity.
2. Cell-mediated immunity.

Red Flag Alert: Autoimmune Disease

If the immune system does not recognise 'self markers' on normal host cells, it will lead to autoimmune disease – an inappropriate immune response against host cells. An example of autoimmune disease is type 1 diabetes.

Antibody-mediated Immunity

Antibody-mediated or 'humoral' immunity, named due to antibodies being present in 'humours' or body fluids; in this case, lymph and blood. Antibodies produced by the B cells are distributed around the body, where they bind to antigens, first making them inactive, preventing them from entering a normal cell and causing harm, and second, marking them for destruction by phagocytes or complement.

As well as the antibodies being distributed, the B cells will also display the antibody they produce on their cell membrane, which acts as an 'antigen receptor'. When an antigen binds to the receptor, the B cells will enlarge and divide, producing two different B cells: memory B cells and plasma cells. This division of cells is known as clonal expansion.

- *Memory B cells* provide immunity from an antigen by memorising it and responding when exposed to the same antigen again.
- *Plasma cells* produce large number of antibodies that target the antigen that initially triggered the B cell. Unlike the memory B cell, they only live for a very short time.

Antibodies are Y-shaped proteins. They bind to antigens, which marks them as targets for destruction (Figure 16.17). Each antibody recognises one antigen. The tip of each 'Y' contains a binding site that locks in the antigen and neutralises it to prevent it from causing further harm, while waiting for destruction. There are five main types of antibodies or immunoglobulins (Table 16.4).

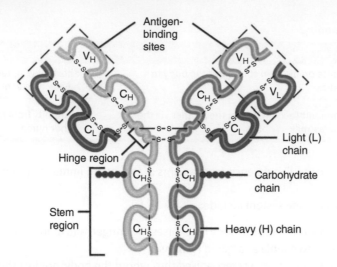

FIGURE 16.17 Model of an antibody. Source: Peate and Evans (2020)/John Wiley & Sons.

TABLE 16.4   Immunoglobulins.

Antibody	Function
IgG	The most common and the one that lives the longest. It provides the majority of antibody mediated immunity due the wide range of pathogens it attacks. Crosses the placenta to give temporary passive immunity to the fetus
IgA	Prevents antigens from crossing the epithelium. Found in mucosal areas such as the gut, respiratory and urogenital tract and in bodily secretions such as saliva, tears and breastmilk and colostrum. Important in preventing neonatal gut infections in babies who are breastfed
IgE	Found on the cell membrane of mast cells and basophils; often binds to antigens that can trigger an allergic reactions by releasing histamine
IgM	The principal antibody produced in an initial response to an antigen and activate complement
IgD	Little is known about this antibody except that it is found on the cell surface of B cells and acts as an antigen receptor

Ig, immunoglobulin.

Cell-mediated Immunity

Cell-mediated immunity is an immune response that does not involve antibodies.

T cells (Table 16.5) originate in the bone marrow and mature in the thymus. Once mature, they circulate around the body, mainly in the lymphatic vessels. They have a 'T cell receptor' on their surface; however, unlike B cells, they cannot detect an antigen themselves. Instead, they have to wait and be presented with the antigen on the membrane of another cell, an antigen-presenting cell (Figure 16.18), before they can respond.

Macrophages are an important link between the innate and adaptive immune systems. Macrophages will initially detect and destruct bacteria and other harmful organisms systematically but, having broken it down, they will then display part of the antigen on the surface if their membrane, which they can present to T cells that recognise that particular antigen. This in turn activates the T cell. Once activated, the T cell, like the B cell, will the divide and proliferate (clonal expansion) into four different T cells.

TABLE 16.5 **The adaptive system – T cells.**

T cell type	Function
Killer (CD8+)	Cytotoxic, which means that they are able to directly kill virus-infected cells, as well as cancer cells
Helper (CD4+)	Activate the memory B cells and killer T cells, which leads to a greater immune response
Regulatory	Prevent immune cells from inappropriately reacting against its own cells (self), otherwise known as suppressor cells
Memory	Provide immunity from an antigen, by memorising it and responding when exposed to the same antigen again

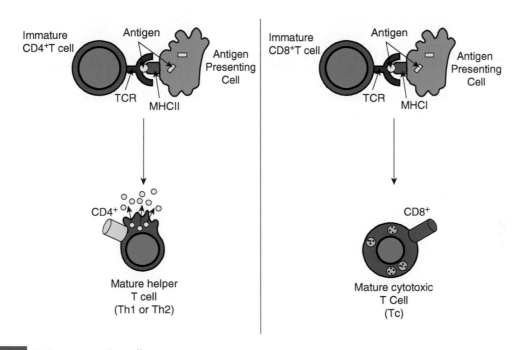

FIGURE 16.18 Antigen-presenting cell.

Physiological Changes to the Immune System in Pregnancy

The maternal immune system plays a vital role in establishing and maintaining a healthy pregnancy. During pregnancy, there needs to be a balance between protecting the fetus from rejection while still protecting the maternal system from infection. Although these changes have a protective effect for the fetus, they may also increase maternal risks and the severity of some autoimmune diseases, such as systemic lupus erythematosus, while having little or no effect on others (e.g. rheumatoid arthritis) or even providing temporary improvement in conditions such as Graves' disease. An overview of the immune system in pregnancy is shown in Box 16.1.

BOX 16.1   **Overview of the Immune System in Pregnancy**

- An increase in NK cells post ovulation plays a critical role in preparing the endometrium for pregnancy and in regulating trophoblast invasion.
- Immune cells accumulate in the endometrium.
- There is an increase in complement activity.
- Eosinophils and basophils counts are not altered in pregnancy.
- There is a decrease in T cells but an increase in regulatory T cells in pregnancy to prevent fetal rejection due to higher levels of oestrogen and progesterone.
- Human chorionic gonadotrophin stimulates neutrophil production.
- Reduced resistance to localised Gram-negative bacteria due to corticosteroid collections around the placenta and fetus, which supress phagocytic activity.
- NK cell activity around the uterus is supressed by prostaglandins, which reduce fetal rejection but will also reduce resistance to other pathogens (e.g. toxoplasmosis and listeriosis).

Increased Vulnerability to Infection in Pregnancy

Owing to the altered balance between T cells and regulatory T cells in pregnancy, there is an increased vulnerability to some infections during pregnancy, including:

- Listeriosis
- Herpes
- Influenza
- Rubella
- Chickenpox (varicella)
- Human papillomavirus
- Hepatitis
- Pertussis.

Box 16.2 shows some clinical considerations for vaccination in pregnancy.

BOX 16.2   **Clinical Consideration: Vaccinations in Pregnancy**

Influenza

- Influenza is an acute viral infection affecting the respiratory tract.
- Symptoms include pyrexia, sore throat, muscle pain, headache, runny nose.
- Complications:
  - Mother – bronchitis and pneumonia.
  - Baby – premature birth, low birth weight and increased risk of stillbirth.

Vaccination

- Active artificial immunity (Table 16.3) to protect against the risks of influenza-associated morbidity and mortality; recommended for people in high-risk clinical groups in the UK since the late 1960s.
- Pregnancy was added to the list in 2010 and vaccination is routinely offered to all pregnant women.

Whooping Cough

- Whooping cough is a bacterial infection affecting the respiratory tract.
- Symptoms include cold-like symptoms initially then a mucus cough develops with a high-pitched wheeze – 'whoop' sound.
- Complications: symptoms can be severe in babies under six months old and can lead to dehydration, breathing difficulties and pneumonia.

Vaccination

- Active artificial immunity (Table 16.3).
- The whooping cough vaccine was introduced for pregnant women in 2012, as babies cannot receive their first whooping cough vaccine until around eight weeks of age.

Fetal Tolerance

Normally, foreign or 'non-self' cells would be targets for the maternal immune system, provoking an immune response to tag and destroy them. However, despite half of the fetal antigens originating from the father, the maternal immune system appears tolerant and allows the fetus to develop and grow without rejection.

Reflective Learning Activity

With regards to fetal tolerance, why is the presence of the fetus accepted?

It is clear that the maternal–fetal immune interaction is complex and it is still not fully understood. However, there are several mechanisms involved that provide safe coexistence for the mother and fetus.

The maternal immune system is primed during unprotected sexual intercourse, when it is exposed to major histocompatibility complex proteins in seminal fluid. This allows the maternal immune system to become exposed to paternal antigens, enabling regulatory T cells to recognise, bind to and tolerate them.

During implantation, the trophoblast cells invade the decidua but may act as a barrier, preventing the maternal immune cells and antibodies from entering the fetal circulation. Although some trophoblast cells will invade the spiral arteries to enable remodelling to accommodate the increase blood flow needed in the placenta, these extravillous trophoblast cells do not seem to provoke an immune response. This may be due to the presence of human leucocyte antigens (HLA). Trophoblast cells inhibit the cytotoxicity of T cells and NK cells, as well as increasing the number of regulatory T cells.

Specialised NK cells found in the placenta differ from the NK cells that normally patrol the body. They have key roles throughout pregnancy to support and maintain the placenta and fetus. Specialised NK recruitment to the uterus is trigger by rising level of oestrogen and progesterone (Table 16.6).

TABLE 16.6 Role of specialised natural killer cells throughout pregnancy.

Trimester	Action	Purpose
First trimester	Proinflammatory	To help establish a healthy endometrium
Second trimester	Anti-inflammatory	To support placental and fetal development
Third trimester	Proinflammatory	Induce parturition

The Placenta and Membrane Barrier

The placenta and membrane unit acts as an effective barrier between mother and fetus in the transmission of most immune cells and antibodies. However, immunoglobulin (Ig) G can cross the placental barrier via active transport at low levels from approximately 20–22 weeks, increasing throughout pregnancy, with the highest levels crossing from around 34 weeks of gestation to full term. IgG gives temporary passive immunity to the fetus. This immunity is important, as it provides protection from antigens that the maternal system has encountered, provoking an immune response and giving rise to temporary immunity from the same antigens after birth. Until the neonatal immune system matures, IgA, IgM and IgD do not cross the placenta but are transported in colostrum.

Red Flag Alert: Risk of Infection

Neonates who are at higher risk of infection are:

- Preterm infants – as they will receive lower levels of IgG from the mother.
- Babies who are small for gestational age – placental dysfunction reduces the transfer of IgG.

The fetus is at risk from viral and some bacterial pathogens causing infections. Although many viruses and bacteria are able to cross the placental barrier, relatively few will do so, due to maternal immune cells accumulating in the endometrium, which are triggered to respond to the antigens, detecting and destroying them before they are able to cross the placental barrier.

The physical barrier of unbroken membranes protects the fetus from infection, while the liquor has bacteriostatic properties, preventing the growth of bacteria, and bactericidal properties, which will destroy bacteria. The fetus is also protected from ascending infection by the thick mucoid plug in the cervix, which contains antimicrobial proteins. Following spontaneous rupture of membranes, the physical barrier is disrupted. If this is either premature or prolonged, the risk of maternal infection is increased, which may in turn increase the risk of fetal or neonatal sepsis (Table 16.7).

Group B Streptococcus

Group B Streptococcus (GBS) is a gram-positive bacterium. Between 20% and 30% of adults including pregnant women are colonised with GBS in the gastrointestinal and genitourinary tracts and are asymptomatic carriers. However, GBS can cause severe infections in newborn infants and is a leading cause of infectious neonatal morbidity and mortality.

TABLE 16.7 Neonatal sepsis.

Onset	Definition	Causative organisms
Early	Usually defined as infection in the first 72 hours after birth, although many present in the first 24 hours following birth	Predominantly those that may colonise the vagina or lower gastrointestinal tract in the mother and acquired by the neonate around the time of birth including group B Streptococcus and Gram-negative bacteria
Late	Usually defined as infection between 72 hours of birth and 28 days of age	Gram-positive bacteria – *Staphylococci*
		Gram-negative bacteria – *Pseudomonas*
Hospital-acquired (nosocomial)	Invasive procedures, intravenous lines, catheters or passed via people or equipment	Gram-negative bacteria – *Staphylococci*
		Fungi – *Candida albicans* and *Candida parapsilosis*

Red Flag Alert: Early-onset Neonatal Infection

Risk factors for early-onset neonatal infection include:

- In a multiple pregnancy, suspected or confirmed infection in another baby.

Other risk factors include:

- Invasive GBS infection in a previous baby or maternal GBS colonisation, bacteriuria or infection in the current pregnancy.
- Preterm birth following spontaneous labour before 37 weeks of gestation.
- Confirmed rupture of membranes for more than 18 hours before a preterm birth.
- Confirmed prelabour rupture of membranes at term for more than 24 hours before the onset of labour.
- Intrapartum fever higher than 38°C if there is suspected or confirmed bacterial infection.
- Clinical diagnosis of chorioamnionitis.

For further information, see National Institute for Health and Care Excellence guideline (NICE 2021).

Medications Management: Antibiotics

An antibiotic is a substance that works against bacterial life; 'anti' meaning 'against' and *bios*, the Greek word for life Antibiotics work by destroying, disabling or slowing the growth of targeted bacteria. Antimicrobial is a broader term for substances that are active against all microbes that cause infection (e.g. viruses and fungi), as well as bacteria.

Use of Antibiotics

Antibiotics may be offered to reduce the risk of neonatal infection, for example (RCOG 2017):

- Preterm spontaneous rupture of the membranes (before 37 weeks) but not in labour.
- GBS in a previous pregnancy.
- In labour with known GBS.
- GBS found in the urine prelabour.
- Prolonged rupture of membranes.
- Maternal pyrexia in labour.
- Signs of infection in the neonate.

Colostrum and Breast Milk

Human milk is not only able to nourish but also provides the neonate with passive immunity. The immune properties of colostrum and breast milk include:

- *Immunoglobulins*: IgA is the most important of these, as it lines the surface of the gut mucosa to protect against harmful gut pathogens such as salmonella, *Escherichia coli*, Staphylococci and Streptococci.
- *Lactoferrin* is a protein which can break down the cell wall of a microbe, causing its destruction, and also binds to iron, which makes it unavailable for microbial growth.
- *Macrophages and neutrophils* detect and destroy pathogens. They are found in high levels in the early production of breast milk, with levels reducing from about 10 days postpartum.
- *Bifidobacterium* (Bifidus) is a Gram-positive bacterium that colonises the intestinal flora and reduces Gram-negative bacterial growth, such as *E. coli*, Salmonella and *Hemophilus influenzae*, which can cause meningitis.
- *Lysozyme* is a bacteriolytic protein which can break down the cell wall of a microbe, causing its destruction.

Sepsis

Sepsis is the immune system's overreaction to an infection or injury. Normally, the immune system fights infection but sometimes the body's overwhelming and life-threatening response to infection can lead to tissue damage, organ failure and death, as the body attacks its own organs and tissues. Sepsis requires urgent medical treatment to reduce and reverse the damage. Sepsis may become 'severe' when there is organ damage, resulting from the body's inflammation and may result in 'septic shock'. Sepsis may require care in a high-dependency unit and considerations need to be made regarding fetal surveillance or neonatal care, observing for fetal or neonatal sepsis.

Red Flag Alert: Sepsis

Management of sepsis – the 'sepsis six':

1. Oxygen
2. Cultures
3. Antibiotics
4. Fluids
5. Lactate measurement
6. Monitoring urine output.

With implementation within one hour – the 'golden hour' (Daniels and Nutbeam 2019).

Orange Flag Alert: Sepsis

Psychological considerations – ideally, the separation of mother and baby due to treatment for sepsis needs to be avoided where possible. However, if care is needed in a high-dependency unit that it not part of the labour ward or neonatal unit, then the risk of separation anxiety and stress needs to be managed carefully.

Snapshot 16.1   Group B Streptococcus

Sameenah is in spontaneous labour at 39^{+2} weeks gestation with her second baby. She was found to be GBS positive during her first pregnancy. The current pregnancy has been uneventful; however, during labour she develops a pyrexia of 38.1°C.

- What are your considerations for both mother and baby?
- What is your plan of care and why?

Take Home Points

- The body protects and adapts to harmful pathogens by using the innate and adaptive immune systems.
- Specialised NK cells found in the placenta have a key role in pregnancy to support and maintain the placenta and fetus.
- Influenza and whooping cough vaccinations are offered during pregnancy, providing active artificial immunity.
- Human milk provides a neonate with passive immunity.

Summary

The immune system is a complex defence system made up of organs and cells, continually protecting the body against harmful microbes with the potential to cause infection and damage to the body. The pathogens we come into contact with are also constantly changing and evolving and with it the immune system has to continually adapt, to protect against current as well as future threats. Pregnancy brings its own challenges to the immune system, which is a fine balance between, not only protecting against, but playing host to foreign tissue, whilst allowing the fetus to grow and develop, safe from infection.

References

Coico, R. (2021). *Immunology: A Short Course*, 8e. Chichester: Wiley.

Daniels, R. and Nutbeam, T. (2019). *The Sepsis Manual*, 5e. Birmingham: United Kingdom Sepsis Trust.

Delves, P.J., Martin, S.J., Burton, D.R., and Roitt, I.M. (2017). *Roitt's Essential Immunology*, 13e. Chichester: Wiley.

NICE (2021). *Neonatal Infection: Antibiotics for Prevention and Treatment*. NICE Guideline NG195. London: National Institute for Health and Care Excellence https://www.nice.org.uk/guidance/ng195.

Peate, I. and Evans, S. (2020). *Fundamentals of Anatomy and Physiology For Nursing and Healthcare Students*, 3e. Chichester: Wiley.

Peate, I. and Mitchell, A. (2022). *Nursing Practice: Knowledge and Care*, 3e. Chichester: Wiley.

Peate, I. and Nair, M. (2016). *Fundamentals of Anatomy and Physiology For Nursing and Healthcare Students*, 2e. Oxford: Wiley-Blackwell.

RCOG (2017). *Prevention of Early-onset Neonatal Group B Streptococcal Disease*. Green-top Guideline No. 36. London: Royal College of Obstetricians and Gynaecologists.

Further Reading

Bamfo, J.E.A.K. (2013). Managing the risks of sepsis in pregnancy. *Best Practice & Research. Clinical Obstetrics & Gynaecology* 27 (4): 583–595.

Edwards, J.M., Watson, N., Focht, C. et al. (2019). Group B Streptococcus (GBS) colonization and disease among pregnant women: a historical cohort study. *Infectious Diseases in Obstetrics and Gynecology* 2019: 5430493.

Hanna, J., Goldman-Wohl, D., Hamani, Y. et al. (2006). Decidual NK cells regulate key developmental processes at the human fetal-maternal interface. *Nature Medicine* 12 (9): 1065–1074.

Hoang, H.T.T., Leuridan, E., Maertens, K. et al. (2015). Pertussis vaccination during pregnancy in Vietnam: results of a randomized controlled trial pertussis vaccination during pregnancy. *Vaccine* 34 (1): 151–159.

Hughes, E. (2001). Skin: its structure, function and related pathology. In: *Dermatology Nursing: A Practical Guide*, vol. 15 (ed. E. Hughes and J. Van Onselen), 30–33. Edinburgh: Churchill Livingstone.

NICE (2018). *Flu Vaccination: Increasing Uptake*. NICE Guideline NG103. London: National Institute for Health and Care Excellence www.nice.org.uk/guidance/ng103.

Nigam, Y. and Knight, J. (2020). The lymphatic system 2: structure and function of the lymphoid organs. *Nursing Times* 116 (11): 44.

Sherwood, L. (2016). *Human Physiology: From Cells to Systems*, 9e. Boston, MA: Cengage Learning.

Standring, S. and Adams, M.A. (2016). *Gray's Anatomy: The Anatomical Basis of Clinical Practice*, 41e. Saint Louis, MO: Elsevier.

Swartz, M.A. (2001). 'The physiology of the lymphatic system', advanced drug delivery reviews. *Advanced Drug Delivery Reviews* 50 (1): 3–20.

Wilson, M.E. (2019). *Antibiotics: What Everyone Needs to Know*. New York, NY: Oxford University Press.

Zhang, X. and Wei, H. (2021). Role of decidual natural killer cells in human pregnancy and related pregnancy complications. *Frontiers in Immunology* 12: 728291.

Online Resources

European Federation of Immunological Societies: https://www.efis.org
An umbrella organisation for European immunology societies.
National Institute for Health and Care Excellence: www.nice.org.uk
NICE's role is to improve outcomes for people using the NHS and other public health and social care services.
Royal College of Obstetricians and Gynaecologists: www.rcog.org.uk
A professional association 'working to transform women's health and reproductive care'.
UK Sepsis Trust: https://sepsistrust.org/professional-resources/sepsis-e-learning
Provides excellent professional resources and e-learning for clinical staff.
World Health Organization: https://www.who.int
A specialised agency of the United Nations responsible for international public health.

Glossary

Active immunity	Immunity acquired as a result of exposed to an antigen.
Adaptive/acquired immunity	Immunity acquired through life when the body comes into contact with different infectious agents.
Agranulocyte	A white blood cell that does not contain granules.
Antibody	A Y-shaped protein; also called an immunoglobulin.
Antibody-mediated immunity	Also known as humoral immunity; part of the adaptive immune system.
Antigen	A protein found on the surface of a pathogen that can provoke an immune response.
Basophil	A white blood cell which releases histamine, responsible for inflammatory responses.
B cell	A lymphocyte cells that produces antibodies.
Bone marrow	A spongy substance found in the central cavity of long bones that produces stem cells.
Cell-mediated immunity	Part of the adaptive immune system response that does not involve antibodies.
Complement	A group of proteins that initiate a response that enables the removal of antigens.
Cytokine	Protein that stimulates or communicates with another cell.
Dendritic cell	A type of fixed macrophage cell, found in the epidermis and dermis.
Granulocyte	White blood cell consisting of granules containing proteins.
Heparin	An anticoagulant.
Histamine	A chemical involved in local immune responses.
Immunoglobulin	Also known as an antibody.
Inflammatory response	A physiological response to damaged cells or invasion of the physical barriers.
Innate	Inborn or natural.
Leucocytes	Another term for a white blood cell (*leuco* = white, *cyte* = cell).
Lymph	A clear watery fluid similar to plasma.
Lymph node	Small, bean-shaped structure containing fixed macrophages.
Lymphatic system	A system containing organs and vessels containing lymph.
Lymphatic vessel	A one-way transport system for fluid called lymph.
Lymphocyte	The main type of white blood cell found in lymph.
Macrophage	Specialised white blood cell involved in phagocytosis and antigen presentation.

Mast cell	Cell that releases histamine and heparin within the immune response.
Monocyte	A phagocytic white blood cell.
Neutrophil	White blood cell that is an effective phagocyte.
Natural killer (NK)	Lymphocyte that patrols the body in search of abnormal cells or harmful cells.
Oedema	Swelling caused by fluid.
Passive immunity	Immunity acquired from a donor or acquired via the placenta or breastmilk.
Pathogen	A disease-causing microbe.
Phagocytosis	*Phago* = to eat and *cyte* = a cell; therefore, a cell that eats!
Plasma cell	Cell that develops from B cells and produces a large number of antibodies.
Pyrexia	A rise in the body's temperature above the normal level.
Sepsis	The immune system's overreaction to an infection or injury.
Spleen	An oval-shaped organ of the immune system.
T cell	A lymphocyte cell that is a major component of the cell-mediated immune system.
Thymus	A bilobed organ of the immune system.

Multiple Choice Questions

1. Antibodies are produced by which cells of the immune system?
   a. Mast cells
   b. Basophils
   c. B cells
   d. T cells

2. Which circulating innate immune cells contains granules of histamine?
   a. Macrophages
   b. Dendritic calls
   c. Basophils
   d. Monocytes

3. Which of these is <u>not</u> an organ of the lymph system?
   a. Spleen
   b. Thymus
   c. Pancreas
   d. Lymph nodes

4. Which of these is not a normal effect of the inflammatory response?
   a. Pain
   b. Localised swelling
   c. Pus formation
   d. Shivering

5. Which is the most common antibody and provides the majority of antibody-mediated immunity?
   a. IgA
   b. IgG
   c. IgD
   d. IgM

6. Which of the following T cells is cytotoxic?
   a. Killer
   b. Helper
   c. Regulatory
   d. Memory

7. What is an antigen?
   a. A cell of the immune system
   b. A protein found on the cell of a pathogen
   c. A chemical involved in the immune response
   d. A disease-causing microbe

8. Which of these is not part of the innate immune system?
   a. Complement
   b. Vaccines
   c. Lysozyme
   d. The epidermis

9. Which antibody crosses the placental barrier giving temporary passive immunity to the fetus?
   a. IgM
   b. IgD
   c. IgG
   d. IgA

10. Which type of specialised immune cell can be found in the placenta?
    a. B cell
    b. Regulator T cell
    c. Killer cell
    d. Plasma cell

Conditions Associated with the Immune System

The following is a list of conditions that are associated with the immune system. Take some time and write notes about each of the conditions. Think about the related anatomy and physiology that may need to be considered in the conditions below. Remember to include aspects of patient care. If you are making notes about people you have offered care and support to you must ensure that you have adhered to the rules of confidentiality.

Group B Streptococcus

Toxoplasmosis

Chorioamnionitis

Sepsis

Whooping cough

SARS-CoV-2 virus (COVID-19)

Chapter 1

1. c
2. c
3. b
4. a
5. c
6. c
7. b
8. c
9. d
10. b

Chapter 2

1. c
2. c
3. d
4. c
5. b
6. a
7. d
8. a
9. d
10. b

Fundamentals of Maternal Anatomy and Physiology, First Edition. Edited by Ian Peate and Claire Leader.
© 2024 John Wiley & Sons Ltd. Published 2024 by John Wiley & Sons Ltd.

Chapter 3

1. a
2. b
3. d
4. c
5. b
6. a
7. a
8. b
9. c
10. b

Chapter 4

1. c
2. c
3. b
4. a
5. b
6. c
7. a
8. b
9. d
10. c

Chapter 5

1. c
2. a
3. b
4. a
5. b
6. a
7. d

8. c

9. a

10. a

Chapter 6

1. c

2. c

3. a

4. a

5. b

6. d

7. a

8. d

9. b

10. b

Chapter 7

1. c

2. c

3. c

4. d

5. d

6. d

7. b

8. c

9. b

10. c

Chapter 8

1. c

2. a

3. b

4. c

5. d

6. b

7. d

8. d

9. a

10. c

Chapter 9

1. a

2. b

3. c

4. c

5. c

6. a

7. a

8. b

9. d

10. a

Chapter 10

1. b

2. a

3. c

4. d

5. b

6. c

7. b

8. c

9. a

10. b

Chapter 11

1. b
2. c
3. b
4. d
5. b
6. c
7. d
8. a
9. d
10. a

Chapter 12

1. a
2. c
3. a
4. d
5. c
6. b
7. d
8. b
9. a
10. b

Chapter 13

1. c
2. c
3. d
4. b
5. a

6. a

7. d

8. c

9. a

10. b

Chapter 14

1. a

2. d

3. c

4. c

5. a

6. b

7. b

8. c

9. b

10. d

Chapter 15

1. d

2. c

3. b

4. a

5. d

6. b

7. a

8. b

9. c

10. b

Chapter 16

1. c
2. c
3. c
4. d
5. b
6. a
7. b
8. b
9. c
10. c

Index

Fundamentals of Maternal Anatomy and Physiology, First Edition. Edited by Ian Peate and Claire Leader.
© 2024 John Wiley & Sons Ltd. Published 2024 by John Wiley & Sons Ltd.